43.85

369 0240974

Workplace Mental Health Manual for Nurse Managers

Lisa Y. Adams, PhD, MSc, RN, is a course instructor at Athabasca University, Alberta, Canada, and MacEwan University, Alberta, Canada. She has 23 years of experience in progressive leadership roles such as nurse manager, clinical nurse specialist, professional practice consultant, and project leader in the fields of mental health and addictions. Her research and academic interests lie in mental health nursing for seniors, corrections/forensics, addictions, and criminology, and she is currently working in a postdoctorate program bridging mental illness and corrections. Dr. Adams has completed and/or published several peer-reviewed research studies and articles. She is an active volunteer in her community for a variety of organizations, such as the Canadian Cancer Society, the Canadian Mental Health Association, and the Seniors' Resource Center; is an active member of several professional organizations, including Sigma Theta Tau International and the Canadian College of Health Leaders; is chapter president of the Canadian Gerontological Nurses Association; and is a volunteer peer reviewer for *Aging and Mental Health, Health and Social Care in the Community*, and *Healthcare Management Forum*. She is also an editorial board member for *Healthcare Management Forum*. This is her first book.

Workplace Mental Health Manual for Nurse Managers

Lisa Y. Adams, PhD, MSc, RN

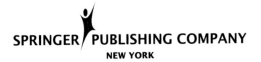

SPRINGER PUBLISHING COMPANY
NEW YORK

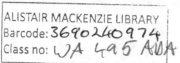
Copyright © 2015 Springer Publishing Company, LLC

All rights reserved.

No part of this publication may be reproduced, stored in a retrieval system, or transmitted in any form or by any means, electronic, mechanical, photocopying, recording, or otherwise, without the prior permission of Springer Publishing Company, LLC, or authorization through payment of the appropriate fees to the Copyright Clearance Center, Inc., 222 Rosewood Drive, Danvers, MA 01923, 978-750-8400, fax 978-646-8600, info@copyright.com or on the Web at www.copyright.com.

Springer Publishing Company, LLC
11 West 42nd Street
New York, NY 10036
www.springerpub.com

Acquisitions Editor: Margaret Zuccarini
Composition: Amnet Systems

ISBN: 978-0-8261-3745-6
e-book ISBN: 978-0-8261-3746-3

14 15 16 17 18 / 5 4 3 2 1

The author and the publisher of this Work have made every effort to use sources believed to be reliable to provide information that is accurate and compatible with the standards generally accepted at the time of publication. Because medical science is continually advancing, our knowledge base continues to expand. Therefore, as new information becomes available, changes in procedures become necessary. We recommend that the reader always consult current research and specific institutional policies before performing any clinical procedure. The author and publisher shall not be liable for any special, consequential, or exemplary damages resulting, in whole or in part, from the readers' use of, or reliance on, the information contained in this book. The publisher has no responsibility for the persistence or accuracy of URLs for external or third-party Internet websites referred to in this publication and does not guarantee that any content on such websites is, or will remain, accurate or appropriate.

Library of Congress Cataloging-in-Publication Data

Adams, Lisa Y., 1968– author.
  Workplace mental health manual for nurse managers / Lisa Y. Adams.
    p. ; cm.
  Includes bibliographical references and index.
  ISBN 978-0-8261-3745-6 (print : alk. paper) — ISBN 978-0-8261-3746-3 (e-book)
  I. Title.
  [DNLM: 1. Mental Health Services. 2. Occupational Health Services. 3. Nurse Administrators. 4. Psychiatric Nursing—methods. 5. Workplace. WA 495]
  RC440
  616.89′0231—dc23
                                                                                    2014010942

Special discounts on bulk quantities of our books are available to corporations, professional associations, pharmaceutical companies, health care organizations, and other qualifying groups. If you are interested in a custom book, including chapters from more than one of our titles, we can provide that service as well.

For details, please contact:
Special Sales Department, Springer Publishing Company, LLC
11 West 42nd Street, 15th Floor, New York, NY 10036-8002
Phone: 877-687-7476 or 212-431-4370; Fax: 212-941-7842
E-mail: sales@springerpub.com

Printed in the United States of America by Gasch Printing.

I dedicate this book to my husband of 11 years, Shannon Gerard Adams. Your support, patience, and humor during this challenging but exciting journey have made me smile when I needed to; you picked me up when I was feeling discouraged, and you were the wind beneath my wings when I was flying low. You were and always will be my pillar of strength and the solid foundation of what completes me. As well, to my mom and dad, Barbara and Hedley Clarke, for your support and encouragement, and for steering me in the right direction in life.

Contents

Foreword

Workplace mental illness, the absence of basic human caring, and stress are all growing realities in our culture and our time. This workplace mental health text provides a comprehensive overview, if not thesis, of the contributing factors to workplace stress and how to revisit our work life and our own mental health. The book also offers new insights and constructive approaches to issues that are otherwise overwhelming to consider or address.

How can nurses and health care workplaces expect to offer health and healing when such basic foundational human dynamics of mental health are not addressed? This work opens the door to both the dynamics and the deep dimensions of the root issues facing humanity and our places of work and play.

Workplace Mental Health Manual for Nurse Managers seeks to provide answers to personal and professional challenges and to offer solutions to the problems of postmodern violence and incivility, which are the very absence and antithesis of human caring and health.

Jean Watson, PhD, RN, AHN-BC, FAAN
Distinguished Professor and Dean Emerita
University of Colorado Denver, College of Nursing
Founder, Watson Caring Science Institute

Preface

During 15 years of leadership experience in nursing, including mental health and professional nursing practice, and experience as a manager and professional practice consultant, I have faced many challenges and been privy to requests for help from nurses encountering difficult and complex situations. As nurses learn in their fundamentals of nursing course, mental health spans the continuum of nursing, regardless of the setting; perhaps more importantly, it is not restricted to patients.

Today's health care landscape has brought many changes, challenges, and even turmoil for nurses. The changes, challenges, and turmoil can threaten nurses' mental health. As a nurse leader, I have seen the effects of these threats and have personally traversed some of this landscape. I have witnessed situations in which nurses were subjected to assault, harassment, addictions, violence, and bullying, which unnecessarily added stressors to the day's regular workload of managing complex patient care. In several of these situations, a lack of work–life balance contributed to these unwarranted "attacks." With nurses having nowhere to turn, no one to understand, and no policies for support or direction, I insistently raised awareness of these issues from a professional practice standpoint by preparing and offering regular presentations, with a particular focus on workplace bullying. The demand was overwhelming, and what began as sessions for one group of nurses quickly grew into a weekly schedule of presentations.

Throughout my professional nursing journey, bullying in different forms reared its ugly head at unexpected times and from unexpected corners of the profession. As a novice nurse, I was yelled at publicly and bullied by another nurse; in graduate school, I was belittled and slammed, and I was the target of derogatory remarks.

The book is organized into four parts. Part I, "The Importance of Achieving a Healthy Work Environment," establishes the importance of creating a healthy work environment. Part II, "Creating and Fostering a Respectful Workplace Environment," describes the roles and responsibilities of health care institutions, workplace managers, and individual employees in creating, fostering, and continuing healthy workplace attitudes and respectful behaviors. Part III, "The Issues That Challenge One's Mental Health," investigates the variety of situations within a workplace environment that can erode mental health among coworkers, including the effects on coworkers of bullying, violence, addictions, and unethical behavior. Part IV, "Strategies for Managing the Mentally

Unhealthy Workplace," explores various approaches at the personal, professional, and organizational levels that can influence change from an unhealthy to a healthy workplace environment.

For all nurses who have experienced cronyism, blatant disregard, and disrespectful treatment, this book is written for you. No nurse or nursing student should be subjected to unprofessional, disrespectful behavior on the part of workplace colleagues, and it is my hope that you will never have to endure it. It is my aim to arm you with the knowledge and know-how to enable you to confront troubling, tormenting, conflicting situations and individuals appropriately, and to arm you with the values, ethics, and knowledge and practices needed for you to confidently move forward in your career. May you always treat your colleagues with respect and strive to protect your character, integrity, and self-value, so that they do not unfold or weaken in the grasp of a bully or from the unkind comments or actions of a jealous intimidator. Carry yourself and your accomplishments proudly and with courage, and raise your head high.

Lisa Y. Adams

Acknowledgments

I would like to acknowledge and credit the most significant role models and mentors in my life: my two PhD thesis supervisors at the University of Alberta, Dr. Priscilla Koop and Dr. Colleen Norris, and my current director, Ms. Colleen Simms, whom I have known for many years. Each of you has shown a passionate interest in my undertakings, a patience that excels beyond compare, and a respectful collegiality that makes me feel valued for what I do—something I will never forget. You all have a very compassionate core, a genuine presence, and a professional integrity that are admirable, respected, and motivating—true nursing leadership attributes that seem a rarity at times, and that touch many a life, more than you will ever know. Thanks as well to the staff and management at Springer Publishing Company, particularly Margaret Zuccarini, whose energy and support made this book become a reality and a dream come true. Bless you all.

1

Stress, Mental Health, and Mental Illness 101

The world we have created is a product of our thinking;
it cannot be changed without changing our thinking.
—*Albert Einstein*

LEARNING OBJECTIVES

By the end of this chapter, the learner will be able to:

1. Understand the meaning of stress, mental health, and mental illness.
2. Discuss the physiological processes and behavioral responses that occur as a result of stress.
3. Identify and discuss the differences between the good, the bad, and the ugly of stress.
4. Highlight epidemiological trends of stress and how stress can impact nursing students in particular.

Mental health and mental illness are everyone's business. Mental health is defined by the World Health Organization (WHO) and the Centers for Disease Control and Prevention (CDC) as "a state of well-being in which the individual realizes his or her own abilities, can cope with the normal stresses of life, can work productively and fruitfully, and is able to make a contribution to his or her community" (CDC, 2011b). It is not simply the absence of a diagnosable mental illness (Mental Health Foundation, 2013). In essence, mental health is like a package that helps describe our social, emotional, and psychological well-being. When we are mentally healthy, we are able to enjoy our life and environment, and the people in it. We can be creative, learn, try new things, and take risks. We are better able to cope with difficult times in our personal and professional lives, and we have feelings of increased self-esteem and self-confidence. We feel the sadness and anger that can come with the death of a loved one, a job loss, or relationship problems and other difficult events, but in time, we are able to get on with and enjoy our lives once again (Canadian Mental Health Association [CMHA], 2013a).

With good mental health, you can typically perform many functions and activities of life without undue heartache or stress. These include the ability to learn;

to feel, express, and manage emotions; to build relationships with others; to cope; and to have a sense of contentment, as well as a zest for living, laughing, and having fun. In doing so, you create resiliency, adaptability, high self-confidence, high self-esteem, good work–life balance, meaning and purpose in life, and optimism to see the glass as half full, not half empty (Elements Behavioral Health, 2013; Mental Health Foundation, 2013).

At the opposite end of the spectrum, however, when alterations to one's mental health occur, a mental illness can develop. Mental illness refers collectively to "disorders generally characterized by dysfunction of mood, thought, and/or behavior," as recognized by the *Diagnostic and Statistical Manual of Mental Disorders, Fifth Edition (DSM-5;* American Psychiatric Association, 2013). The development of mental health concerns and/or disorders has great potential to infringe on all those activities of living first identified.

The ways in which we maintain our mental health or are susceptible to the development of a mental illness is highly individualized. Being mentally healthy does not necessarily translate into the absence of mental illness. Unequivocally, one can still have a mental illness and be considered mentally healthy. For example, you may have depression and cope quite well in society and still consider yourself mentally healthy. Likewise, what causes you anxiety, stress, and challenges to your mental health may be well accepted or tolerated by others. Similarly, what coping mechanisms work for you to handle stress may or may not work for someone else. In all likelihood, if you do have good mental health, you are able to cope with the stressors and demands that life has placed upon you, you are able to strive to fulfill your utmost potential—no matter what that potential may be, and you in some way play a valuable contributing role with your family, friends, workplace, and community (Mental Health Foundation, 2012).

While much emphasis and even health system dollars are directed to address physical illnesses (Institute of Health Economics, 2008), mental illnesses are just as important as physical illnesses. In fact, mental illnesses and physical illnesses have a reciprocal relationship whereby inadequacies in the management of one can exert a direct impact on the development or exacerbation of the other. Just like physical illness, mental illness operates on a continuum. For example, people who experience impaired mobility, such as results from a broken leg or fractured hip, are prevented from being involved in the activities they previously enjoyed, like running, walking, swimming, shopping, or whatever may have brought them pleasure and purpose. As a result, they may become depressed, anxious, or both.

Before we get into more detail about mental illness, let's first allay some myths that you have most likely heard. For example, mental illness is not a sign of weakness of character; all human beings are born with the genetic vulnerability to mental illness, which indiscriminately strikes all segments of society. Second, mental illness is not an old person's disease; in fact, depression, in particular, is concentrated among men and women in their prime working years and in their children, with those between 15 and 24 years of age most likely to experience a mental disorder. Like a diabetic coma, a heart attack, a stroke, a concussion, or breast cancer, depression and posttraumatic stress disorder (PTSD) have physical, physiological, and psychological effects (Royal Canadian Mounted Police [RCMP], 2010).

HISTORY OF MENTAL ILLNESS

To better understand mental illness, the role it can play in the workplace, and why it is often viewed negatively, it helps to know where it came from and how it evolved to what we understand it to be today. The history of mental illness helps put the negativity surrounding it into perspective. In the workplace, this understanding is essential for all nurses so they can be better prepared to identify, educate, and support individuals and colleagues with mental illness. Mental health and mental illness are covered in nursing educational curricula and span the continuum across all medical, surgical, and community settings; however, this does not guarantee that all nurses understand it, identify it, or are able to support colleagues and others who have it. Although nursing professes to be a "caring" profession in the delivery of health care, it should never be assumed that all nurses and nursing staff are aware of the intricacies of mental illness.

The history of mental illness in the world today has experienced a significant societal evolution. Having had the ground shaken beneath its feet, in a tsunami sort of way, society still battles the ripples, stereotypical undercurrents, and flood of criticism and stigma created by mental illness. From the prehistoric depths and darkness of evil, demonic possession, witchcraft, and sorcery to the power of religion and magic and then onward to supernatural phenomena, sources of mental illness have been many, but at every step along the way, the one common thread that repeatedly occurs is that of punishment, fear, the unknown, and societal misfit. Predating ancient civilizations to prehistoric times, to 10,000 BCE, there was little or no definitive division between medicine, magic, religion, and spirituality. Later, in 5000 BCE, humans predominantly believed that mental illness resulted from supernatural phenomena and represented some form of evil, such as demonic possession, witchcraft, and sorcery. Others believed it occurred as a result of God inflicting punishment for sinful behaviors.

The mentally ill were treated horrifically and were often shackled to the walls of dungeons in cold, cramped, concrete quarters with iron cuffs and collars, treated barbarically like animals, and subjected to bloodletting, abuse, torture, and starvation. They were displayed as sideshow freaks for public amusement and hidden away in pigpens and cellars by ashamed families. Furthermore, exorcisms, incantations, prayer, atonement, and torture under the pretext of surgical intervention in the form of lobotomies, often performed experimentally with trephination (chipping a hole in the skull), were all used to help drive out the evil spirits.

As we try to combat the stigma associated with mental illness, a continuous battle ensues in which it becomes highly conceivable why we need to better understand the concept of mental illness, particularly in our workplace, where we spend much of our working life. Furthermore, the horrific history of mental illness reinforces why overcoming the stigma and stereotypes surrounding mental illness is difficult—all the more reason to write this book and address the matter among working nurses head-on.

ETIOLOGY OF MENTAL ILLNESS

To begin a discussion of mental health and mental illness, let's first focus on what causes mental illness. There are many different etiologies of mental illness, and again, all are individualized depending on the person experiencing it. Although the exact cause of mental illness has been debated for years, it remains a gray area. When we talk about causes of mental illness, we typically focus in on core sources, such as biological, psychological, and environmental factors, and on life's lived experiences, or some combination thereof.

Biologically, key sources include the biochemistry of the brain, injury, infections, and genetics. As developing or aspiring nurses, we have learned and are still learning about the existence and function of neurotransmitters in the brain and the chemical imbalances that can occur. These chemicals of the brain, or neurotransmitters, keep the brain in check and functioning optimally; however, when an imbalance of neurotransmitters occurs, neurons fail to communicate with each other, neuronal transmission and messages sent and received are disrupted, and signs and symptoms of mental illness occur. Today's advances in research and knowledge of mental illness have even pinpointed specific areas of the brain that are linked with the occurrence of particular mental illnesses. In some cases, even hormonal imbalances can affect mental health (Mayo Clinic, 2013).

Brain injury has also been linked to the development of mental illness. This injury may occur as a result of prenatal or delivery trauma, substance abuse by an expectant mother, or injury to the adult brain may occur as a result of intrinsic or extrinsic trauma or force (Katz, 2012; Mayo Clinic, 2013). For example, a prenatal loss of oxygen to the brain of the fetus has been linked with the occurrence of autism in children (Katz, 2012). Furthermore, the expectant mother who uses or abuses illicit drugs and substances compromises the development of the fetal brain and precipitates the development of anxiety, depression, and paranoia (Katz, 2012). Babies born to mothers who take methadone during pregnancy are typically born with symptoms of withdrawal from addiction.

Infections, genetics, and poor nutrition can either precipitate the development of a mental illness or worsen the presentation of mental illness symptomology. For example, as suggested by Katz, "a condition known as pediatric autoimmune neuropsychiatric disorder (PANDA) associated with *Streptococcus* bacteria has been linked to the development of obsessive-compulsive disorder and other mental illnesses in children." Genetically, people who have family members with a particular mental illness are increasingly likely to develop the mental illness themselves as a result of inheriting the same genetic traits. Poor nutrition can also impact the development and normal functioning of one's brain and good mental health (Katz, 2012).

Psychologically, many factors have been credited with contributing to the development of mental illness. These range from neglect to abuse, creating low self-esteem and confidence. For example, a child subjected to psychological trauma, such as emotional abuse, physical abuse, and/or sexual abuse, has increased susceptibility to the development of a mental illness. Neglect, the early loss of a parent, poor ability to relate to others, feelings of inadequacy, anxiety, low self-esteem, low confidence, anger, and loneliness can all predispose one to the development of a mental illness (Katz, 2012).

Normal life events that occur in our immediate environments can also increase risk for mental illness, such as the death or loss of a loved one (Katz, 2012; Mayo Clinic, 2013), changing jobs or schools, substance abuse by parents, and dysfunctional family life. Growing up in a family in which there is history of sexual or physical abuse leads to low self-esteem and confidence and unhealthy patterns of thinking linked to mental illness, such as pessimism and distorted ways of thinking. Furthermore, exposure to toxins and struggles to meet social or cultural expectations, such as those that occur in a society that positively associates thinness and dieting fads with beauty, fame, and fortune, can cause mental illness to arise (Katz, 2012).

EPIDEMIOLOGY OF MENTAL ILLNESS

According to the National Comorbidity Survey Replication, 26% of American adults aged 18 and older have a diagnosable mental disorder in any given year (Kessler, Chiu, Demler, & Walters, 2005). Furthermore, nearly 50% of U.S. adults will develop at least one mental illness during their lifetime (CDC, 2011b). Americans are clearly suffering. Globally, this growing trend occurs in Canada (CMHA, 2013b), Australia (Australian Institute of Health and Welfare, 2013), and Europe (WHO, 2013); these organizations report rates of mental illness at 20% (4.5 million) Canadians, 20% (3.2 million) Australians, and 27% (83 million) Europeans, respectively.

These rising epidemiological trends produce a significant financial cost to society. According to the WHO, mental illness results in more disability in developed countries than any other group of illnesses, including cancer and heart disease (CDC, 2011a). More specifically, it costs countries millions and billions in health care costs and overall economic burden. In the United States, for example, a staggering $300 billion was spent in 2002 (CDC, 2011a), while the United Kingdom spent $1.3 billion U.S. (European Commission, 2004). Similarly, Canada and Australia spent $18.9 billion U.S. (The Conference Board of Canada, 2012) and $18.6 billion U.S. (Australian Bureau of Statistics, 2013), respectively. Regardless of the country or geography, one of the primary sources of mental illness is stress.

UNDERSTANDING STRESS

It is futile to talk about mental health and mental illness without including the topic of stress. As a nurse or aspiring nurse leader, you probably don't need me to get into much detail around the topic of stress, as you have most likely already experienced and lived it yourself. However, we often need reminders of how stress impacts us, and maybe by understanding the impact we can become more motivated to identify it, address it, and prevent it. Nurses are actually one group of people in society who, because of their past learning in social sciences, pathophysiology, and anatomy, feel they "know better" how to keep the harmful effects of stress at bay and that this will never happen to them (Moola, Ehlers, & Hattingh, 2008). For those who are nursing students, your recent involvement in your anatomy and physiology courses will be of much value; for those nurses who have graduated, a trek down memory lane is in store for you, only this time we focus on "you" and how stress impacts you. This section, therefore, will provide for you a brief overview of stress and its common concepts, with a particular emphasis on its physiological and psychosocial impact.

TABLE 1.1   Ways to Express Stress in Various Languages

LANGUAGE	PHRASE USED
German	Ich fühle mich gestresst
French	être stressé
Australian	Wound up tight
Turkish	aşırı stresli
American	Spun out
Dutch	Benadrukt
Arabic	شعور بالاجهاد
Chinese	我今天很累
Japanese	私はストレスがたまっています
Spanish	estoy estresado
Canadian	I feel stressed

Stress is one of those concepts that is open to interpretation, as individuals experience and perceive it quite differently. By definition, stress is "the pattern of specific and nonspecific responses an organism makes to stimulus events that disturb its equilibrium and tax or exceed its ability to cope" (American Psychological Association [APA], 2012). It is a "condition of the mind–body interaction" with an individualized expression. It is not just the dramatic stressful events that exact their toll, but also the many events of daily life that elevate and sustain activities of physiological systems and cause sleep deprivation, overeating, and other health-damaging behaviors, producing the feeling of being "stressed out" (MacEwan, 2006). Despite its various meanings for various people, stress has found its way to be expressed universally. As seen in Table 1.1, the phrase "I'm feeling stressed" or "stressed out" has many universal translations.

Short-lived situations such as leaving home to go to work and getting stuck behind road construction, making you late for work, create stress, but over the long term, dealing with a difficult colleague at work who repeatedly refuses to pull his or her own weight and help out with the workload of the nursing unit/setting also creates long-standing stress. In any event, it is important to recognize the point at which stress can become dangerous. When stress begins to infringe upon your own normal performance, such as living a normal routine life, freely engaging socially with others, and feeling good about going to work and loving your job, it becomes a more serious issue. Furthermore, stress can play havoc with your emotions, thus causing you to feel easily irritated and fatigued, lose concentration, and be short with others (APA, 2012). The body's initial response to stress is a universal one and typically depicts the flight-or-flight response and the work of Hans Selye (1974).

Stressors, or key sources of stress, are unequivocally just as important to acknowledge. Stressors are defined by the APA (2012) as "an internal or external event or stimulus that induces stress." In essence, a stressor is any event or situation that an individual perceives as a threat; stressors can be negative or positive.

Stressors are what actually precipitate either adaptation to or the stress response itself and represent the demands placed on the body. Stressors for nurses in the workplace, for example, can be demanding patients, existing conflict with colleagues, and the level of busyness and workload in the nursing setting/unit.

Job stress is what we hear people refer to when work is overwhelming and infringing on their lives in general. Everyone has a certain amount of stress while working or completing family responsibilities. However, having stress for unnecessary or unknown reasons can adversely affect mental health. As a rule, many of us don't acknowledge our own strengths, values, and potentiality, or how much they are worth. It is this self-underestimation that can lead to an inferiority complex, which causes serious psychiatric problems in the future. While some stress can energize and motivate us to do a good job, when job demands are excessive, don't match our abilities, allow little control, or provide little support, stress can negatively affect us (Pfizer, 2013).

Job stress is widely experienced and so pervasive that it affects people from all industries, ranks, and socioeconomic levels. Because so much of our lives are spent at work, job stress can create stress in other areas as well. For example, when people are stressed at work, they may have less patience and less energy, so relationships suffer; they let exercise go by the wayside and possibly experience burnout or depression. Because of the close link between job stress and general chronic stress, both can take a significant toll on overall health and wellness (Scott, 2010).

The most common cause of stress in the workplace is lack of time and excessive workloads, followed by poor interpersonal relations and the risk of accident and injury. Depending on your situation, stress can also be caused by many factors, such as boredom, repetition, unrealistic deadlines, adapting to change, starting a new job or being in a dead-end job, fear of layoffs, noisy or unsafe work environments, office politics, difficult personality types, or even bullies. In addition to very real external factors, a contributing factor in feeling stressed is your internal response to outside events. For example, if you receive criticism from your boss, you could interpret that as your boss's dissatisfaction with you and become upset or pessimistic about it, or you could see it as a positive suggestion to help you improve and succeed. (Pfizer, 2013)

Regardless of the cause, stress is a very real problem that can lead to a range of physical, emotional, and behavioral problems and infringe on every aspect of life (Pfizer, 2013).

In recent years, we have been hearing a lot about workplace events, such as disrespectful workplaces, bullying (Stokowski, 2010), and even violence (Green, 2013; Ricciardi, 2014) in the nursing profession. All of these have been identified as significant sources of stress for nurses that impact not only their levels of stress, but also their overall mental health, work performance, and work satisfaction. Learning about perpetrators, who they are, how they work, what they do, and the impact they can have on the nurse is a rising research interest in nursing and holds some very important information that you should be aware of. Bullying and violence are discussed in Chapters 7 and 8, respectively.

THE BODY'S RESPONSE TO STRESS

Your body's stress response kicks in when you feel under threat, whether that threat is real or perceived. Mammals have evolved a superb mechanism to ensure we have the best possible chance of survival when faced with a life-threatening situation. Almost everyone is familiar with the physical symptoms of intense stress: racing heart, sweaty palms, "butterfly-filled" belly. It is also possible to experience low-grade, ongoing stress without those immediate symptoms. The chemicals that the body produces are the same and can negatively affect the body at the cellular level. "Your heart beats faster, your blood pressure increases, and you breathe faster, pumping maximum oxygen and energy-rich blood to your muscles. Your liver releases more sugar into your blood, ready for action" (Your Amazing Brain, 2014). All nonessential body functions, such as digestion and writing your papers, cease as you divert all energy to your muscles and brain. We don't have control over stressors that create a real or imagined stress for us, but we can work to control our reaction to help manage stress for our own good and for the good of our workplace.

No matter what the sources of stress you are experiencing, there is a universal response process that our body produces. Founded on the ideas of Hans Selye (1974), the "flight-or-fight" response best describes for us how the body responds to acute stress. The flight-or-fight response works to help protect our bodies and our minds; however, we still have to be careful because it can actually heighten stress levels even more and precipitate a cycle that may never get resolved. Therefore, by being aware, recognizing, knowing, and understanding your style under stress, you can start making positive changes to help address it (Selye, 1974). This complex physiological process that occurs involves primarily the brain, nervous system, and endocrine system. These systems realistically control and influence your cognition, experience, emotions, and behaviors (MacEwan & Gianaros, 2010).

The adrenocorticotropic hormone (ACTH) also stimulates the inner core (medulla) of each of the two adrenal glands so that epinephrine (adrenalin) is released. Epinephrine causes the body's response to the stress, such as increased respirations, dilated pupils, increased pulse, and increased heart rate. Accompanying and complementing the flight-or-fight response is what is known as the general adaptation syndrome. This system response comprises alarm, resistance, and recovery/exhaustion phases and represents the whole impact of stress on the body, be it short-term, acute, or chronic stress (Selye, 1974).

The brain releases endorphins to relieve pain, heart rate increases and heart increases its strength of contraction to pump more blood, blood pressure rises, digestion slows so the much needed blood may be diverted to muscles, salivation and mucous secretion decreases and you get a dry mouth feeling, pupils dilate so that you have a more sensitive vision, senses of sight, hearing, smell, and taste are heightened, ready to identify any threats, sweating increases to flush waste and to cool down the body, blood clotting increases to prevent bleeding to death during physical threat, sugars and fats are released into the blood stream to supply fuel, adrenaline and other hormones are released into the bloodstream to provide energy, muscle tension increases to prepare for action in the shortened time, bronchi dilate, allowing for more air into the lungs, breathing gets shallow and faster to supply more oxygen to the muscles and body tissue. This reaction is pure stress and is a result of a cascade of hormones that starts as soon as your brain realizes that a demand is being made on your body. These physiological effects of stress are meant to be short term. Once the danger passes, the body should return to its state of homeostasis, the state of internal equilibrium when all the body systems function smoothly and are balanced. (Stress Relief Tools, 2012)

What was described previously as the "flight-or-fight" response depicts primarily the "alarm" phase of the general adaptation syndrome. Here, your body is preparing for action by releasing a series of chemicals that was just described. However, there are other physiological processes that continue from this phase, and these we will refer to as the resistance and the recovery/exhaustion phases. After the body is alarmed and readied that action may be needed, it then has a capacity built up to resist the stressor and its effects, so that homeostasis or the body's equilibrium can be maintained. When the body is successful at keeping the person safe or out of harm's way, homeostasis is achieved, and the body is able to restore itself physiologically in equilibrium and recovery. These stress mechanisms aim to help the body cope and are protective in nature, as they try to promote short-term adaptations, known as allostasis (MacEwan & Gianaros, 2010).

In the event that the body is not able to recover and restore itself to equilibrium, exhaustion may occur. Exhaustion occurs when the body's resources and energy stores become depleted and the body loses its ability to adapt to the stressful event and the turmoil of bodily processes that were triggered. Here, the body's protective mechanisms fail, potentially leading to "long-term" dysregulation or allostasis, as identified above, and "maladaptive wear and tear on the body and brain under chronically stressful conditions" (MacEwan & Gianaros, 2010). The exhaustion of your body and the negative impact it can create may not be immediately visible to you or others. However, it is during the exhaustion phase that the negative harmful effects of stress make their debut. As the body constantly attempts to respond and adjust to higher and higher levels of stress, wear and tear result and set the body up for failure in the areas of the cardiac, cardiovascular, immune, and digestive systems, in particular.

THE PATHOPHYSIOLOGY OF STRESS

Many of us don't realize the full impact that stress has on our bodies. It is of little wonder, then, that stress is often referred to as the "silent killer." From the research obtained to date, I want to walk you through what happens physiologically when you are dealing with stress, particularly for prolonged periods of time. By the time I am finished here, I hope you realize that it would be a prudent exercise to let the stress go. Don't let it take control of your life. You have to remember that you and only you are always in control of your life. You are the one who has total control over what you do, what you say, and how you respond to stressful events and objects. We are all going to experience stress, some perhaps at higher levels than others, because life would not be life without it. However, the key here is up to you, in how you perceive it, respond to it, cope with it, and let it take control of you, your thoughts, and your behaviors. To help you determine the extent to which you perceive it, cope with it, and control it, we will first discuss its impact physiologically.

The stress response itself is not harmful or even potentially pathological in nature. It is just the body using any and all of the resources it has to respond to actual or potential threats. However, when stress becomes demanding, prolonged, and sustained, the homeostasis of the body and the brain becomes threatened, and health becomes endangered (Fuchs & Flügge, 2003).

Stress exerts many effects on various parts of the body. Some of these vital parts or organs include the brain, the heart, the gastrointestinal system, and the immune system. Furthermore, the impact on the brain is what significantly contributes to the development of mental illnesses in general, or at least enrich the foundation on which they can become precipitated. With the brain as a starting point, very soon the effect of long-term stress begins to permeate systemically to other body organs as well. Through the sympathetic nervous system pathway, every organ in the body is affected by yet another hormone, adrenalin, which is released once stress occurs (Fuchs & Flügge, 2003). Because one of the main outcomes of stress is altered mental health, it is worthwhile to become familiar with the process that occurs and the altered chemical balances that can precipitate the development of a mental illness. As suggested by MacEwan and Gianaros (2010), "the brain is the key organ of stress activity, coping and recovery processes."

The Brain

Stress exerts significant effects on the brain. The brain serves many functions and has much neuronal plasticity and flexibility to respond to the internal and external pressures place upon it (Fuchs & Flügge, 1998). "The brain is the key organ of the response to stress because it determines what is threatening and, therefore, potentially stressful, as well as the physiological and behavioral responses which can be either adaptive or damaging" (MacEwan, 2007). Once the body is subjected to stress, there are several neuronal processes that trigger the release of several other subsequent effects, starting with the brain. "Stress and stress hormones produce both adaptive and maladaptive effects on this brain region throughout the life course. Even early life events influence lifelong patterns of emotionality and stress responsiveness and alter the rate of brain and body aging" (MacEwan, 2007).

Over time, stress causes disruptions to neural circuitry, neurotransmitter metabolism, neuroendocrine function, and synaptic plasticity (Salim, Chugh, & Asghar, 2012). The main brain structures involved are the limbic system, hypothalamus, and pituitary gland as well as their interconnecting neuroendocrine systems. As described by Fuchs and Flügge (1998), "limbic and hypothalamic brain structures integrate neuroendocrine, autonomic, emotional, and cognitive inputs and determine the magnitude and duration of behavioural, neural, and hormonal responses to stressful experiences" (p. 295). In particular, "the hippocampus, amygdala, and prefrontal cortex undergo stress-induced structural remodelling, which alters behavioral and physiological responses" (MacEwan, 2007). "Dr. Rajita Sinha, a professor of psychiatry and neurobiology at Yale University School of Medicine and director of the Yale Stress Center, reports in the journal *Biological Psychiatry* that even among healthy individuals, adverse life events that cause stress can lead to shrinkage in parts of the brain responsible for regulating emotions and metabolism." Furthermore, "it's not individual traumatic events that have the most impact, but the cumulative effect of a lifetime's worth of stress that might cause the most dramatic changes in brain volume" (Park, 2012).

Sinha adds that even "very recently affected subjects showed smaller grey matter in their brains in the prefrontal cortex, a region that is responsible for self-control, emotions and physiological functions such as maintaining proper glucose and insulin levels." Furthermore, it is "important for top-down regulation of our emotions, cognition, desires, and impulse control. As nerve tissue in this region disappears due to constant battering from repeated stressful events, our ability to counteract potentially dangerous desires, such as for addictive substances, or control our impulsive behaviors to do dangerous things, may wane" (Park, 2012).

The death and dying of neurons is a significant event for how stress impacts the brain. The death of neurons and neuronal atrophy that occurs in the limbic, hypothalamic, and even the whole prefrontal cortex can shrink significantly in size, infringing on one's memory and learning process ability. Its neuronal synapses and synaptic activity are all compromised, potentially causing increased aging of the brain. In addition, with glucocorticoid hormones as one of the key mediators in this process, their high levels following stress can actually cause the death of neurons (Fuchs & Flügge, 1998). The steady release of cortisol, for example, causes the brain to become battered with stress and not only leads to a great deal of wear and tear on the brain (MacEwan, 2007) but also can literally excite neurons to death. Structurally, the brain itself begins to change in response to these alterations/events.

Functionally, from a nurse's perspective, critical thinking and decision making become jeopardized (Starcke & Brand, 2012); reliance on memory for knowledge and past practices becomes challenged (Fuchs & Flügge, 1998); the capacity for new learning of practice skills, research, and knowledge becomes limited (Fuchs & Flügge, 1998); and the nurse's ability to cope with adversity is lowered (Park, 2012). Finally, one's measure of impulse control and level of aggression can also change, leading detrimentally to the development of addiction disorders and varying degrees of emotional dysfunction and turmoil.

The interconnectedness between neurons and the endocrine system is made possible by a structure in the brain, the hypothalamus (which is responsible for producing hormones that control body temperature, hunger, mood, sex drive, sleep, thirst, and the release of hormones from many glands, especially the pituitary gland). The hypothalamus sits directly above the pituitary gland, which is primarily responsible for regulating the endocrine system. When an individual faces a stressor or some form of threat, the hypothalamus synthesizes and releases two main chemicals, vasopressin and corticotropin-releasing hormone (CRH), which stimulate the pituitary to release ACTH. ACTH in turn stimulates the release of cortisol, which helps to control the body's metabolism of fats, carbohydrates, sodium, potassium, and protein as well as blood pressure. ACTH then travels via the bloodstream to reach the adrenal glands. The outer layer of the adrenal glands, the cortex, is stimulated to release stress hormones (corticoids), which help the body increase its energy stores as well as raise blood pressure.

Through a cascade of reactions, cortisol causes neurons to admit more calcium through channels in their membrane, so that the neurons become overloaded with calcium, causing increasingly frequent firing of signals and literally exciting brains cells to death. Contrary to traditional ideas, the adult brain does make new neurons, but only in very restricted areas. For example, the hippocampus of an adult rat makes between 5,000 and 10,000 new neurons each day. However, the effects of stress on the brain don't stop there.

What occurs is a metamorphosis of the brain in which remodeling and/or modifications of the brain occur in response to the stress (MacEwan, 2007), modulation of cytokine production occurs, and neuro-inflammation and aberrant behaviors affiliated with the outcomes of depression, anxiety, and cognitive dysfunction can occur, something now termed *oxidative stress theory* (Salim et al., 2012). Even everyday stress can lead to changes in the brain that make us more vulnerable to mental as well as social disorders ranging from depression (MacEwan, 2007; Park, 2012) to addiction and behavioral conditions (Park, 2012), anxiety (Salim et al., 2012), and cognitive impairments (MacEwan, 2007; Salim et al., 2012).

Long-term stress, anxiety, and depression have been linked with an increased risk for dementia and Alzheimer's disease because they stimulate the growth of the proteins that may cause Alzheimer's disease and hence memory loss. Overeating, drinking alcohol, and smoking cigarettes are among the negative informal stress management approaches that people use.

Antidepressant drugs that increase serotonin levels (e.g., selective serotonin reuptake inhibitors, including Prozac) boost the rate at which new neurons are made. Perhaps depression or recovery from it may be related to the formation of new neurons. It's quite clear that chronic stress is related to depression. A common feature of depression is an excess release of cortisol into the blood. Some now suggest that the major changes in serotonin and other neurotransmitters seen in depression are not the cause of depression, but rather are secondary to changes in the stress response.

The Heart

The impact of stress on the heart as well is significant to recognize. Physiologically, as a result of stress, the heart rate increases, and the force with which the blood is pumped and the volume of blood or cardiac output also increase, blood vessels become damaged, blood thickens, coagulation increases, blood platelets increase, and fatty deposits in the arteries increase, which along with increased circulating levels of cholesterol all precipitate and create a ripe environment for the development of atherosclerosis and hence hypertension and heart disease.

The Gastrointestinal System

The gastrointestinal system does not escape the effects of stress. According to the Harvard Medical School (2010), "The relationship between environmental or psychological stress and gastrointestinal distress is complex and bidirectional: stress can trigger and worsen gastrointestinal pain and other symptoms, and vice versa. This is why psychological therapies are often used in combination with other treatments—or even on their own—to treat functional gastrointestinal disorders." As blood is diverted to the body's muscles to prepare for the stress of fight or flight, it is moved away from other, less important areas, such as the gastrointestinal system. Stress causes the gastrointestinal system to literally shut down, peristalsis is reduced, sphincters close, the release of acidic juices decreases, intestinal tone decreases, and hence digestion slows (Harvard Medical School, 2010). Manifestations of such events can lead to health issues such as chronic constipation, stomach acid dysfunction, and ulcers—yet even more stressors for the already stressed nurse. Furthermore, as found by Suarez, Mayer, Ehlert, and Nater (2010), symptoms of gastric disorders "were significantly predicted by increased levels of perceived chronic stress, dispositional stress reactivity, and use of maladaptive coping strategies," and the importance of stress-related factors in individuals with gastrointestinal problems indicates that stress-reducing interventions may be beneficial in these patients.

The Immune System

The impact of stress continues into the body's immune system, where many of the long-term effects of stress reside. When stress occurs and the body proceeds to increase the release of adrenal hormones, such as adrenalin, the production of T-lymphocytes, one of the body's main defenses against viruses, bacteria, fungi, and cancer cells, becomes suppressed. A weakened body leads to delayed healing of wounds and other infections and an increasing susceptibility to bacterial and viral infections and other health-related problems, such as asthma and even cancer (Segerstrom & Miller, 2004).

The impact of stress on the body then is very significant and serious and can precipitate or exacerbate many serious health problems. As nurses are most often working in disease-rich environments, their immunity as well as their cardiac, digestive, and immune systems are paramount to their overall health and well-being. As stated by Segerstrom and Miller (2004), the relationship between stress and the immune system is a significant one. The more a stressor deviates from normal parameters and becomes more chronic, the more components of the immune system become affected in a potentially detrimental way.

THE GOOD, THE BAD, AND THE UGLY OF STRESS

The concept of stress represents each domain of the good, the bad, and the ugly. Although stress is often nonspecific in nature, it requires individuals to make some change to how they normally cope with issues and is often thought of as one of life's greatest mysteries; however, it is in fact a normal and very useful process for all animal species, including humans. We use and even "need" stress for our everyday survival; however, stress can and does create some measure of disruption to our everyday equilibrium. When the effects of dealing with stress surpass what we can handle and our body's efforts to restore homeostasis, we endure a whole different balancing act altogether, only this time it needs to be about what is best for "you." The recipe for success in handling stress really revolves around the ideas of recognizing it, responding to it, coping with it, and addressing it, whether it is good or bad. However, recognizing and appreciating the good kinds of stress must be balanced with being proactive to address the bad stress.

As we have learned, there are numerous outcomes of stress. The development of anxiety is one very common example. We all experience anxiety in our everyday life, both at home and at work. However, just as with stress, how one responds to anxiety also varies. Because anxiety presents in various forms that depend on the degree of stress perceived and experienced, it is worthy here to highlight the general characteristics and various levels of anxiety. As individuals and practicing nurses, it is important for you to recognize and identify how you are responding to various stressors, your level of anxiety, and how you can best incorporate them into the different coping mechanisms you use to address or curtail them. The APA (2012) defines anxiety as "an intense emotional response caused by the preconscious recognition that a repressed conflict is about to emerge into consciousness." Perhaps more significant are the disorders that can arise from prolonged experiences of anxiety, which are characteristically marked by physiological arousal, feelings of tension, and intense apprehension without apparent reason (APA, 2012).

The general characteristics of anxiety are quite diverse. Anxiety is an outcome of stress that manifests itself in many different ways, which include a body state and/or energy that is not directly observable but behaviors that are, a subjective experience, and a holistic experience impacting many dimensions of one's life, and that has no one single specific object, source, or event as the main precipitating factor. As anxiety occurs in many different forms, the degree to which it is experienced by an individual is also on a continuum. This continuum ranges from mild to moderate levels of anxiety and then further to severe and even panic forms of anxiety, all of which we present here as the good, the bad, and the ugly of stress.

Good Stress

In mild to moderate levels, stress is an integral function of our everyday life. We actually call this type of stress "eustress." Eustress, originally explored in a stress model by Richard Lazarus (1966), is "the positive cognitive response to stress that is healthy, or gives one a feeling of fulfillment or other positive feelings." Furthermore, this is the good stress that keeps us feeling vital, alive, and excited about living (Scott, 2010). This type of stress is actually necessary for our everyday survival and growth. It is what gives you the additional fuel and energy that enable you to swerve to avoid a car accident on your way to work, to respond to a "999" call or emergency hospital call, and to intervene quickly in the operating room setting when things start to go wrong. In addition to avoiding some negative events, good stress can also be channeled into making us more productive at what we do, whether it is work or otherwise. It increases our productivity, our motivation, our commitment, our strength to continue, and the acute ability to think on our feet, critically analyze our surroundings, and make accurate decisions. Stress helps us to learn, adapt to change, act effectively, intervene when needed, and foster the growth and development of others, as well as ourselves. Unlike distress, to be discussed next, we view eustress very positively, and it often represents something we look forward to with enthusiasm, excitement, and vigor, and that has much meaning attached to it for us.

In nursing, stress helps to assist in the development not only of our own physical health but also of our mental and psychological health. It is an entity that allows us to perceive, recognize, respond, and cope with any internal and external threats that are made against us. In a positive manner, moderate levels of stress energize our strength, our dedication, and our ability and capacity to be productive, to grow, and to cope with whatever life throws our way.

In response to good stress, people typically manifest a mild form of anxiety. Mild anxiety occurs in response to everyday regular life events. These are the activities you engage in as part of your normal activities of daily living. This is the level of anxiety that is implied above, through stress that is able to exert many positive aspects. In a state of mild anxiety, you would experience an increased energy, alertness, and perception. Some of these positive aspects, identified above as well, include increased motivation, productivity, growth, creativity, and learning.

As nurses function in a state of mild anxiety, they are experiencing an increased energy, motivation, and physiological functioning. It enables them to deal with the little everyday stressors of working, such as the morning coffee break that you didn't get and now you are very hungry, or the interaction with the physician who was having a bad day but left you feeling temporarily uncomfortable. Cognitively, mild anxiety facilitates and enhances critical thinking, acute problem solving and responses, and differential decision making.

Bad Stress

Bad stress often presents itself as acute stress that can go as quickly as it comes. This stress is not necessarily harmful at the outset and can often be resolved with regular coping mechanisms and defenses, enough to return you to a nearly normal state. This type of stress often comes from conflicted relationships, overpacked schedules, and, yes, stressful jobs (Scott, 2010).

Stress has indeed developed a bad rap, particularly in nursing. However, it did so for very good, sound reasons. Bad stress can impact your physical and mental health as well as your overall emotional well-being. This bad stress, often referred to as "distress," is defined as persistent stress that is not resolved through coping or adaptation and so may lead to anxiety, withdrawal, and depressive behavior (Selye, 1974). As a result, it can interfere with one's ability to accomplish a job (Fevre, Kolt, & Matheny, 2006) or complete the tasks of one's daily living needed for functionality and survival.

In some cases, trying to avoid bad stress only propagates more stress. An example would be saying yes and taking on a heavier patient load than you know you can realistically manage, rather than dealing with the guilt you know you will feel by saying no and declining the heavier workload. As suggested by some (CMHA, 2010), bad stress at work occurs when the demand (e.g., deadlines, expectations, etc.) exceeds the level of control (little choice, little freedom to complete) and the nurse has to deal with it. Similarly, bad stress can occur when the amount of effort (physical or mental) exceeds the amount of reward (compensation, status, financial gain, or career enhancement) received for completing the task(s). What results is an imbalance that causes one to experience stress. Bad stress serves only to lower morale among staff nurses (CMHA, 2010), strain interprofessional relationships at work and relationships at home, infringe upon one's personal life, and cause nurses to question their actions, competencies, and abilities. Nurses who experience bad stress are probably unhappy in their current positions, have a low sense of self-esteem and confidence, and are beginning to have a low sense of self-worth in all that they do in spite of their good intentions.

Sometimes, when you are having a very busy day at work, you have received two acutely ill patients from the emergency department, two of your postop patients are taking a turn for the worse, and the doctor you are working with is not cooperative at all, stress levels are running high. Now add to this scenario that you are a new mom who has just returned to work after maternity leave, your 10-month-old little girl was not feeling well when you left home this morning, and your husband has gone out of town on a business trip for about 2 weeks. This scenario is perhaps not that far-fetched compared with what many nurses actually face.

In the case of moderate anxiety, the nurse is still very functional, but some often insidious periods of time or occurrences may create more frequent episodes of "pause for thought," or you perhaps slow down and think things through more carefully than you normally practice. This level is also considered quite a "normal" experience to endure.

As a nurse experiencing bad stress and moderate anxiety levels, you are probably not seeing the "broader" picture of what your patient needs. You are not dysfunctional at this point, as you are still very able to solve problems, provide care, and troubleshoot; you may just need some direction or prompting to do so. This level of anxiety is not yet a threat to your competency, knowledge, or practice but is cautionary in nature because you are dealing with the lives of highly vulnerable people, your patients. With moderate anxiety, perception is starting to become significantly narrowed because you are so focused on the possible cause of your anxiety. The nurse needs a little more direction and encouragement here to accomplish nursing tasks and can easily lose focus and attention to the detail or task at hand. Your physical and emotional health and level of discomfort can become compromised and may even be accompanied by increased nausea, vomiting, and/or dizziness in its extreme form.

Ugly Stress

When we become overburdened with all the demands placed upon us, our bodies become overwhelmed; we find it difficult to cope with these stressors, and they begin to take their toll on our bodies. This can occur when our stress response is triggered again and again and in the recovery mode our bodies fail to return to normal. This leads to the development of "ugly" and/or chronic stress over a period of time that doesn't resolve with coping strategies.

Ugly stress can result in health problems and diseases such as anxiety and depression, a higher prevalence of addictions, and a greater susceptibility to infectious diseases, to name a few. When such a severe reaction to stress occurs, our bodies become overwhelmed and debilitated to a certain degree. We are no longer able to function optimally as we once did, and our thought processes decline, concentration suffers, focus narrows, and memory becomes jeopardized and altered, so what was once looked on or judged to be safe and normal may not be. Nurses who encounter severe forms of prolonged stress have triple the rate of cardiovascular diseases (CMHA, 2010).

GENERAL SIGNS AND SYMPTOMS OF STRESS

There are generally many different signs and symptoms of stress. Some can be obvious, although most are very subtle and unnoticeable. Perhaps the most immediate symptomology that characterizes the body's response to stress includes such signs as physiological tachycardia, palpitations, tremors, muscle tension, diarrhea, frequent urination, diaphoresis, dry mouth, cold and clammy skin, pallor, and dilated pupils. Psychologically, tension, apprehension, indecisiveness, oversensitivity, tearfulness, agitation, irritability, dread, panic, powerlessness, a low sense of self-worth, and poor reality testing in the form of delusions and hallucinations can occur.

More subtly, signs and symptoms of stress can be characterized by hyper- or hypoglycemia (Milutinovic, Golubovic, Brkic, & Prokes, 2012), increased anti-inflammatory response and infections, decreased immunity, and cardiac complications.

Furthermore, as a result of increased central nervous system stimulation, confusion, disorientation, and thought disturbances can occur. Nurses vary in their perceptions of signs and symptoms. Some of the recognized signs and symptoms that were perceived differently among nurses were headache, insomnia, fatigue, despair, lower back pain, mood swings, hypertension, mental illness, stroke, and diabetes mellitus (Milutinovic et al., 2012). Anguish, anxiety, and gastrointestinal signs were also noted (Violante, Benso, Gerbaudo, & Violante, 2009).

Beyond moderate levels of anxiety and bad stress comes ugly stress in the forms of severe anxiety and panic. In severe anxiety, the individual is not very functional, struggles to perform activities of daily living, and is fraught with extreme worry and exaggerated degrees of fear over events that have or have not yet occurred. Severe anxiety or the cycle of constant worry tends to override the functions of the body to the point that physical symptoms begin to affect the person. This level of anxiety can potentially compromise a nurse's prudent, competent, and accountable practice as well as jeopardize patient safety and care. The nurse becomes engulfed by unreasonable concerns about financial status, personal safety, and/or health. As a practicing and licensed health care professional providing care to vulnerable patients, the nurse has difficulty concentrating and focusing on tasks at hand, to a more severe degree than is experienced with moderate anxiety. The nurse also has great difficulty relaxing and sleeping and may even begin to experience symptoms such as headaches, nausea, muscles aches, shortness of breath, heart palpitations, and hot flashes. This nurse would be seen as someone who is irritated, absent-minded, and even frantic at times because of feeling so overwhelmed by perceived fear and apprehension that something is going to happen. What were once perceived as easy nursing tasks are now difficult to complete and unravel because focus and concentration are lost, and even with prompting and reminders, completion of tasks is difficult. Because your perception is narrowed and you are so focused on your own thoughts and trying hard to complete your tasks, you can lose sight of patients' needs. Connecting the dots between the details of care, treatment, and assessment begins to impair your clinical judgement and therefore patient care, as some details assume exaggerated importance while other, significant pieces of information are missed.

The ultimate negative outcome of ugly stress is panic-level anxiety and is the most detrimental state of anxiety. During panic-level anxiety, the individual experiences brief but intense periods of apprehension, fear, and terror. There is an overall sense of impending doom, and the perceptual field is narrowed significantly. Symptomology at this level of anxiety can be characterized by trembling, shaking, confusion, dizziness, nausea, and trouble breathing. The sense of panic can arise abruptly, peak in only minutes, and last for many hours before starting to subside. The outcome of a panic state can be damage to one's health, eventual exhaustion, and even death if it is prolonged. When episodes of severe or panic anxiety occur frequently, even when the source of the anxiety has passed, one may be characterized as having an anxiety disorder.

When nurses experience feelings of panic, again, similar to what occurs in severe anxiety, the delivery of patient care and the quality of that care are at higher risk for being jeopardized. Panic drastically impairs their functioning in every respect. In this state of mind, nurses experience great difficulty in thinking, communicating, functioning, and concentrating on currents tasks and responsibilities. They are unable to think rationally and therefore competently, and they may even begin to depersonalize themselves from reality. They can begin to find comfort in a false sense of reality that can even manifest as delusions or hallucinations. Failure at being able to cope in its worse form can result in pathological behaviors.

In cases in which anxiety continues for prolonged periods of time, the possibility of a chronic anxiety disorder may occur. Characterized by a generalized feeling of apprehension and nervousness, chronic anxiety can significantly impact the body and its normal physiological processes. These individuals always seem to be waiting for something terrible to occur. They are what you and I would sometimes refer to as "worry warts," only in a much more extreme form. Similar to an unwanted wart or growth that won't go away, your life is forever anxious and never fully enjoyed or appreciated because you are so busy ruminating over what has occurred, why something happened, what should have occurred, or what needs to occur.

STRESS IN NURSING AND HOW IT IS PERCEIVED

The issue of stress among nurses is highly prevalent. Much of the research on nurses focuses on the topic of stress and how it impacts their quality of work life and job performance (Adriaenssens, de Gucht, & Maes, 2012; Nahm, Warren, Zhu, An, & Brown, 2012). Many different sources of stress have been identified for nurses that range from the environmental context (Chen, Lin, Wang, & Hou, 2009; Kawano, 2008) to patient populations (Adriaenssens et al., 2012) and even to their own coping mechanisms, self-care behaviors, and perceptions (Nahm et al., 2012). Chapter 2 will cover in depth nurses' sources of stress. Stress exists for nurse leaders as well.

In one study, Roffey Park (2005) found that "78% of managers are suffering from work-related stress."

The experience of stress for nurses, then, is obviously not a new phenomenon. A typical day at work can often resemble a rollercoaster ride as nurses scurry around attending to their patients' needs and their family concerns and complaints, giving 150% of themselves, working with physicians and collaboratively with other health professionals, engaging in astute and timely documentation, and mentally processing all other demands placed upon them. As health care providers who spend much of their time at work thinking, processing knowledge on their feet, and translating research into practice in an expedited manner, nurses work in one of the most physically and mentally challenging jobs in health care and often do so in 12-hour shift increments, outside the parameters of the nocturnal clock. For nurse leaders, looming deadlines, staffing issues, fiscal obligations, schedules, patient care issues, organizational bureaucracies, and ongoing accountability and responsibility to executive management are many of the stressors that can impact their performance. Furthermore, nurse leaders remain committed to and abreast of their front-line nurses to help alleviate, intervene, and buffer some of the stressors so that patient safety and quality of care are maintained. As stressors and various levels of stress differ according to the nurse setting, as well as the urgency and critical nature of care provision, it is safe to say that nurses often experience similar stressors, depending on their own perception of the stressors, of course. Therefore, we will select and discuss common nursing stressors in general so that we can all relate to the examples provided.

As we work through this book, we will discover the intricacies of stress among nurses and how stress impacts on a nurse's mental health. We will also discover the sources, costs, and strategies that you as a person and nurse, as well as nurse leaders and organizations, can engage in both proactively and reactively to promote the mental well-being of nurses and prevent mental illness.

A NEW NORMAL

Stress is not something nurses fail to recognize in general. We talk about it a lot and complain about it a lot, and some of us try to do something about it to help it go away; however, it still seems to consume much of our day and life. It is not unusual for a nurse to be overheard saying, "I am so stressed out today," or "I don't work well under stress." There are two ends of a continuum that are concerning in which the confrontation of stress can become a "normal" entity. At the lower extreme, nurses brush off the day's insignificant stressors and say, "Oh, that will go away," and they choose to ignore it and shrug off their racing pulses and insomnia and constant angst as nothing unusual (Park, 2012). On the flip side, nurses can become inured to stress and its increasing levels, so that they just adapt, adjust their approach, and move on, almost to the point that it goes unnoticed, but unknowingly to them it still accumulates and compounds the effects of all other stressors. Nurses are so caught up in doing their job and caring for others that they often fail to take care of themselves. Therefore, what happens is that they keep putting off or forgetting about their own stressors and stress levels, and stress starts to become a normal part of functioning.

MEDICAL STUDENT SYNDROME

Whatever stage you may be at in your nursing career, you may be susceptible to what is known by many as medical student syndrome, now commonly called "medicalstudentitis," which is a form of hypochondriasis (Collier, 2008). I include this phenomenon here because it truly reflects how we as humans can become so engrossed in what we learn and process, and become so stressed and anxious about it that it begins to alter our cognitive processes and even infringe on our own mental health. Medical student syndrome presents itself as a constellation of symptoms (psychosomatic symptoms, I might add) of the very disease a student is studying. This syndrome dates back to 1908, when Boston neurologist Dr. George Lincoln Walton described the condition in his 1908 book, *Why Worry?* (Collier, 2008). Later, studies from the 1960s suggested that more than 70% of medical students contract phantom illnesses (Lewis, 1966), and even later, in 2001, the trend continued; however, it was now suggested that "it should be considered a normal effect of their education, not a form of hypochondriasis" (Moss-Morris & Petrie, 2001).

Although initially recognized as occurring among medical students who were studying about body processes and pathophysiological change, the same phenomenon can equally apply to nursing students because they too engage in studies of the intricacies of the body, diseases, symptomology, and outcome, and they begin to think that this very symptomology and disease presentation apply to them and that they have some such diseases.

Later, in Chapter 6, we will discuss the whole notion and value of perception, and it is in no truer form than when it presents itself in nursing students who are convinced that they manifest symptoms of the very diseases they are studying. Anecdotal accounts of nursing students experiencing what I will refer to here for all intents and purposes as "nursing student syndrome" are many. So intense have these experiences become that the students have really worked themselves into an anxious or depressive state, again illustrative of how their mental status has become altered. For example, students of the health care professions begin to diagnose in themselves such entities as digoxin toxicity (even though they did not take digoxin; Bossman, 2012), kidney failure (Bossman, 2012), Lou Gehrig's disease, and depression (Collier, 2008) merely based on the signs and symptoms that are characteristic of such diseases and the most probable diagnoses.

In spite of their hyperawareness and past lecture maladies and worries, students should be encouraged to seek help for these phantom illnesses. As psychiatrist Dr. Derek Puddester suggests, "If people are becoming very preoccupied with something they heard (and/or read) and it's bothering them, they need to see their family doctor" (Collier, 2008).

It would be most prudent to also discuss the specialties that students often choose, which is sometimes fundamentally related to their own past histories and experiences or those of a loved one, such as a family member or friend. We choose our speciality in nursing for various reasons, very often because we ourselves had a lived experience in that particular area or we know of a family member or friend who experienced some challenges in this area. Even among psychology students, according to the *Canadian Medical Association Journal*, those planning to major in psychology "reported more worry about their psychological health than those planning to major in some other field." Also, students who reported a history of psychological treatment were more likely to intend to pursue an advanced degree in counseling or psychotherapy (Hardy & Calhoun, 1997).

For example, I chose the area of psychiatric nursing as an interest of mine because I wanted to advocate for one of society's most vulnerable populations: those with mental illness. At a personal level, I had an uncle who had what was called back in the 1960s "severe mental retardation," a term that I wish to replace today with "developmental disability." Although many don't associate a developmental disability with mental illness, it is actually classified as such in the *DSM-5* (American Psychiatric Association, 2013). In any event, psychiatric nursing represented someone to whom I was close to and someone from my young viewpoint who was not able to talk, walk, or feed, toilet, and dress himself—a very vulnerable person from my perspective.

SUMMARY

This chapter provides a succinct but important overview of mental health, mental illness, and stress. Understanding the physiological underpinnings of stress, how it manifests itself even though it may not always be visible to the naked eye, and how these processes can impact and alter one's mental health is critical as nurses draw on their skills, knowledge, and expertise to provide optimal, safe, and quality care to patients and collegial support to one another.

DISCUSSION QUESTIONS

1. Discuss the meanings of stress, mental health, and mental illness.
2. What physiological and bodily processes occur as we respond to stress?
3. What happens when our bodies experience stress repeatedly over a long period of time?
4. What are the differences between the good, the bad, and the ugly of stress?
5. Discuss the epidemiological trends of mental illness.

REFERENCES

Adriaenssens, J., de Gucht, V., & Maes, S. (2012). The impact of traumatic events on emergency room nurses: Findings from a questionnaire survey. *International Journal of Nursing Studies, 49*(11), 1411–1422.

American Psychiatric Association. (2013). *Diagnostic and statistical manual of mental disorders* (5th ed.). Retrieved from http://www.psych.org/practice/dsm

American Psychological Association. (2012). *Glossary of psychological terms*. Retrieved from http://www.apa.org/research/action/glossary.aspx

Australian Bureau of Statistics. (2013). *Feature article 2: Mental health*. Retrieved July 5, 2013, from http://www.abs.gov.au/AUSSTATS/abs@.nsf/Lookup/1301.0Chapter1108 2009%E2%80%9310

Australian Institute of Health and Welfare. (2013). *Mental health*. Retrieved July 1, 2013, from http://www.aihw.gov.au/mental-health

Bossman, U. P. S. (2012). *Nursing student syndrome finally got me.* Retrieved March 12, 2013, from http://allnurses.com/general-nursing-student/nursing-student-syndrome-788850. html

Canadian Mental Health Association. (2010). *Workplace mental health promotion.* Retrieved from http://wmhp.cmhaontario.ca/workplace-mental-health-core-concepts-issues/issues-in-the-workplace-that-affect-employee-mental-health/stress

Canadian Mental Health Association. (2013a). *Mental health: Benefits of good mental health.* Retrieved June 2, 2013, from http://www.cmha.ca/mental_health/benefits-of-good-mental-health

Canadian Mental Health Association. (2013b). *Fast facts about mental illness.* Retrieved July 1, 2013, from http://www.cmha.ca/media/fast-facts-about-mental-illness/#.UfbsB6OneSo

Centers for Disease Control and Prevention. (2011a). *Mental illness.* Retrieved from http://www.cdc.gov/mentalhealth/basics/mental-illness.htm

Centers for Disease Control and Prevention. (2011b). *U.S. adult mental illness surveillance report.* Retrieved from http://www.cdc.gov/Features/MentalHealthSurveillance

Chen, C. K., Lin, C., Wang, S. H., & Hou, T. H. (2009). A study of job stress, stress coping strategies, and job satisfaction for nurses working in middle-level hospital operating rooms. *Journal of Nursing Research, 17*(3), 199–211.

Collier, R. (2008). Imagined illnesses can cause real problems for medical students. *Canadian Medical Association Journal, 178*(7), 820. doi:10.1503/cmaj.080316

Elements Behavioral Health. (2013). *How to promote good mental health.* Retrieved from http://www.elementsbehavioralhealth.com/mental-health/how-to-promote-good-mental-health

European Commission. (2004). *The state of mental health in the European Union.* Retrieved July 1, 2013, from http://ec.europa.eu/health/archive/ph_projects/2001/monitoring/fp_monitoring_2001_frep_06_en.pdf

Fevre, M., Kolt, G. S., & Matheny, J. (2006). "Eustress, distress and their interpretation in primary and secondary occupational stress management interventions: which way first?" *Journal of Managerial Psychology, 21*(6), 547–565. doi:10.1108/02683940610684391

Fuchs, E., & Flügge, G. (1998). Stress, glucocorticoids and structural plasticity of the hippocampus. *Neuroscience and Biobehavioral Reviews, 23*(2), 295–300.

Fuchs, E., & Flügge, G. (2003). Chronic social stress: Effects on limbic brain structures. *Physiology and Behavior, 79*(3), 417–427.

Green, M. (2013). Tougher laws on violence against nurses. *Tennessee Nurse, 76*(3), 1–2.

Hardy, M. S., & Calhoun, L. G. (1997). Psychological distress and the "medical student syndrome" in abnormal psychology students. *Teaching of Psychology, 24*(3), 192–193. doi:10.1207/s15328023top2403_10. Retrieved from http://www.tandfonline.com/doi/abs/10.1207/s15328023top2403_10

Harvard Medical School. (2010). *Stress and the sensitive gut.* Retrieved from http://www.health.harvard.edu/newsletters/Harvard_Mental_Health_Letter/2010/August/stress-and-the-sensitive-gut

Institute of Health Economics. (2008). *How much should we spend on mental health.* Retrieved from http://www.ihe.ca/documents/Spending%20on%20Mental%20Health%20Final.pdf

Katz, M. (2012). *Web MD: Causes of mental illness.* Retrieved July 4, 2013, from http://www.webmd.com/anxiety-panic/mental-health-causes-mental-illness

Kawano, Y. (2008). Association of job-related stress factors with psychological and somatic symptoms among Japanese hospital nurses: Effect of departmental environment in acute care hospitals. *Journal of Occupational Health, 50*(1), 79–85.

Kessler, R. C., Chiu, W. T., Demler, O., & Walters, E. E. (2005). Prevalence, severity, and comorbidity of twelve-month DSM-IV disorders in the National Comorbidity Survey Replication (NCS-R). *Archives of General Psychiatry, 62*(6), 617–627.

Lazarus, R. S. (1966). *Psychological stress and the coping process.* New York, NY: McGraw-Hill.

Lewis, C. E. (1966). The interesting student syndrome. *Journal of Medical Education, 41*(10), 991–992.

MacEwan, B. S. (2006). Protective and damaging effects of stress mediators: Central role of the brain. *Dialogues in Clinical Neuroscience, 8*(4), 367–381.

MacEwan, B. S. (2007). Physiology and neurobiology of stress and adaptation: Central role of the brain. *Physiological Reviews, 87*(3), 873–904.

MacEwan, B. S., & Gianaros, P. J. (2010). Central role of the brain in stress and adaptation: Links to socioeconomic status, health, and disease. *Annals of the New York Academy of Sciences, 1186*(2), 190–222.

Mayo Clinic. (2013). *Mental illness: Causes.* Retrieved July 4, 2013, from http://www.mayoclinic.com/health/mental-illness/DS01104/DSECTION=causes

Mental Health Foundation. (2012). *What is mental health?* Retrieved from http://www.mentalhealth.org.uk/help-information/an-introduction-to-mental-health/what-is-mental-health

Mental Health Foundation. (2013). *What is good mental health?* Retrieved January 28, 2013, from http://www.mentalhealth.org.uk/help-information/an-introduction-to-mental-health/what-is-good-mental-health

Milutinovic, D., Golubovic, B., Brkic, N., & Prokes, B. (2012). Professional stress and health among critical care nurses in Serbia. *Arhiv za higijenu rada i Toksikologiju, 63*(2), 171–180.

Moola, S., Ehlers, V. J., & Hattingh, S. P. (2008). Critical care nurses' perceptions of stress and stress-related situations in the workplace. *Curationis, 31*(2), 77–86.

Moss-Morris, R., & Petrie, K. J. (2001). Redefining medical students' disease to reduce mortality. *Medical Education, 35*(8), 724–728.

Nahm, E. S., Warren, J., Zhu, S., An, M., & Brown, J. (2012). Nurses' self-care behaviors related to weight and stress. *Nursing Outlook, 60*(5), e23–31.

Park, A. (2012). *Stress shrinks the brain and lowers our ability to cope with adversity. Feeling stressed by family and work woes? It could be taking a toll on both your brain and your body.* Retrieved June 20, 2013, from http://healthland.time.com/2012/01/09/study-stress-shrinks-the-brain-and-lowers-our-ability-to-cope-with-adversity/#ixzz25MXqR2Xc

Pfizer. (2013). *Stress-busting tactics for any workplace.* Retrieved from http://www.morethanmedication.ca/en/article/index/stress_busting_tactics

Ricciardi, R. (2014). Violence prevention: A nursing issue. *Journal of Pediatric Health Care, 28*(1), 4.

Roffey Park. (2005). *Failure to manage change heightens stress, harassment and conflict at work, survey claims.* Retrieved from http://www.trainingreference.co.uk/news/bp050128.htm

Royal Canadian Mounted Police. (2014). *RCMP mental health strategy 2014–2019.* Retrieved from http://www.rcmp-grc.gc.ca/fam/strat-eng.htm

Salim, S., Chugh, G., & Asghar, M. (2012). Inflammation in anxiety. *Advances in Protein, Chemistry and Structural Biology, 88*, 1–25.

Scott, E. (2010). *Chronic job stress is a risk factor for heart disease.* Retrieved from http://stress.about.com/od/stresshealth/a/jobstress.htm

Segerstrom, S. C., & Miller, G. E. (2004). Psychological stress and the human immune system: A meta-analytic study of 30 years of inquiry. *Psychological Bulletin, 130*(4), 601–630. doi:10.1037/0033-2909.130.4.601

Selye, H. (1974). *Stress without distress* (p.171). Philadelphia, PA: J.B. Lippincott Company.

Starcke, K., & Brand, M. (2012). Decision making under stress: A selective review. *Neuroscience and Biobehavioral Reviews, 36*(4), 1228–1248. doi:10.1016/j.neubiorev.2012.02.003

Stokowski, L. A. (2010). *A matter of respect and dignity: Bullying in the nursing profession.* Retrieved from http://www.medscape.com/viewarticle/729474

Stress Relief Tools. (2012). *Your body and the physiological effects of stress.* Retrieved from http://www.stress-relief-tools.com/physiological-effects-of-stress.html

Suarez, K., Mayer, C., Ehlert, U., & Nater, U. M. (2010). Psychological stress and self-reported functional gastrointestinal disorders. *The Journal of Nervous and Mental Disease, 198*(3), 226–229.

The Conference Board of Canada. (2012). *Mental illness imposes high costs on the Canadian economy.* Retrieved July 5, 2013, from http://www.conferenceboard.ca/press/newsrelease/12-07-19/mental_illness_imposes_high_costs_on_the_canadian_economy.aspx

Ulas, T., Buyukhatipoglu, H., Kirhan, I., Dal, M. S., Eren, M. A., Hazar, A., Demir, M. E., et al. (2012). The effect of day and night shifts on oxidative stress and anxiety symptoms of the nurses. *European Review for Medical and Pharmacological Sciences, 16*(5), 594–599.

Violante, S., Benso, P. G., Gerbaudo, L., & Violante, B. (2009). Correlation between job satisfaction and stress factors, burn-out and psychosocial well-being among nurses working in different healthcare settings. *Giornale Italiano di Medicina del Lavora ed Ergonomia, 31*(1 Suppl. A), A36–A44.

World Health Organization. (2001). *Strengthening mental health promotion (fact sheet no. 220).* Retrieved from http://www.cdc.gov/mentalhealth/basics.htm

World Health Organization. (2013). *Facts and figures: Prevalence of mental disorders.* Retrieved from http://www.euro.who.int/en/what-we-do/health-topics/noncommunicable-diseases/mental-health/facts-and-figures

Your Amazing Brain. (2014). *Stress: your brain and body.* Retrieved from http://www.youramazingbrain.org/brainchanges/stressbrain.htm

2

Understanding Workplace Mental Health

*It's up to you today to start making healthy choices. Not choices that are
just healthy for your body, but healthy for your mind.*
—Steve Maraboli

LEARNING OBJECTIVES

By the end of this chapter, the learner will be able to:

1. Discuss the value of work in one's life.
2. Identify and discuss some of the significant sources of stress in one's personal life.
3. Identify and discuss some of the significant sources of stress in one's professional life as a nurse.
4. Identify and discuss some of the significant sources of stress that can arise from an organization and impact a nurse's life.
5. Discuss the significance of attitude in workplace mental health.

It goes without saying that health care organizations are in the business of promoting, educating, and trying to address individuals' and society's optimal health. Then why does it seem that the health of the employees of the organization at times is not a priority? While large organizations busy themselves preparing the health promotion and disease prevention plan for its catchment population and society at large, the health of employees can very often become overlooked and not addressed. An organization is only as good as the people that run it, and given that nurses comprise a significant portion of an organization's workforce, maintaining good mental health of nurses (as well as of all other employees) should be a priority. Organizations need policies and programs that can keep staff healthy and functioning well to meet the needs of the patients they serve.

During any single working day, nurses can endure a lifetime of actual lived and vicarious experiences through the struggles and sickness of their patients and the patients' families. Nurses will often sit tirelessly through the night with a dying patient who has no family, work a double shift, have their patient load double because a colleague has called in sick with no relief obtained, accompany a single mother through her labor and delivery experience, receive three to four patients from the operating room in any given shift, get told off by a family member who is displeased with the care his or her mother is receiving, get punched in the face by a traumatically head-injured patient, or worry about a mentally ill patient with a day pass who has not yet returned from a "promised" outing. In any event, nurses are perhaps the most integral caregivers in health organizations and settings, and they can be subjected to many increased stressors merely as a result of the context in which they work and the work they provide. Unlike any other health care professionals, nurses are with patients 24-7 and therefore exist as the primary point of contact for the patients and families on any issues and concerns that arise.

Nurses are often the most abundant health care professionals that comprise health care organizations. Nurses are very astute at trying to meet the needs of others and their patients, but very little of their time and efforts is devoted to caring for themselves. In fact, some would even say that nurses are great at taking care of others, but just simply terrible at taking care of themselves. In the absence of such self-care, a nurse's physical and mental health can become compromised.

As alluded to in Chapter 1, it is crucial to remember that there is no health without mental health. As determined and understood globally, mental health and physical health are inextricably linked, one unequivocally exerting an equal and mutual impact on the other (World Health Organization [WHO], 2014a). For nurses who frequently take the lives of others into their own hands, there is no other more important place to understand mental health than in the workplace, regardless of their practice setting.

WHY IS WORK SO IMPORTANT?

Mental health is a state of well-being in which every individual realizes his or her own potential, copes with the normal stresses of life, works productively and fruitfully, and is able to make a contribution to the community (WHO, 2014a). Internationally, work is an indicator of one's mental health. We spend approximately 30% to 60% of our life at work, so it is bound to have an impact on who we are as people. The very reasons why work is so important to us are comparatively similar to why work is so valuable to our mental health. We have already seen why good mental health is critical to our everyday life; mental health in the workplace is just as vitally important from personal, professional, and organizational perspectives. Every aspect of work and what it does for us makes us who we are today and is why workplace mental health is such a critical component to discuss.

Today's work climate is increasingly seeing an emphasis on the psychological health of the employee. From a time when nurses used their backs as their main work tool and occupational health and safety and workers' rights were limited primarily to physical injuries incurred on the job, the work climate has changed (Scott-Clarke, 2011). Today, we have become a more educated society about workers' rights and responsibilities, as well as increased organizational responsibility and accountability and the need for respectful workplaces. Furthermore, noticeably increasing in frequency are the costs of absenteeism, disgruntled employees, workplace bullying, and harassment.

Both on and off the job, work has an effect on us, and we in turn affect our work. We talk, complain, celebrate, and struggle (Briscoe, 2013). Our relationship with work is not only economic and social; it is cultural and spiritual as well. In a society that has become more independent, expressive, and competitive in culture, our work has become significantly integrated with our lives and who we are as individuals.

We live in an age of choice, and as far as our working lives are concerned, we are no longer satisfied with just any old job. Our jobs have to have meaning for us, they have to play a positive role in our existence, and they have to add value to our lives. This is particularly the case with those younger than 30, who have grown up with a far greater sense of autonomy and personal awareness than any previous generation (Freedman, 2009).

We spend 30% to 60% of our life at work, and there are many fringe benefits that we receive by working or being employed. These benefits involve various domains of our lives and provide many key activities we need to achieve fulfillment of the different domains of our physical, social, personal, psychological, and spiritual well-being. Theoretically, in an ideal world work helps people address all of those basic hierarchal needs identified by Abraham Maslow (1962). In order of priority and importance to survival, they are physiology (air, food, water, sleep, sex, homeostasis, and excretion); safety and security (employment, housing, family, health, and property); love and belongingness (friendship, family, and sexual intimacy); self-esteem (confidence, achievement, respect); and self-actualization (creativity, problem solving, spontaneity, lack of prejudice, and acceptance of facts).

Physically

Physically, work fulfills many of life's purposes. It gives you a place to go outside of your home, a change of scenery, and a place away from the monotony of home life, as a diversion. As well, it physically enables you to buy the things in life you need for survival or even those things you enjoy, such as the smaller, finer luxuries of life. The little sports car you always dreamed of owning, the cruise trip every Easter that helps to break up the winter blues—all are niceties that make working worthwhile for you and your family. Most importantly, however, working gives you the ability to survive, puts a roof over your head, provides a shelter that gives you a sense of safety and security, pays for the electricity that gives you warmth against the harsh winter or stormy elements, and enables you to put food on the table. From the perspective of Maslow (1962), the physical benefits provided by work primarily target the first two levels of Maslow's pyramid, those being one's need to satisfy hunger and thirst and one's need to survive. Further, it gives people a significant reason to get up every day, stay motivated, keep active, and participate as a valuable member of society, hence a strengthened mental health.

Spiritually

Work also brings many people meaning from a spiritual perspective. According to Wong (2013), a "healthy dose of spirituality and meaning in the workplace is good for business." Initiated by the negative forces of workplace violence, globalization, scandals of unethical behaviors, and threats of terrorism, work can help to complete our inner meanings and fulfillment, as well as resolve internal conflict and threats to our security. Wong suggests that spirituality can improve morale, productivity, loyalty, and job satisfaction and even gives a competitive edge with integrity. Furthermore, as organizations permit and encourage private places at work for prayers, meditation, and yoga, business leaders seek moral and spiritual guidance in how they conduct business and increase productivity. This holistic approach helps to recapture a sense of community at work, cooperation, and empowerment, and it increases passion, purpose, and respect. Furthermore, it can help eliminate fear, animosity, and conflict.

Socially

Socially, work provides many fringe benefits for nurses and influences their persona and overall quality of life. The work itself, work environment, and even the organizational beliefs and values contribute significantly to the social role and behaviors we develop and exhibit. For our personal and professional development, work provides valuable networking media, a social venue to develop relationships and sources of social support, and fulfills a typical human need for social contact, social inclusion, and social connectedness; we are after all social beings. A supportive networking platform at work enables us to laugh, cry, vent, and just listen. In addition, it provides another source of leisure activities, such as occurs at a staff holiday function, a summer barbecue, or celebratory events that surround a colleague's retirement or baby shower. Work serves to counteract loneliness for one who is single, divorced, or widowed; is a source of developing lifelong friendships; and can represent an escape from a difficult home life (Gold & Shuman, 2009). In essence, work is a valuable source of social fulfillment. From the perspective of Maslow (1962), the social fulfillment work provides helps us to achieve a sense of belongingness and love, a persona and better overall quality of life, and a significant sense of belonging to a community (Hansen & Keltner, 2012). In spite of the evolution of electronic social media, people still "crave" and need a place where they can meet people, form relationships and friendships, and "experience a sense of community," to give people meaning. Furthermore, they then feel valued, recognized, and needed for the contributions they make (Hansen & Keltner, 2012). Work also provides people with a fringe benefit of autonomy, giving nurses independence and freedom to work at their own pace while using their own skill set.

Personally

Personally, work provides much value to individuals. There are many fringe benefits of work as well that support the growth and development of one's personal self. These benefits revolve around the enjoyment and personal satisfaction people get from going to work, so that they are able to keep active, challenged, and personally fulfilled. Humans are creatures of habit, and work provides a routine lifestyle and interest that they are comfortable with, as they know what is expected of them and gives them a reason to get up every day, stay motivated, and keep active to participate as a valued member of society. Furthermore, it provides room for personal growth and development and enables people to expand their knowledge, foster their personal goals, and broaden their horizons. It is a source of pride, strength, and determination and symbolizes strong moral character and integrity (Gold & Shuman, 2009, p. 44).

Work shapes our lives. When we meet others, the first question we ask is "what do you do?" to understand one of the most important ways we define ourselves (Briscoe, 2013), which is an integral and essential part of our career. Work provides for people an opportunity for learning and self-realization. Some organizations have built their reputations on taking an interest in their staff and advancing their learning, such as Procter & Gamble (Hansen & Keltner, 2012). This company offers staff members opportunities to learn, expand their horizons, improve self-awareness, increase self-confidence and self-esteem, and achieve a greater sense of self, all for the purpose of promoting personal growth and meaning.

At work you are not only provided with the opportunity to do things but also do things to obtain a sense of accomplishment, recognition, self-worth, and greater satisfaction; when recognized, you aspire to do and accomplish more, not just for yourself but for others as well. In nursing, for example, you achieve a greater sense of self-satisfaction by doing good for others at this vulnerable time in their lives and grasping an opportunity to help others.

In terms of prestige, status, and power, work continues to help provide many personal benefits. For example, an organization that confers respect, recognition, and a sense of worth on employees provides them meaning at work (Hansen & Keltner, 2012). A doctorate in nursing from Harvard University is a source of great status for some individuals. In terms of power, work provides a venue for building, acquiring, and exercising power.

From the perspective of Maslow (1962), work helps to fulfill the need for belongingness, self-esteem, and any potential for self-actualization, as individuals derive a significant degree of self-satisfaction, motivation, comfort, and strength of character to achieve any goals they set.

Work defines who we are as humans and gives us a sense of identity. It gives us a sense of recognition of who we are and what we enjoy doing in life. For example, we often introduce ourselves by saying I am a plumber, a journalist, or a teacher, and for nurses it would possibly be I am a nurse, a nurse manager, a professor, or a chief nurse officer. The nursing profession is more than just a career, it is an identity. Nursing represents something a person is rather than something a person does, and it is the attributes that nurses possess that distinguish the nursing discipline from others. For both our families and society at large, it makes a statement about who we are and reflects our contributing values to society and fosters a sense of creativity.

As suggested by Freedman (2009), our careers are our lives, and "because we value the freedom to choose personal satisfaction and economic prosperity, we are drawn towards a world in which we require our economic activity to be both satisfying and chosen." Work provides for us a sense of purpose, an opportunity for increased experience, expertise, and a broader knowledge base, and it makes people feel good about themselves and something everyone has a right to, socially, ethically, and legally.

Psychologically and Mentally

The mastery of new tasks, exciting challenges, and regular thought-provoking stimulation that we get from working all contribute to our sense of self-worth, self-concept, self-esteem, and self-image. Psychologically, work serves many dimensions of our psychological and mental health and well-being. Work produces great benefits, such as increased self-esteem, confidence, sense of identity, sense of purpose, self-worth, autonomy, competence, independence, achievement, and an overall increased quality of life, satisfaction, and accomplishment (McDaid, 2008), all of which feed into one's keen positive sense of self and integrity.

Psychologically, work is a source of pride, strength, and determination. As a nurse, you are given the opportunity to enhance the lives of others and put them on the road to recovery. Mentally, the cognitive stimulation and interaction provided by work tasks, skills, and responsibilities and the rewards of succeeding all fuel our motivation and produce psychological growth of self and a nurturance of increased knowledge, creativity, and intellect.

Even for those employees with mental illnesses, work promotes adaptation, decreases stigma in society, and provides them with an income to participate more fully in society (McDaid, 2008).

From the perspective of Maslow (1962), work provides much psychological and mental health value for level 4 and level 5 needs, where work helps to fulfill people's need of social esteem and self-respect and increases their potential for self-actualization, so that they have an "efficient perception of reality, acceptance of self and others and spontaneity, a strong focus, autonomy, and independence and are capable of doing things for [themselves] and making decisions on [their] own, are in tune with [the] world around them, and are sensitive to the needs of others, enjoy humor, are not hostile, creative, [have] strong individuality and strive to keep learning" (Boyum, 2013). To further attest to the value that work provides for one's mental health, employment in particular is one proven valuable form of therapy that helps individuals with mental illness integrate back into society (Kinoshita et al., 2013; Marshall et al., 2013). In fact, employment serves as a critical component in their rehabilitation, recovery, and vocational functioning. People with mental illness often have great difficulty obtaining a job. In fact, the rates have been reported to be as high as 70% to 90% (Reiersen Thompson, 2004). This clearly indicates the value of employment, especially for those with mental illnesses or mental health concerns.

WHAT IS A PSYCHOLOGICALLY SAFE WORKPLACE?

A psychologically healthy workplace is one in which employees have the ability, freedom, and comfort level to think, feel, and behave in a manner that enables effective performance in all areas of life and work. This type of environment is where employees feel safe, respected, and appreciated by their leader and the organization, which in turn enhances productivity and morale, increases positive work attendance records, and creates fewer short- and long-term disability claims.

Respect is a very important piece of a psychologically safe workplace. The conversation around workplace mental health cannot occur in the absence of a discussion of respect. Workplace mental health is very much contingent on respect, for without respect one's mental health at work can become a catastrophe, as it sometimes does. As we move through this book, you will quickly realize how valuable respect in the workplace is and what stress, incivility, turmoil, and even violence can occur in its absence. Disrespect in its extreme form in the workplace can exert devastating consequences on nurses and their families, friends, patients, and employing organization.

Workplace mental health is important for many professionally related reasons. Every time a nurse works, he or she takes the lives of many into her care and responsibility. Work is an important source for building and maintaining professional networks that include and support all workers, help avoid conflict among colleagues, multitask, increase focus and concentration, and promote patience and respect with colleagues and patients (Advisory, Conciliation, and Arbitration Service, 2013).

A psychologically safe workplace is one that works to reduce the risk of injury to employee mental well-being, takes precautions to avert injury to psychological health, and provides workplace accommodations when necessary. A workplace that is psychologically safe is one absent of bullying, harassment, and stigma around mental illness. It is a workplace that aims to address and resolve mental health issues in the workplace and to ensure the psychological health of its employees. The interconnection between psychological health and safety is evident—a workplace needs a psychologically safe environment to ensure the psychological health of its employees (Craig-Broadwith, 2012).

There are several principles and/or concepts that are important for the sustainability of good workplace mental health. These principles range from the promotion of good mental health to the prevention of mental illness or concerns and all activities in between to make a mentally healthy workplace become a reality. These principles include making information available, developing or enforcing standards and best practices, supporting early intervention, ensuring fair and equitable claims practices, promoting mental health services, offering and enhancing educational efforts, having supportive people at work whom you can talk to and who will help you, open communication, and a positive work culture. An integrated management approach is needed. A primary focus on needs; recognition that health is determined by many interdependent factors; promotion of employee and employee joint responsibility; and assessment, evaluation, and continued quality improvement are integral (National Quality Institute, 2012).

Most of us cannot help but wonder if work actually causes mental health disorders. However, there is no simple answer to this question because the outcome is really contingent on the person involved and many other extraneous variables, such as the person's coping style, perceived stressors, past experiences, and so forth. Burton (2010) suggests that many different workplace factors may contribute directly to the development of mental distress (demoralization, depressed mood, anxiety, burnout, etc.); however, while mental distress may not be a direct cause of and reach the level of a diagnosable mental disorder, it can still be a significant source of considerable suffering for the employee, productivity loss for the employer, and legal consequences if "toxic work conditions" are judged to have contributed to an employee's suffering and disability. Hence, a supportive workplace can reduce the onset, severity, impact, and duration of a mental health disorder.

Mental health problems, such as depression, anxiety, substance abuse, and stress, are common, affecting individuals, their families and coworkers, and the broader community. In addition, they have a direct impact on workplaces through increased absenteeism, reduced productivity, and increased costs. Mental health problems are the result of a complex interplay between biological, psychological, social, and environmental factors. There is increasing evidence that both the content and context of work can play a role in the development of mental health problems in the workplace (Burton, 2010).

Society today is talking more and more about mental health, and we have made great strides from when mental health was a taboo issue. In this competitive world, people have to face multiple challenges. These challenges may be occupation- or family-related or financial matters. The great challenge is protecting mental health from these challenges (Williams, 2012).

In a recent report for the Mental Health Commission of Canada, "The Road to Psychological Safety: Legal, Scientific and Social Foundations for a National Standard for Psychological Safety," Shain argues that "normal" resilient people can be brought to the brink of mental distress and even pushed over the edge by conditions at work (Williams, 2012). Organizations that make the effort to identify psychosocial risks and to create a psychologically healthy workplace reap benefits in productivity, sustainability, and growth.

Respect is a word that carries much meaning. Respect is one of the key attributes that promotes an optimally functioning society and one of the main threads that weaves, promotes, and sustains the tapestry of relationships, particularly at work. The profession of nursing and the intricacies of relationship potential is one example. In fact, it is professions like nursing that should be fueled by respect, dignity, caring, and humanistic behaviors. Although we see notions of respect, dignity, and caring threaded through nursing standards of practice, operational documents, position statements, and vision/mandates, respect applies primarily to the therapeutic nurse–patient relationship. As Johnstone (2012) points out, although a critical element in nursing, "the imperatives of respect in the nurse–nurse relationship and workplace environments have received comparatively little attention in the nursing literature" (p. 31).

Respect is perhaps one of the most valued attributes a workplace can possess. The advantages that respect among nurses and nursing colleagues bring are truly immeasurable. Nurses need to feel valued and respected for who they are, what they do and offer, what they say, and how they have made or can make a difference to others. The care they provide, the efforts and energies they exert, and the knowledge they illuminate need to matter and be recognized, acknowledged, and appreciated. As most nurses spend about one third of their life at work, the portrayal and receipt of respect by colleagues is vital for their optimal functioning and work performance. Although Huston and Brox (2004) suggest that health care professionals should not have to be reminded of respectful practice at work, they do. As they suggest, "As external pressures increase to meet the 'bottom line' in the business of health care, human frailties will often creep into the workplace, and questionable behavior can exhibit itself in the most subtle of ways. This behavior can range from favoritism, intimidation, and bullying to actually breaking the law, all under the guise of management and leadership" (Huston & Brox, 2004, p. 268).

The presence of respect in the workplace brings a multitude of benefits. It benefits not only the nurse as a person and professional, but also the nurse's colleagues, the patients, and the organization as a whole. The benefits for the nurse as a person are far-reaching. When nurses are shown respect, they tend to have a much more relaxed yet motivated demeanour. They are made to feel content and welcome in a warm manner, their presence feels affirmed, they feel listened to and rewarded for what they do and are doing, and they are self-assured for what has been done (Bournes & Milton, 2009). Respect also positively correlates with improved health and well-being (Laschinger, Leiter, Day, Gilin-Oore, & MacKinnon, 2012).

The Nurse as a Professional

Professionally, respect fosters a greater sense of self, and nurses tend to feel confident with their competencies, like colleagues, secure in their workplace, and a valued player and team member (Johnstone, 2012). Collegial relationships also need respect to be functional. According to Johnson (2009), the fundamental lack of respect between doctors and nurses is a huge problem that affects every aspect of their jobs. Staff morale, patient safety, and public perception of the industry all suffer as a result. Although criminal behaviors such as throwing scalpels and squirting a used syringe in a coworker's face have occurred, it is often the day-to-day putdowns that can be the most harmful. "The worst behavior problem is not the most egregious," wrote one participant. "It's the everyday lack of respect and communication that most adversely affects patient care and staff morale."
Many nurses end up leaving their current positions because they are experiencing some level of dissatisfaction or discontent with their colleagues or supervisor/superior that arises from disrespect (Hayes et al., 2006).

For patients receiving nursing care, the benefits of a respectful workplace continue. There is an enhanced level of safe and quality care (Johnstone, 2012). As well, benefits of shorter length of stay and decreased organizational costs have been found to occur. The retention of a stable, consistent, and satisfied nursing workforce helps to ensure that a high level of quality patient care and safety can be maintained (Institute of Medicine, 2004).

The Organization

Respectful and collegial workplaces for nurses produce many positive spin-offs for the organization. A supportive and empowering workplace is important because it promotes the retention of nurses (Laschinger et al., 2012). An organization that values good mental health for its employees has much to boast about with respect to operational success. Such an attitude impacts not only the organization's financial bottom line but also public relations, staff engagement, and respect. For example, good mental health in a workplace boosts business productivity; goals and strategic directions for economic growth and global competitiveness; general population health goals; the business's reputation; employee morale, loyalty, and commitment; corporate responsibility; a valued-based culture; reasonable workload and stress levels; recruitment and retention success; and an upbeat and stimulating managerial style. Unequivocally, it decreases absenteeism costs as well as the risk for liability and legal suits. Taking care of employees' psychological well-being is crucial for the long-term success of any organization. A healthier and happier employee is a more productive, engaged, and motivated employee. Thus, ensuring the psychological health and safety of your employees makes good business sense (Craig-Broadwith, 2012). About 69%

of employees report that work is a significant source of stress, and 41% say they typically feel tense or stressed out during the workday (American Psychological Association [APA], 2009).

Achieving Respect

Johnstone (2012), in her well-focused and admirable article, outlines a recipe for how respect can be achieved successfully in a nurse's workplace (p. 2). First, it is important to acknowledge an individual's moral worth and dignity because each nurse has his or her own set of values and positive attributes, so be mindful of these. You need to work with, not against, your colleagues. Second, attention is needed as you focus on what they are saying and what message they are trying to get across, so don't block out their presence and dialogue attempts with belittling remarks, negative innuendos, or patronization. Third, be mindful and empathetic with attuned listening, and take them seriously by showing you are genuinely concerned and listening attentively. Fourth, be supportive. Your colleagues need to know you are there for them and supportive of their beliefs and values. Fifth, you need to save face and preserve the relationships you have built and established. Trust needs to be maintained, nurtured, and strengthened, so avoid the pollution of gossip, rumours, intimidation, humiliation, and destruction and the toxicity it can bring to the workplace. It is disrespect that falters and threatens the morale and humanism so often admired and achieved in nursing.

Sources of Stress at Work That Can Impact Our Mental Health

The American Institute of Stress (2013) states that "numerous studies show that job stress is far and away the major source of stress for American adults and that it has escalated progressively over the past few decades." In a 2012 survey, 83% of Americans report they experienced increased workplace stress and a sense of being "frazzled" (Globe News Wire, 2013). Similarly, the American Nurses Association (2011) found that 74% of nurses cited the acute and chronic effects of stress. Globally, workplace stress has no boundaries. Over half (51%) of Canadian employees say they experience a great deal of stress at work (The Health Communication Unit, University of Toronto, 2004).

Sources of stress at work are often the very factors that impact the development of a mentally healthy workplace. In whatever form it may appear, stress is the key precipitator of poor or deteriorating mental health and comes from a myriad of sources. These can be categorized on three levels as personal, professional, or organizational.

Personal

Means of Survival

People work so they can obtain the necessities of life, such as shelter and food. Nurses are no different from anyone else when it comes to working to make ends meet. Oftentimes, nurses work more than one job (Trinkoff, Geiger-Brown, Brady, Lipscomb, & Muntaner, 2006) to achieve the basic necessities of living. I was once in that situation myself, when I was a young, single girl and worked three jobs because I wanted to live comfortably, needed transportation, and had to pay for graduate school. Hence, financial and economic factors can exert a significant impact on our experienced stress levels (National Institute for Occupational Safety and Health [NIOSH], 2008). According to the Centers for Disease Control and Prevention (CDC; 2013), "the ability to identify major depression in the workplace is complicated by a number of issues such as employees' concerns about confidentiality or the impact it may have on their job that cause some people to avoid screening."

Other realistic sources of nurse stress included "high workloads, unavailability of doctors, unsupportive management, human resource issues, interpersonal issues, patients' relatives, shift work, car parking, handover procedures, no common area for nurses, not progressing at work, and patient mental health" (Happell et al., 2013).

Social Support

Social support and capital play a major role in how we as humans perform our daily activities and deal with life's challenges and stressors. Social support is what can make or break your reaction to stressors. Social support provides a vital element for individuals who are faced with challenges in life and work. In essence, it is a supportive mechanism that people use to cope. Social support serves to provide encouragement, boost our sense of self, and enhance our self-esteem in all that we do.

Not only did a low level of social support predict the occurrence of common mental disorders (Scott, 2010), but increasing social support was negatively associated with mental health problems (Mark & Smith, 2012). As stated by Read (2013), "Attributes of nurses' workplace social capital included networks of social relationships at work, shared assets and shared ways of knowing and being" where communication, trust, and positive leadership practices helped to build this. The existence of social capital for nurses is associated with positive consequences for nurses, patients, and the organization.

Unhappy With Current Position

There is nothing worse than working at a job with which you are not happy or content. As a result, you are then not only stressed with the external environment of the job that is not satisfying and the workplace and perhaps people you come to dislike, but you are also now struggling with an inner turmoil of why you haven't yet done anything to change it. In this case, we think of the old adage that "a change is as good as a rest," and that is so true on many fronts. Known as an old proverb of British origin, specifically the genteel English middle class, it basically means just that—you can get as much good from changing the work you do as from having a rest (Cambridge Dictionaries Online, 2014).

Psychological Demands

The psychological demands of nursing are many. Perhaps the very impetus of this chapter is a focus on many of the demands that produce psychological impacts (Scott, 2010). As you read on throughout this chapter, you will focus on each of these individually, with specific examples to help illustrate.

Ethical Conflicts

Ethical conflicts that occur for nurses at work can add to their stress levels (Ulrich et al., 2007). Given that this topic is covered very well in Chapter 8, it will be omitted here.

Job Prestige

The status of one's position can also create stress for nurses. In fact, subjects with higher-status jobs were less likely to have job stress-related metabolic syndrome than were those with lower-status jobs (Scott, 2010).

Physical Exertion

Nursing is often referred to as a very demanding and physically challenging yet rewarding job. We go into nursing knowing the tasks that have to be completed, the knowledge base that is needed, and the types of populations to which we will provide care. Teamwork and taking a collaborative approach of working with one another help alleviate some stress. Lifting, pulling, and pushing beds, equipment, wheelchairs, and stretchers, and yes, even lifting patients, are physically demanding tasks that can place a great deal of stress on the nurse's body. We all know proper body mechanics, but we often forget ourselves in the rush of work and continue to bend, lift, and pull against best practices. Remaining cognizant of those body mechanics, particularly for our backs, is something nurses need to take seriously so as to avoid job strain (Scott, 2010). Therapeutic interventions with total-care patients who may be bedridden, combative, confused, or psychiatrically unstable can be physically challenging. Repetitive tasks such as the simple action of pulling up a patient in bed can also be physically demanding.

Job Insecurities

Government and organizational cuts can threaten nurse job security, as they fear layoffs, redundancies, and forced job change. Given that many nurses hold temporary, part-time, float, or casual call-in positions, job insecurity can be a constant worry (Boya, Demiral, Ergor, Akvardar, & De Witte, 2008; Ruokolainen, Mauno, & Cheng, 2013), so much so as to pose mental health challenges (Scott, 2010). As found by Boya et al., perceived anxiety and depression were significantly associated with qualitatively and quantitatively measured job insecurity in nurses. Although job insecurity is a rather permanent stressor among nurses nowadays (Boya et al., 2008; Ruokolainen et al., 2013), age and dedication have a significant role to play. A younger age and a low level of job dedication both acted as protective factors against the negative effect of a high level of job insecurity. Furthermore, while a high level of job dedication protected younger nurses from the negative effects of job insecurity on work, family conflict, and parental stress, older nurses who reported a low level of job dedication showed better well-being in the presence of a high level of job insecurity.

Starting a New Job or Position

Starting a new job or position can be very daunting; a new position in a different facility or setting with new colleagues and new roles, responsibilities, and competencies can be stressful, particularly if you have worked in one place for a lengthy period of time. According to Arcurs (2014), while elation and excitement are first experienced, they are quickly followed by nervousness, panic, and anxiety. However, with the right approach, perception, and values, beginning a new job can be more generally positive and enjoyable and not as stressful as many make it seem to be.

One's Own Coping Mechanism or Lack Thereof

Coping falls into two categories: problem-focused coping strategies and emotion-focused coping strategies (Kelly, 2010). Problem-focused coping directly targets the task at hand, what it is we are physically trying to achieve, whereas emotion-focused coping is the strategy we employ to help us deal with our feelings of stress, distress, or anxiety that may arise as a result of the stressor or task we are facing. Because of the emotional rollercoaster ride on which we often find ourselves, many suggest that problem-focused coping is the most effective means to deal with stress (Kelly, 2010). However, nurses can very easily fall into poor coping practices. The recognition of one's own destructive coping strategies, such as addictions, is one such example (Chen, Lin, Wang, & Hou, 2009; Violante, Benso, Gerbaudo, & Violante, 2009).

Job Satisfaction

Another significant source of stress for nurses is the level of job satisfaction they feel with the organization and work they do. As stated by Moneke and Umeh (2013), nurses' job satisfaction is a key issue to consider in the retention of critical care nurses. For operating room nurses as well, work rewards, administrative management of job satisfaction, and the operating room environment allow more effective coping strategies (Chen et al. 2009). Organizational commitment for some was found to be the strongest predictor of job satisfaction (Moneke & Umeh, 2013) and was a protective factor against job dissatisfaction (Violante et al. 2009). As found by Ward (2011), factors such as greater patient acuity, unpredictable and challenging workspaces, violence, increased paperwork, and reduced managerial support all contributed to decreased nurse work satisfaction.

Gossip and Rumors

Unlike assumptions, in which individuals focus on what they, themselves, believe to be true, rumors and gossip also occur to impact significantly on the workplace and people's overall mental health therein. Although the impetus of gossip and rumors is predicated on the fact that knowledge is power, that does not necessarily translate into a positive use of knowledge or the generation of productive power. Although gossip and rumors can be negative or positive, we will focus here on the negative, as this is what seems to be most prevalent in the workplace, is more interpersonally focused, and so has the greatest potential to do more damage. Furthermore, whereas gossip pertains exclusively to people, rumors may involve events as well (Foster &

Rosnow, 2006). For the purposes of this discussion, we will refer to both gossip and rumors as one in the same because they both exert very similar potential effects in the workplace.

We have all experienced it—the whispers in the corridor that cease when you walk by and the clique of people huddled together in a corner making periodic glances at those around them and passing by to see if anyone is close enough to possibly overhear the conversation taking place.

Gossip is initiated for a variety of reasons, many of which rest solely with the person and the character or lack thereof of that person. Reasons include a need to feel superior, the promotion of one's own self-interest, a need for attention or to fit in and belong socially, envy and jealousy, the need for control and power, and simple boredom.

The need to feel superior is a common root for gossip. For reasons such as having a low level of self-esteem, feeling sorry for yourself, engaging in socially unacceptable habits or behaviors that you know are wrong, or perceiving an inadequacy in yourself (e.g., not liking your weight, your physical appearance, or just wishing you could be more loud-spoken), rumors begin. In attempts to inflate their own self-esteem and confidence and to overcome their own perceived inadequacies, people generate false, socially unacceptable, and distasteful information about others, so that others will, they hope, feel as low as they feel about themselves.

The desire or need to fit in and be socially accepted is also a reason why gossip begins. Beginning or perpetuating gossip gives one a sense of acceptance by a specific group. These individuals are perhaps not loud-spoken, are timid and even shy to speak up and say much or to express an opinion, but engaging in gossip, they believe, places them at a higher level of being accepted and included in a group of others. Unfortunately, the very person who is being gossiped about is typically left out of the group for the exact same reason you are now being let into it. In all likelihood, this was you some time ago, someone who didn't fit in and is now gossiping to just "belong."

Attention seeking is another well-known reason for gossip to prosper. This often occurs when you believe you have a piece of information that no one else is aware of, and the sharing of this "juicy" piece of information with others automatically makes you the center of attention, although the attention is very short-lived. You time the delivery of this information when the most people will be present to hear it, so as to receive the utmost of your purpose and desired result.

Another reason for engaging in gossip stems from the desire for increased control and power. By the propaganda of rumors and gossip, you seek out to indiscreetly hurt others and their self-esteem by inflating your own image. This often occurs in terms of popularity; your desire to climb that leadership ladder would receive a boost by your deflating the esteem and confidence of others, thus making yourself seem like a much better person and candidate.

Sadly, another reason that gossip begins is jealousy or envy of another person. For any one of a number of reasons, such as knowledge, prestige, personal attributes, or scholarships, others feel threatened and use gossip in an effort to again make others feel inferior. They often have something or have received some sort of accomplishment or recognition that may be just a dream to others. The ultimate aim is to hurt another person and to damage that person's reputation and to do so noticeably, so that others witness it and a decrease in the person's popularity or personal sense of self will result.

Regardless of the reason for initiating gossip, the people who start it are often the less powerful people in an organization and are already dealing with issues of inferiority themselves. In their attempts to move ahead, they create and circulate gossip and rumors about others, thus making themselves look like superior leaders who know lots and are falsely confident with an elevated sense of self-esteem—all at the expense of someone else's reputation, character, and integrity.

The damage of gossip can be either short- or long-term, but in any event, it is destructive, has malicious intent, is personally demeaning, and creates a very tense atmosphere. For nurses, it is a direct hit to their character, their integrity, and their self-worth. The fault finding that occurs plays on their vulnerabilities, breaches their privacy, and can destroy their reputation. Their integrity and trust in others are destroyed, as are their self-esteem and confidence, putting them at increased risk for mental illnesses such mood disorders and anxiety disorders, all because they have been victims of gossip. How they feel about themselves has plummeted, and their upbeat and positive motivation and spirit that once were are now no more.

Gossip creates a tense and negative workplace atmosphere, decreasing the comfort level of many. Interpersonal and professional relationships have been sabotaged, reputations have been tarnished, morale has been destroyed, and the quality care that was once provided is now repeatedly questioned and scrutinized because of one's questioning of self. Gossip in the workplace wastes a significant amount of time that the organization is on the hook for, with great costs in lost productivity, divisions, and conflicts.

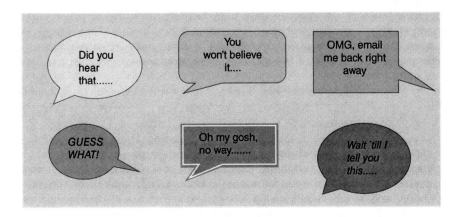

Professional

There is much detail about sources of stress that can jeopardize a nurse's mental health. Many of these stressors can cumulatively impact you as a licensed health care professional and a practicing nurse. The end result can be detrimental to your livelihood, which is to practice nursing, and to the patients you serve, and it can also add to your own personal stressors. This section will highlight some sources of potential stress for you, the nurse, as a practicing professional.

A professional nurse's prudent, astute, and competent practice is what produces good-quality and safe patient care. A nurse who is subjected to many undue, uncontrollable stresses is highly likely to jeopardize patient care, breach the expected standards of nursing practice, and violate organizational policies and procedures. These stresses include work overload, patient acuity and demands, interpersonal conflicts and strained relationships, unsupportive managers, and poor communication that often fosters the development of rumors and gossip. Other factors revolve around organizational bureaucracies, uncertainty of change, lack of staff engagement, contagion of negativism, societal impact, poor leadership, complacency, and poor communication.

Physical Environment

The physical environment can play a significant role in creating stress among nurses (WHO, 2014b). The physical environment can be noisy and uncomfortable (Daft, 2011; Tomey, 2009), and it can also impose an increased risk for developing health problems (NIOSH, 2008). Environmental hazards as well, including chemical hazards (e.g., waste anesthetics, hazardous drugs, cleaning compounds) and airborne and blood-borne pathogen exposure (Geiger-Brown & Lipscomb, 2010) impact nurses' stress levels.

Mahmood, Chaudbury, and Valente (2011) found that "inadequate space in the charting and documentation area, lengthy walking distances to patient rooms, insufficient patient surveillance, lack of visibility to all parts of the nursing unit, small size of the medication room, inappropriate organization of medical supplies, high noise levels in the nursing unit, poor lighting, and lack of privacy in the nursing stations" were all workplace environmental stressors. They suggest that the work nurses perform is already physically and psychologically intense, and a poor design and layout of the physical work environment only escalate stress levels more.

From a nurse setting perspective, there are many considerations to be aware of. Nurses who work in highly acute nursing settings endure some of the greatest stress in the workplace (Adriaenssens, de Gucht, & Maes, 2012; Milutinovic, Golubovic, Brkic, & Prokes, 2012; Violante et al., 2009), but it varies. Whether stress is a result of repetitive exposure to trauma, such as in the emergency department or on the front-line battlefield, hectic working conditions (Adriaenssens et al., 2012), or nurse shortages, all represent key sources of stress for nurses. Continuous movement while providing, responding, and performing lifesaving actions, and at the same time trying to create a good relationship with patients and their next of kin, is extremely stressful for nurses (Elmqvist, Fridlund, & Ekebergh, 2012). However, the greatest stressor and most traumatizing event for most nurses is the death or serious injury of a child or adolescent (Adriaenssens et al., 2012). Whether you are a nurse working in the emergency department, in home care (Violante et al., 2009), at a naval/military base, or as "street" nurse, significant sources of stress are present (Chen et al., 2009). Even specifics between units exist; Morelius, Gustafsson, Ekberg, and Nelson (2013) found that the stress levels of nurses working in child and adolescent psychiatry were significantly higher than they were for neonatal intensive care unit nurses with respect to poorer general health and higher burnout scores.

Let us not forget the nurses who are working in war-torn areas. Some of us who work in clean, well-resourced hospitals probably don't appreciate how good we have it. As Tschudin and Schmitz (2003) remind us, modern nursing actually evolved out of war. If you recall the times of Florence Nightingale and the valuable role she played in the Crimean War, you will begin to see the significance. Just as important, however, is what nurses working in war-torn countries face on a daily basis. We have already learned and seen many mental illness effects of working in combat (Capehart & Bass, 2012; Wall, 2012). Nurses are no exception. The devastation, the dying, and the wretchedness of destruction all take a toll on nurses' mental health and well-being (Gaylord, 2006).

Whether noise levels, poor lighting, uncomfortable temperature, or tight spaces, they can all impact the ease with which a nurse can complete the job. For critical care nurses, the greatest stressors seem to be the physical and psychological work environment. The dimmed work environment causes sensory deprivation, lethargy, and depression that can further potentiate one's stress. The small, poor layout and long, narrow corridors; lack of storage space; poor lighting; overcrowded units; absence of windows and a quiet staff lounge that is comfortable; and curtains that don't give much privacy while patient care is provided are other stressors in critical care settings. Old crank-up beds; faulty, aged equipment; background noise; inadequate temperatures; and poor lighting on the unit really impact nurses. The social working environment was least stressful for critical care nurses (Milutinovic et al., 2012).

Finally, the very nature of the work is also call for concern. While much benefit is derived from being a nurse and helping people get on the road to recovery from illness, there also come some concerns merely from the nature of the work being done. These concerns often manifest themselves as stressors, as nurses can experience worry about being exposed to infectious diseases, such as those of their patients (NIOSH, 2008), accident and/or injury, as would occur in needle sticks (Daft, 2011; NIOSH, 2008; Tomey, 2009), exposure to infectious and hazardous substances in the workplace, and, as we will cover in much greater detail in Chapter 8, exposure to work-related violence or threats (NIOSH, 2008).

Resource Shortage

A shortage of nurses in all sectors of nursing has been a recognized concern for all countries (WHO, 2003). For novice nurses, nursing students, and aspiring nursing students, this is good news because once you finish your academic program, you will perhaps more easily obtain gainful employment. An aging workforce, an aging demographic, and the looming costs of unsustainable health care systems have significantly contributed to this trend. Under the direction of executives, nurse leaders are tasked with cutting back and saving money where and when possible. Sadly, what can result is inadequate staffing (NIOSH, 2008; Yoder-Wise, 2011), which places additional stress on the nurses who are working as replacements for those calling in sick or on leave. For example, shortages of nurses result in unsafe patient care, increased expense, and increased stress levels among other nurses (Moneke &

Umeh, 2013). Furthermore, organizational constraints can be predictors of nurses' stress (Kath, Stichler, Ehrhart, & Schultze, 2013).

Aging Workforce in Nursing

Like many other occupations and/or careers, nursing is experiencing an aging workforce. As baby boomers near retirement, junior nurses may be worried about losing a great deal of skill, knowledge, and expertise that the more senior nurses had to share (McHugh & Lake, 2010). Secondly, research suggests that as nurses near their retirement, they may not be as eager or ambitious to take on new challenges, new roles, and new tasks as they were in their junior years. This applies particularly to senior nurses acting as mentors (also referred to as job shadowing) as nursing students fulfill required clinical placements in hospitals and health care agencies.

Complacency

There is nothing worse than working with people who do not pull their own weight. In other words, you are teamed up with someone or a team of people whom you know from past experiences have no interest in working in the nursing profession. As an ambitious nurse, you like to get into work, provide the care needed and desired by the patient, and do so in a timely and efficient manner. You also like to practice and see compassion woven through that caring experience along the way. When you don't have that equal counterpart to achieve the tasks and care at hand, complacency can become a significant stressor for you in the workplace.

Gaining commitment from employees should be the primary goal of every company. Once a spirit of allegiance is achieved, employees become motivated to fulfill the organization's mission while working toward achieving its vision.

Poor Job Fit

Nurses working in jobs that don't fit their interests and skills are certain to become more and more stressed over time (Smith, Segal, & Segal, 2013). You need to choose a job that is right for you, that suits your skills, interests, and career goals, and that will encourage you to do your job well, remain interested in your work tasks, enjoy going to work each day, and to stay in your chosen occupation over the long term.

Workload

Excessive workload that is characterized by not enough time, support, or resources to complete the tasks at hand is a significant course of stress, and sometimes the biggest stressor in the workplace (NIOSH, 2008; Yoder-Wise, 2011, p. 553). Patient demands (Violante et al., 2009), role overload (Kath et al., 2013), monotony and/ or chaos (Smith et al., 2013), patient acuity (Yoder-Wise, 2011, p. 553), unrealistic deadlines and demands (Williams, 2012), and work intensity (The Health Communication Unit, University of Toronto, 2004) are all sources of stress and potential threats to a nurse's mental health that can lead to anxiety disorders, mood disorders, and job burnout (Jasperse, Herst, & Dungey, 2013; Rodwell & Martin, 2013; Smith et al., 2013).

Poor Leadership

Nursing leaders play an integral role in how smoothly a nursing setting operates and in how quality and efficiency of care are handled. A common source of impaired workplace mental health for nurses is the people who are positioned to be their managers. Research has found that unsupportive managers are a significant source of tension and anxiety in a nurse's workplace (Rodwell & Martin, 2013). Poor leadership can permeate an organization, resulting in poor workplace mental health. Poor leadership is evidenced by complacency, poor morale, uncertainty, animosity, and increased conflict. Again, its undercurrent can filter down to front-line nurses, resulting in poor morale, anxiety, and frustrations. In the absence of good leadership, the operation of a nursing unit/setting, the quality of service provided, and the relationships among staff can suffer. For example, unfair management practices (NIOSH, 2008), poor communication with supervisors (The Health Communication Unit, University of Toronto, 2004), worry about administrative feedback (Chen et al., 2009), refusal to allow employee discretion over methods of work (Williams, 2012), and low levels of support from coworkers and supervisors (Jasperse et al., 2013; NIOSH, 2008: Smith et al., 2013) all add significantly to a nurse's stress level on the job. Jasperse et al. (2013) add that this lack of manager support can also lead to job dissatisfaction, stress, and burnout.

Estes (2013) found that "targeted subordinates reacted with noncompliance with significant organizational performance norms. The incidence of abusive supervision was 46.6%, with 36.6% of the nurses reporting negative influence on performance and compliance. Supervisory abuse is a problem to the healthcare organizations because of the counterproductive behaviors that resulted. Concern is specifically suggested regarding possible negative influences to patient satisfaction."

As found by Sveinsdóttir and Blöndal (2013), low job satisfaction, little praise from nurse managers, and performing unprofessional work often prompted nurses to leave their workplace. Factors contributing to nurses' intention to leave may result in a lack of interest in work, low morale, and ultimately unsafe patient care. "Employees who rate their managers as 'sensitive' miss an estimated 3.7 days of work, whereas employees whose managers are rated as 'non-sensitive' miss approximately 6.2 days of work" (MacBride-King & Bachmann, 1999).

Finally, poor nursing leadership can stem from issues within the nurse managers themselves. Nurse leaders too can become overwhelmed because they are the middle persons between directors, executives, and front-line nurses. While they play a pivotal role in creating work environments that retain staff nurses, they too have several variables impacting their perception of stress, some of which include "people and resources, tasks and work volume, and performance expectations" (Shirey, McDaniel, Ebright, Fisher, & Doebbeling, 2010). Although nurse managers use more effective coping strategies than novice nurses do, perhaps merely from their lived professional experiences, they too can exhibit poor work performance and leadership as a result of increased stress levels.

The nature of nursing and the giving of oneself to help others can be very physically and emotionally demanding for a nurse. You are dealing with acute and serious illness (Yoder-Wise, 2011), difficult patients and/or trauma (NIOSH, 2008), and you are also dealing with death on a sometimes daily basis (Yoder-Wise, 2011, p. 553).

Poor Staff Engagement

The engagement of staff is also a critical contributing factor impacting the workplace mental health of an organization. Engaged workers have a lot of energy, are very enthusiastic about their jobs, and are absorbed by their work (Van Bogaert, Wouters, Williams, Mondelaers, & Clarke, 2013). While staff engagement aims to motivate, inspire, and increase commitment, its absence causes poor morale, decreased motivation, and decreased productivity.

In an organization that offers little or no incentives for a job well done or opportunities to further oneself, either personally or professionally, staff engagement is problematic. In their study on the readiness of graduate nurses and its impact on job satisfaction, work engagement, and their intention to stay, Walker and Campbell (2013) found that the dimensions of work readiness, inclusive of organizational acumen, clinical competence, and social intelligence, predicted job satisfaction and work engagement and mediated the relationship between organizational acumen and intent to stay.

Neville and Cole (2013) found that engagement in health promotional behaviors may contribute to nurses' well-being in counteracting compassion fatigue, burnout, and dissatisfaction. In addition, it is impacted by status, certainty, autonomy, relatedness, and fairness (Tillott, Walsh, & Moxham, 2013) and symbolizes the rudimentary underpinnings of staff engagement.

As Van Bogaert et al. highlight, nurse work engagement is needed to help ensure workforce stability and quality of patient care. When nursing teams perform well, nurses tend to be more engaged and satisfied with their jobs and are more willing to stay in their positions and report better quality of patient care (Van Bogaert et al., 2013). However, nurses' engagement is often jeopardized by increased workload, increased overtime, and other factors that negatively affect workplace culture (Greco, Laschinger, & Wong, 2006; Yamada, 2008).

Work–Life Conflicts

Conflict in the workplace can wreak havoc with your stress levels. In an environment that needs your total attention and concentration, conflict can jeopardize the necessities of delivering safe and quality patient care. For a nurse, sources of conflict can emerge from one's personal as well as professional life. A mismatch in values can occur if personal values differ from the way an organization does business or handles employee grievances; it will wear on employees (Smith et al., 2013). Although conflict with professional colleagues in the workplace is a common occurrence, one of the most difficult conflicts is that between work and family (NIOSH, 2008; The Health Communication Unit, University of Toronto, 2004). Nurses feel so pressured to complete large amounts of work that they do not have a balance between work and personal life.

New Nurses and Novice Nurses

Entering a practice setting for the first time can be very stressful and mentally draining for new and novice nurses. As found by Maddalena, Kearney, and Adams (2012), "Although novice nurses are highly motivated to provide quality patient care, they encounter many sources of stress, including 'difficult person-alities,' inadequate orientation and mentoring, and horizontal violence from nursing and medical colleagues. Although these stressors are compounded by staffing shortages and heavy workloads, supportive mentoring and adequate orientation are key factors to successful transition." French (2011) adds that all new nurses "go through a 'breaking-in' stage" when they first enter their work-place that is accompanied by what she calls "an unfathomable stress." As a new nurse speaking from experience, French feels that novice nurses are often not prepared for the pressure they will encounter and are often reluctant to talk about it.

Threat of Violence or Bullying

It is recognized that violence in the workplace is a significant factor impacting stress and the increased disposition to the development and/or exacerbation of mental health concerns, so for our purposes it is covered in its entirety in Chapter 9 (Daft, 2011; Tomey, 2009). Similarly, workplace bullying holds the same concerns with respect to workplace stress and mental health concerns for nurses, so it too will be covered in its entirety in Chapter 7.

Organizational Factors

The quality of patient care provided by a hospital may also influence nurse stress. Beliefs about whether the institution provides high-quality care may influence the perceived stress of job pressures and workload because higher-quality care is reflected in greater support and availability of resources. A poor organizational climate that becomes evident through an identified lack of management commit-ment to core organizational values and conflicting communication styles are just two examples of organizational factors that can impact nurses' stress and mental well-being (NIOSH, 2008).

Increasing Roles and Responsibilities

As the profession of nursing evolves, expands, and changes, nurses' roles and responsibilities have also changed and grown. Part of this change and evolution of practice relates directly to the increased technology that has now become a key piece of nursing care (Goldschmidt, 2011).

Changes in procedures, policies, and practices that are constantly being built from evidence-informed research also play a role in increasing the nurse's roles and responsibilities.

As the skill mix, scope, and competencies of nursing practice expand, so too do the roles of advanced practice nurses and nurse practitioners. For example, mentor-ship and shadowing of nursing students is something that is now expected by many jurisdictions of nursing practice, and although a small incentive is offered, it can still add to a nurse's already growing stress level in the workplace. The arrival and use of nurses as physician assistants with increased responsibility and accountability for the work that they do is another example.

Personal and Professional Development Opportunities

Continuing education is increasingly necessary for nurses to keep abreast of rapid changes in patient care because of advancements in knowledge and technology (Berings, 2006). Most countries typically expect their nurses to pursue continuing education as they practice (Flores & Castillo, 2006; Ni et al., 2013). The lack of opportunity to engage in personal and professional development such as training can be a significant source of stress for nurses, as it is often perceived as a missed opportunity for growth and promotion (NIOSH, 2008).

Patients and Families

Nurses deal with people who are possibly going through the biggest significant personal change in life that they will ever encounter. Because stress and the perception of one's stress and stressors is so individualized, stress from patients and their families can be found in any and all nurse practice settings (WHO, 2010). Patients requiring complex care; the acute, critical emergency department; and confused, elderly, or mentally ill patients all have concerns and demands of their own and naturally require a lot of nursing attention. As a result, nurses feels that they cannot provide adequate amounts of care to other patients. This often makes for a very difficult juggling of time and priorities so all patients are treated equally.

Patient Safety and Quality Concerns

A key role of a licensed nurse, as part of a recognized, defined profession, is to protect the public. Therefore, ensuring that safety and quality of care are met is an identified source of stress for nurses (Chen et al., 2009). Van Bogaert et al. (2013) add that "reports of quality of care by the interdisciplinary team were predicted by dedication, absorption, nurse–physician relations, and nurse management."

Pace and Urgency of Care Needed

No matter what the setting in which you work or plan to work in the nursing profession, there is always some degree of urgency in the care needed and issues needing attention (NIOSH, 2008). In acute settings in particular, nurses' readiness to save lives is a stressor of time pressure (Elmqvist et al., 2012). With the hustle and bustle of everyday nursing, the nurse has to also be cognizant of prioritizing patients' care. As already found, workplace stress today is linked to a lack of control over the pace of work (The Health Communication Unit, University of Toronto, 2004).

Changing Technologies

We are inundated today with increasing technology that eases our tasks, promotes longevity, promotes health, and prevents the onset or exacerbation of disease. At the bedside or in our offices at work, we are repeatedly interacting with technology, computers, iPads, electronic documentation, diagnostic imaging equipment, wound-cleaning chemicals, and now even antibacterial pillows. Nurses can feel stressed and bombarded by the new equipment and technology that are becoming necessary to deliver patient care, especially nurses who are not so computer-savvy. Furthermore, for the senior nurses who pioneered nursing practice, the advent of increased technology can be an added stressor, in spite of the fact that this new technology may improve patient care and lessen the nurse's workload somewhat.

But wait; let's move this philosophy to the bedside, where care is given to patients or individuals who are in their weakest and most vulnerable state. The electronic blood pressure cuff that is frequently used has removed the need for this nurse–patient contact. The pulse oximeter and use of the iPad for an assessment and documentation tool as well create a similar outcome of decreasing interpersonal contact. The point being that when you take the human factor out of patient care provision at all levels, a cold and impersonal automation is left to flourish. The organization is so preoccupied with fulfilling its mandate and organizational goals in the most financially responsible manner possible that the people of the organization and hence the patient care ultimately suffer. For any health care organization, this is truly a balancing act to find equilibrium.

The effects of technology creating an impersonal culture are well-known (Barnard & Sandelowski, 2001). Instead of technology freeing the nurse for more patient contact time, an unexpected outcome has resulted. A paradigm shift in society has occurred, and patients now are much more complex in their needs and demands, nursing shortages are experienced, and increasing workloads have only served to decrease human contact and interaction even more.

Schedule

Shift work is often targeted as a source of stress for nurses (Geiger-Brown & Lipscomb, 2010; NIOSH, 2008). While it is an expected part of the nurse's job, much research on the effects of shift work for nurses has shown that this is not necessarily so. Although night shifts have often been touted as being negative for one's health (Berger & Hobbs, 2006), recent research suggests otherwise (Ruggiero, 2005; Ulas et al., 2012). Whether it is 12-hour day shifts or night shifts, the effects were found to be the same. Problems such as fatigue, sleep problems, anxiety, and difficulties trying to maintain regular and healthy lifestyles often occur (Ulas et al., 2012), with neither day nor night shift nurses experiencing any greater effect than the other. Further, regardless of types of shifts worked—findings were consistent across day shifts, night shifts, and rotating shifts—all had general widespread dissatisfaction with their jobs (Ruggiero, 2005). However, in general, shift workers have been suggested to experience much more undue stress than day shift workers. In fact, Matsumoto, Komata, Naoe, Mutah, and Chiba (1996) found that sleep problems after day shifts were worse, as were Zung self-rating depression scale scores, than after night shifts. However, night nurses experience worse sleep problems and fatigue and an increased rate of taking sleep-inducing medications after the first night shift. As found in one study, day shift nurses experienced more migraine headaches; more emotional problems, such as mild depression, anxiety, tension, and insomnia; and were in need of more medical care than were night nurses, while night nurses had increased cholesterol levels and complained more of insufficient time available to spend with children and family and on leisure activities (Portela, Rotenberg, &

Waissmann, 2004). Shift workers also have an increased incidence of gastrointestinal difficulties, disturbed sleep patterns, accidents, anxiety levels, depression, and general dissatisfaction with life compared with regular day nurses. And they actually feel out of "sync" with the world. However, when day and night shift nurses were compared, both inpatient and intensive care unit nurses' total antioxidant status (TAS), total oxidant status (TOS), and oxidative stress index (OSI) and anxiety levels were not significantly different ($p > 0.05$), and all nurses experienced similar effects of day and night shifts (Ulas et al., 2012).

Other scheduling stressors were long hours (Geiger-Brown, 2010; NIOSH, 2008; The Health Communication Unit, University of Toronto, 2004), rotating shifts (Yoder-Wise, 2011, p. 553), and general scheduling practices by management (Ruggiero, 2005).

Lack of Participation and Decision-Making Control in the Workplace

Nurses like and need to have some control in the workplace (WHO, 2005); after all, they are holding very important positions for the delivery of patient care and a high degree of responsibility and accountability. Typically, in the high-pressure and low-control situations in which nurses work, they have an increased risk to their physical and mental well being (Tangri, 2003). When the demands and control at work become imbalanced, stress occurs (Canadian Centre of Occupational Health and Safety [CCOHS], 2012).

Quite simply, employees who have a lack of job control have an increased likelihood of experiencing increased stress levels (NIOSH, 2008; Smith et al., 2013; The Health Communication Unit, University of Toronto, 2004). As highlighted by the low decision latitude of Scott (2010), fewer chances to make choices predict common mental disorders. Smith et al. add that this lack of control brought on by tasks such as hours of work, assignments received, and an inability to control the amount of work they do and how they do it sets the nurse up for significant potential to compromise his or her mental health (Smith et al., 2013; Williams, 2012). Further, job demands and requirements exceeding nurses' skill relate to indicators such as depression, poor commitment, and job dissatisfaction among nurses (Rodwell & Martin, 2013). Physically as well, nurses who have little input into decision making and how their work is organized are 50% more likely to suffer from heart disease, yet another stressor (The Health Communication Unit, University of Toronto, 2004).

Monotonous or Unpleasant Tasks

Blood, guts, and glory all seem to be a normal expectation if you decide to enter nursing. One does not typically envision nursing as boring or involving monotonous and/ or unpleasant tasks, but it can be for some (WHO, 2005), and if you are experiencing this in your job as a nurse, it can actually be a stressor for you. From the University of California, Berkeley, Professors Morten Hansen and Dacher Keltner (2012) suggest that emptiness can occur. If you are spending 30% to 60% of your life at work and fulfilling a job that you dread and do not look forward to because of its monotony, boredom, unpleasantness, and lack of challenge, you are probably doing your body more harm than good, and it literally saps your energy (Hansen & Keltner, 2012).

Change

Change can be a significant source of stress for working nurses. Change is typically perceived with fear, uncertainty, and/or ambiguity because individuals often do not know what to expect as a result of change and how it will impact them, their job, and their livelihood. As we will discuss further in the chapters on the roles of leaders and the organization in helping to promote a mentally healthy workplace change, such change, if effectively managed, can help to eliminate much of this stress for nurses. However, failure to manage change heightens stress, harassment, and conflict at work (Center for Conflict Resolution International, 2013).

Most health care organizations are inundated with change, and change is a vital piece of the success of any organization where treatment, techniques, technology, and approaches change to serve patients better. However, change can come with a price. Although there are many stages to implement change (Kotter, 2014), not always does it translate into a smooth and accepted transition and can often leave a bad taste in people's mouths if it is not done well and involve others (Prosci, 2013). Some of the ripple effects of change that can impact nurses' stress levels and mental health are that it can compromise productivity, retention, communication, routine practice, nurse unity, morale, and commitment. Further, it deters interest from key stakeholders, creates confusion and fatigue, and plays havoc with overspent budgets and missed deadlines, so much so that a project is sometimes abandoned (Prosci, 2013).

Role Ambiguity

Role ambiguity or lack of clarity around one's role in the workplace can place a great deal of stress on individuals experiencing it (NIOSH, 2008; WHO, 2005), particularly nurses (Yoder-Wise, 2011, p. 553). When a nurse is uncertain and not confident about what needs to be done or how to best do it, or even misunderstands the duties or tasks being asked, a great deal of stress, tension, and inner turmoil can arise for the nurse. As suggested by Smith et al. (2013), unclear job expectations such as uncertainty over the degree of authority they have and lacking necessary resources to complete work are some such examples (The Health Communication Unit, University of Toronto, 2004), making role ambiguity one of the best predictors of stress in the workplace (Kath et al., 2013; NIOSH, 2008). As nurses' skill mix and scope of practice continue to evolve and change, so too does their expected degree of accountability. Whether welcomed by you or not, it is a reality and very commonplace in today's nursing profession. As such, it may serve as a stressor to you.

Conflict and Lack of Constructive Conflict Resolution

Conflict, or differences in values, wants, needs, or expectations, is plentiful in workplaces. Although conflict can benefit an organization and create opportunities for creativity, collaboration, and improvement, it can also be costly. The trouble isn't necessarily the fact that conflict exists, it is how we deal with it (Government of Newfoundland and Labrador, 2013). Conflict in the workplace is a significant destructive force that can challenge one's mental health and well-being (WHO, 2005). For example, organizations need nurses to coordinate and oversee patient care, aim for efficiency and cost-effectiveness, and monitor quality control; however, in trying to meet these conflicting expectations, nurses often feel frustrated and distressed (Yoder-Wise, 2011, p. 553; WHO, 2005).

Organizations can often grow to monstrosities, employing thousands of staff across many different facilities, sites, and satellite locations and across large geographical dimensions. Each sector of a health care organization also brings with it the magnitude of various personalities and leadership styles needed to operationalize the organization's goals. The differing opinions, beliefs, and attitudes that accompany those different personalities can impact significantly nurses' mental health. The impact of different personalities, attitudes, beliefs, and behaviors in an organization can optimistically decrease bias and allow a more objective approach and viewpoint in making important decisions or responding to critical events that can occur. However, various personalities can also result in differing opinions, priorities, strategies, and views of what can or cannot work for the organization, or even what is best or not best for an organization. Even at the executive level, the pitfalls of team dynamics can exert a negative impact.

Lack of Recognition and Reward at Work

Reward and recognition serve many functions for employees (WHO, 2005), inclusive of nurses. They foster psychological empowerment (Gkorezis & Petridou, 2011); serve to positively influence recruitment and retention (Spence Laschinger, Leiter, Day, & Gilin, 2009), staff morale (Day, Minichiello, & Madison, 2007), and patient satisfaction (Kennedy, Caselli, & Berry, 2011); and help to build a mentally healthy workplace (CCOHS, 2012). As suggested by Williams (1996), "nurses' validation of professional worth and accolades for a job well done are key to long-term satisfaction."

In the absence of recognition and reward, nurses feel dissatisfied and not valued in an environment inundated with low morale and low patient satisfaction, and they also feel stressed. When there is an effort–reward imbalance, the risk for physical and mental disorders increases (Mark & Smith, 2012; Tangri, 2003). This becomes referred to as a high-effort/low-reward situation, which occurs when the effort given is not proportionately reciprocated with reward and/or recognition; stress and exhaustion can occur (Jasperse et al., 2013; Scott, 2010; Williams, 2012).

Poor Interpersonal Relationships With Colleagues and Multidisciplinary Staff

As health care prides itself on teamwork and collaboration, relationships of nurses with colleagues, staff, and patients are a key component in the workplace where all work together with the common goal of getting the patient well and on the road to recovery. Strained workplace relationships negatively impact employees, such as nurses (NIOSH, 2008; WHO, 2005). It creates a dysfunctional and tense environment, and therefore stress on the nurse, and it can also infringe on a nurse's mental health and potentially jeopardize the standards of nursing practice and the quality and safety of patient care delivery.

For example, poor collegial relations can cause communication breakdown, low levels of colleague support, staff attrition, and discouraging recruitment rates (Cowin, 2013; Smith et al., 2013). Further, it impacts quality and safety of patient care, work satisfaction, and level of nursing professionalism (Cowin, 2013) and impacts nurses' job performance and how they are involved in the decisions about their work and provided with the right resources and adequate support (Van Bogaert et al., 2013). Teamwork in particular, in which the majority of nurses engage, was found to be a significant source of stress because nurses' teamwork impacts nurses' stress levels (Geiger-Brown & Lipscomb, 2010). Furthermore, dysfunctional workplace dynamics, such as bullying and being undermined by colleagues or your boss who micromanages your work, can also threaten nurses' mental health (Smith et al., 2013).

Poor Communication

The sole purpose of communication is to allow the exchange of information, ideas, concepts, emotions, thoughts, and opinions. Communication is a critical component of life and of work as well, and it is key to survival because humans rely upon it to get their needs met. For nurses, communication is a critical piece of getting the job done and providing needed care, and it helps to ensure the safety and security of the patients and colleagues. Clear and open communication to promote the lives and well-being of other, more vulnerable people is needed, but absent it can exert a tremendous amount of stress on the nurse (Geiger-Brown & Lipscomb, 2010; WHO, 2005) because it symbolizes that there are significant measures of responsibility and accountability missing, and hence patient care can become jeopardized. A pilot who flies a plan is in much the same situation because the pilot has in his or her hands the lives of many different people, so as passengers we need that pilot to have a clear mind and open communication. A breakdown in communication can create a less efficient workplace, missed important information, and poor productivity, and it can even be dangerous as safety protocols can get pushed aside. In the case of a nurse, physician, or even an airplane pilot, a breakdown in communication can endanger others' lives (Wolfe, 2013).

Atmosphere

The occurrence of stress that is prolonged and severe enough to precipitate or exacerbate mental health concerns can be positively correlated with negativity in the workplace environment.

As a nurse getting ready to come to work, you begin to feel that it is somewhat of a burden to do so and so something you just don't look forward to. The thought of the bad attitudes, sarcastic remarks, and subtle but nasty innuendos and behaviors of some coworkers coupled with the fact that "you know you might be verbally or professional attacked on any given day" is reason enough to feel this way (Moultry Belcher, 2013). You may even literally fear going to work. Finally, low organizational commitment, job dissatisfaction, reduced self-efficacy, and low levels of workplace peer support in particular can lead to higher levels of cynicism among nurses (Smith et al., 2013). A significant part of that atmosphere is morale. As discussed next, the morale of a workplace can make or break a nurse's experience.

Morale

As today's health care climate evolves, population demographics change, nursing shortages loom, health care budgets shrink, and the competitive race for jobs meets the angst of the recession, governments and organizations struggle to keep morale afloat. As suggested by Kovner & Neuhauser (2004), organizations and its leaders need to seek creative strategies to improve and maintain the high performance of employees, and increased morale is one key strategy that can help. Morale, or the spirit of a person or group as exhibited by confidence, cheerfulness, discipline, and willingness to perform assigned tasks (*American Heritage Dictionary of the English Language*, 2000), can be jeopardized by poor communication, lack of trust, rising layoffs, unclear directions, high rates of staff turnover, and other features (Fink, 2007). Instead of cheerfulness, visible energy, good attendance, attentiveness, and willingness to go above and beyond the call of duty, low morale precipitates increased absenteeism, coworker conflict, insubordination, decreased productivity, disorganized and unkempt work environments, routine complaints about seemingly insignificant work-related issues, and increased patient complaints (Fink, 2007). Low morale can create a great deal of stress in nursing (Kashani, Eliasson, Chrosniak, & Vernalis, 2010) and can be created by and lead to such things as poor communication, lack of empowerment, lack of energizing staff, distrust of management, poor interpersonal relations, and inflexible working conditions (Dye & Garman, 2006). Other influential variables can take the form of departmental layoffs or closures, labor negotiations and contract disputes, high employee turnover rates, changes in leadership, and unclear expectations and corporate direction (Lee, Scheunemann, Hall, & Payne, 2012).

The Weight of Attitude

The relationship between attitude and stress has been well-known for years and is certainly something that people need reminders of. Attitude can have both positive and negative ramifications. In order to appreciate the effects of attitude, it is good to know just how it works and the impact it may have on one's stress level and perception. According to the APA (2014), an attitude is "the learned, relatively stable tendency to respond to people, concepts, and events in an evaluative way." Further, it is a state of mind, feeling, or disposition that involves an expression of favor or disfavor towards a person, place, thing or event. In essence, this is truly a case of "mind over matter." "Everything starts with attitude," and this is so true.

For some, the attitude at work can make or break their desire to be there and the stress levels they can experience therein. Who truly likes going to work with a negative attitude? You know what this is like because you have most likely experienced working with a nurse or other health care professional who regularly has a negative attitude. Your attitude influences your behaviors and responses as well. As nurses interacting daily with other health care professionals and patients, attitude goes a long way in defining who we are and how we perceive stress (Karanikola & Papathanassoglou, 2013). Place yourself in the shoes of a patient who is recovering from illness or surgery. How would you feel if a nurse came into your room in a hurried manner, made no eye contact, didn't smile and did not say good morning, threw a bath towel and washcloth on your bed, grabbed the wash basin, quickly seized and pulled the curtain, and told you to get out of bed? Nursing colleagues have noticed this occurring on a regular basis. For a sick and recovering patient, this attitude from a professional nurse is not acceptable.

Similarly, with a colleague, you walk into the nursing station, you grab a chair that another nurse was just about to sit on, you throw your patient assignment list on the table, you don't smile or greet anyone, and then you proceed to sit with a huge sigh, avoiding eye contact with anyone and staring at the tape recorder that is delivering the patient report. This is not just a one-off, this is what is experienced and observed by others every day you work. These behaviors say a lot about your attitude, which is being impacted by your emotions and perceptions.

We have now seen firsthand how attitude can influence our work environment. The good news is that attitude is something that is often learned and is something that you, yourself, can influence and control. Our attitude is perhaps one of the most important elements that make us who we are, as it illustrates how we respond to the people, events, and circumstances we encounter (Young, 2012).

According to Young (2012), it is our perceptions, choices, and behaviors that define our attitude, whether it is successes in life with a positive attitude or perceived failures in life that form a negative attitude. A positive attitude leads to good morale, good working collegial relationships, and increased productivity (Johnson, 2012). To the contrary, a negative attitude can often lead to work dissatisfaction, poor or unhealthy working relationships, and struggles with work responsibilities.

Nurses' work-related stress might be associated with psychiatric symptoms, leading to altered professional attitudes.

Organizational

Culture

Nurses are not oblivious to the underlying cultures that exist within an organization. Sadly, there are two elements of culture that can threaten organizational goals such as the delivery of safe, competent patient care. One is created by the organization itself, as it strives to achieve its own goals. Second is that which is fostered and built by the nurses on the front line. Both of these cultures can serve to be very counterproductive, not only toward the organizational goals but also to the nursing profession as well.

Health care organizations have a tremendous responsibility for providing safe, quality, and competent care to the people they serve. At the same time, they also have to monitor and guide the work of thousands of employees, meet expected standards of practice and strategic direction for accreditation, and fulfill the organizational mandate and vision under the watchful eye of their board of trustees/directors, all while maintaining an acute sense of responsibility, fiscal stewardship, transparency, and accountability to the public. In some respects, health care organizations can get so caught up with their own agendas that they tend to forget about the front-line workers, particularly the nurses who form much of the backbone that supports and fulfills the main goals of the organization as the human factor often goes unnoticed and underutilized.

It would be prudent for health care organizations to realize that it is the employees who are the most valued asset to the functioning of an organization. A realization is needed by health care organizations that the human or people connection is a valuable resource to an organization if it wants to succeed. The person-to-person contact is what works best and helps to illustrate a genuine interest and desire of an organization to meet the needs of all people; hence, it is one of the best investments that an organization can make.

From a nurse's perspective, a separate culture of its own insidiously grows. This culture is similarly unproductive and can even be detrimental to the goals of the organization. Although an organization seeks to obtain and retain nurses who are knowledgeable, skillful, caring, respectful, and courteous, this does not always ideally occur, and if it does, they can become quickly destroyed by existing rumors.

When this nursing culture is negative and pessimistic, it significantly increases nurses' stress levels (Geiger-Brown & Lipscomb, 2010). In the increased pace of many acute care settings, with risking workloads and lack of manager presence and input, what fosters is a culture of "who cares?" Furthermore, some of the busiest acute units are also the units that experience a high turnover of staff (Applebaum, Fowler, Fiedler, Osinubi, & Robson, 2010). Here, the addition of novice nurses and new hires, who are perhaps reluctant to oppose current bad practices of the unit, can easily slide into and fall prey to the very same behaviors modeled before them, leaving loyalty, dedication, and work ethic behind.

The Power of Politics and Organizational Bureaucracies

Most organizations are defined as being bureaucratic in nature such that the administrative execution and enforcement of legal rules are socially organized. Although bureaucracies are well structured with a human resources personnel system that offers stable, linear careers, a hierarchy among offices, and formal and informal networks connecting people and information, hidden agendas from its players can become an issue of concern. As nurses, we often hear and find out that someone received a favor because of knowing someone up in the hierarchy, and such behaviors often reflect favoritism, an informal buddy system, or a playoff of one staff member against another in return for something good. For lack of a better word, this is what is commonly referred to in layperson's terms as "brownnosing," "sucking up to the boss," or simply "you scratch my back and I will scratch yours." These are the informal networking structures that can literally destroy the morale among nurses who are sometimes more experienced and better qualified for a job or role than the person who got it. However, not much research has been conducted in this area. In most cases, nurses realize it is happening but often sit idly by and speechless because they just don't know how to respond to such behaviors.

Problem Employees

A significant source of stress and deteriorating mental health of nurses can be problem employees. Problem employees make the workplace a very difficult place. Problem employees are people who think they are indispensible and have an astute disconnected sense of their own self-worth, value, and concept (Salpeter, 2013). Although many actually don't even realize they are part of the problem, characteristic behaviors reveal they cannot say no when given a directive from their boss, but it can typically be accompanied by rolling of the eyes, shaking of the head, and the offering of inappropriate and untimely opinions. They cannot take no for an answer, they think they are smarter than everyone else at work, they make excuses for everything, they don't work well in teams because they need to be in control, it's always about them, and they really don't care how others look. Gossip is their favorite pastime so they can be front and center, they never seem to "get it" right the first time, and they repeatedly make mistakes because they don't listen to others. Furthermore, they can sometimes seem like a "loose cannon" and use profanity that people fear. Finally, they live for the weekend and have their own agenda, which does not include an honest day's work.

As a result, a problem employee can make for a very tense workplace that leaves colleagues and leaders with a sense of uncertainty, fear, and intrepidation and an added responsibility of wondering if tasks and patient care are being fully and competently achieved. This prevailing workplace negativity can decrease communication and hence safe, responsible, and accountable care.

SOCIETY

Humans are always a product of their own environment, and the society in which we live contributes significantly to that environment. Societal and environmental influences can cripple a health care organization's workplace mental health. Beyond the confines of an organization and its governance structure and bodies lies a large society that a health care organization has no control over. The recession and threat of terrorism are two such examples.

Much of the recession, as occurred in the United States and many other developed countries in the 1990s to the 2000s and even to the present day, can insidiously infiltrate an organization's business at some point in its operation. Learner (2008), from the National Bureau of Economic Research, defines a recession as "a period of falling economic activity spread across the economy, lasting more than a few months, normally visible in real gross domestic product, real income, employment, industrial production, and wholesale–retail sales." It has great potential to impact people's mental health and can exert long-lasting effects on a person's personal and professional life. Belt tightening of organizations, governments, and countries and decreased transfer payments used to support the work of the organization or health care system and its strategic directions and mandate are commonplace. Such decreases can spark a fire of fear and anxiety among employees as they worry about layoffs, reduced hours of work, and benefits. This same anxiety and fear percolate down to the front lines and ultimately on to the nurse. An event such as this can further increase the amount of rumor mongering and gossip that can occur at the workplace, thus impacting further the mental health of the work environment.

In recent years, the impact of the recession on nurses' mental health as employees has received increasing attention. The year 2009 brought together an international roundtable discussion of many key countries, including the United States, Canada, United Kingdom, Australia, Ireland, and New Zealand, to discuss this very important issue of how the recession could impact workers' mental health (International Roundtable, 2009). This series of meetings began in Canada in August, 2009, and moved to Washington in later 2009 and Ireland in 2010. It was suggested that the negative impact of recessions could last as long as a decade. At a personal level, compounding the actual loss or threat of loss of one's job during a recession are escalated debt levels, reduced property values and savings, as well as reduced services that people can access for help. Furthermore, in tough economic times binge drinking and other addictions increase, smokers are 13% less likely to quit, and there is an increase in heart disease, sleeping disorders, migraines, and hypertension. People forgo buying their much-needed medications, going for checkups, and taking preventative care measures. From a mental health perspective, persons with a large debt have two to three times the rate of depression, three times the rate of psychoses, double the rate of alcohol abuse, and four times the rate of drug abuse compared with the general population. In addition, issues such increased family violence, gambling, crime, family conflict, child neglect and abuse, and spousal abuse increase. Anxiety and suicide are also more likely to occur during a recession or threat of job loss. Recent research suggests that a 1% increase in unemployment equates to a 0.79% increase in the rate of suicide (International Roundtable, 2009). As stated at the International Roundtable (2009), "the psychological impact of economic crisis on individuals and families can easily be compared to the aftermath of a disaster such as Hurricane Katrina" (p. 5).

The threat of terrorism is also a factor that cannot be ignored for how it impacts the lives of nurses, not to mention the whole of the United States, or any other country for that matter. Americans know of terrorism, unfortunately, all too well. The events of September 11, 2001, brought fear, devastation, and compromised mental health for many Americans. As many Americans sat at their desks working in the Twin Towers, little did they know of the catastrophe that awaited them. The understanding of the workplace as a safe, secure, and comfortable place took on new meaning as the Twin Towers became a place of shrieks of terror, anguished cries for help, and blood-splattered confinement with people lying trapped in their offices, stairwells, and corridors.

SUMMARY

The value of work to us as nurses and as human beings is without end. Work serves to fulfill each of our personal, professional, social, physical, and even psychological needs. There are various sources of stress that nurses encounter. Stress is something uniquely experienced by the individual and varies across one's personal, professional, and organizational domains. Whether our personal means of survival, satisfaction or coping strategies, our professional experience of workload, interpersonal conflict or low morale, or an organization's poisonous politics and culture, it is our perception of these stressors that makes them what they are. Although we all differ with respect to how we respond to stress, it is critical to acknowledge and understand what our stressors are. As we come to appreciate the various benefits that our work provides for us, the recognition of such stressors is critical so that we are able to continue doing something that we spend much of life doing—working.

DISCUSSION QUESTIONS

1. Why is work such a valuable component of your life?
2. What are some significant sources of stress in one's personal life?

3. What are some of the significant sources of stress in one's professional life as a nurse?
4. What are some significant sources of stress that can arise from an organization and impact on a nurse's life?
5. What impact can attitude have on workplace mental health?

REFERENCES

Adriaenssens, J., de Gucht, V., & Maes, S. (2012). The impact of traumatic events on emergency room nurses: Findings from a questionnaire survey. *International Journal of Nursing Studies, 49*(11), 1411–1422. doi:10.1016/j.ijnurstu.2012.07.003

Advisory, Conciliation, and Arbitration Service. (2013). *Promoting positive mental health at work.* Retrieved from http://www.acas.org.uk/index.aspx?articleid=1900

American Heritage Dictionary of the English Language (4th ed.). (2000). Definition of morale. Retrieved April 5, 2008, from www.thefreedictionary.com

American Institute of Stress. (2013). *Workplace stress.* Retrieved from http://www.stress.org/workplace-stress/#sthash.ZeOsTo9y.dpuf

American Nurses Association. (2011). *2011 ANA health and safety survey hazards of the RN work.* Retrieved from ENVIRONMENhttp://www.google.ca/url?sa=t&rct=j&q=&esrc=s&frm=1&source=web&cd=8&cad=rja&ved=0CGMQFjAH&url=http%3A%2F%2Fnursingworld.org%2FFunctionalMenuCategories%2FMediaResources%2FMediaBackgrounders%2FThe-Nurse-Work-Environment-2011-Health-SafetySurvey.pdf&ei=TxVbUrOfGM6jkQfqroCACg&usg=AFQjCNHtZZBnMTRYtAR5X5CKaTRM89Ss1g

American Psychological Association. (2009). *Stress in America 2009.* Retrieved from http://www.apa.org/news/press/releases/stress-exec-summary.pdf

American Psychological Association. (2014). *Glossary of psychological terms.* Retrieved from http://www.apa.org/research/action/glossary.aspx

Applebaum, D., Fowler, S., Fiedler, N., Osinubi, O., & Robson, M. (2010). The impact of environmental factors on nursing stress, job satisfaction, and turnover intention. *Journal of Nursing Administration, 40*(7–8), 323–328. doi:10.1097/NNA.0b013e3181e9393b

Arcurs, Y. (2014). *Starting a new job.* Retrieved from http://www.mindtools.com/pages/article/newCDV_29.htm

Barnard, A., & Sandelowski, M. (2001). Technology and humane nursing care: (Ir)reconcilable or invented difference? *Journal of Advanced Nursing, 34*(3), 367–375.

Berger, A. M., & Hobbs, B. B. (2006). Impact of shift work on the health and safety of nurses and patients. *Clinical Journal of Oncology Nursing, 10*(4), 465–471.

Berings, M. G. (2006). *On-the-job learning styles. Conceptualization and instrument development for the nursing profession* (Unpublished PhD thesis). Tilburg University, Tilburg, the Netherlands.

Bournes, D. A., & Milton, C. L. (2009). Nurses' experiences of feeling respected–not respected. *Nursing Science Quarterly, 22*(1), 47–56.

Boya, F. O., Demiral, Y., Ergor, A., Akvardar, Y., & De Witte, H. (2008). Effects of perceived job insecurity on perceived anxiety and depression in nurses. *Industrial Health, 46,* 613–619.

Boyum, R. (2013). *Characteristics of a self-actualizing person.* Retrieved from http://www.self-counseling.com/help/personalsuccess/selfactualization.htm

Briscoe, C. J. (2013). *How social media is playing a great role in our daily life.* Retrieved from http://www.webmasterview.com/2011/12/social-media-role-in-daily-life

Burton, J. (2010). *WHO healthy workplace framework and model: Background and supporting literature and practices.* Retrieved from http://www.who.int/occupational_health/healthy_workplace_framework.pdf

Cambridge Dictionaries Online. (2013). *A change is as good as a rest.* Retrieved from http://dictionary.cambridge.org/dictionary/british/a-change-is-as-good-as-a-rest

Canadian Centre for Occupational Health and Safety. (2012). *Workplace stress.* Retrieved from http://www.ccohs.ca/oshanswers/psychosocial/stress.html

Capehart, B., & Bass, D. (2012). Review: Managing posttraumatic stress disorder in combat veterans with comorbid traumatic brain injury. *Journal of Rehabilitation Research and Development, 49*(5), 789–812.

Center for Conflict Resolution International. (2014). *Workplace conflict.* Retrieved from http://www.conflictatwork.com/conflict/cost_e.cfm

Centers for Disease Control and Prevention. (2013). *Depression.* Retrieved from http://www.cdc.gov/workplacehealthpromotion/implementation/topics/depression.html

Chen, C. K., Lin, C., Wang, S. H., & Hou, T. H. (2009). A study of job stress, stress coping strategies, and job satisfaction for nurses working in middle-level hospital operating rooms. *The Journal of Nursing Research, 17*(3), 199–211. doi:10.1097/JNR.0b013e3181b2557b

Cowin, L. S. (2013). Collegial relationship breakdown: A qualitative exploration of nurses in acute care settings. *Collegian, 20*(2), 115–121.

Craig-Broadwith, M. (2012). *Do you work in a psychologically safe and healthy workplace?* Retrieved from http://calgary.cmha.ca/public_policy/do-you-work-in-a-psychologically-safe-and-healthy-workplace/#.UhNrVdK1G-k

Daft, R. L. (2011). *The leadership experience* (5th ed.). Mason, OH: South-Western Cengage Learning.

Day, G., Minichiello, V., & Madison, J. (2007). Nursing morale: Predictive variables among a sample of registered nurses in Australia. *Journal of Nursing Management, 15*(3), 274–284.

Dye, C., & Garman, A. (2006). *Exceptional leadership.* Chicago, IL: Health Administration Press.

Elmqvist, C., Fridlund, B., & Ekebergh, M. (2012). Trapped between doing and being: First providers' experience of "front line" work. *International Emergency Nursing, 20*(3), 113–119. doi:10.1016/j.ienj.2011.07.007

Estes, B. C. (2013). Abusive supervision and nursing performance. *Nursing Forum, 48*(1), 3–16. doi:10.1111/nuf.12004.

Fink, N. (2007). *The high cost of low morale: How to address low morale in the workplace through servant leadership.* Retrieved from http://www.roberts.edu/Academics/AcademicDivisions/BusinessManagement/msl/Community/Journal/TheHighCostofLowMorale.htm

Flores, P. Y., & Castillo, A. (2006). Factors influencing nursing staff members' participation in continuing education. *Revista Latino-Americana de Enfermagem, 14*(3), 309–315.

Foster, E. K., & Rosnow, R. L. (2006). Gossip and network relationships. In D. C. Kirkpatrick, S. Duck, & M. K. Foley (Eds.), *Relating difficulty: The processes of constructing and managing difficult interaction* (pp. 161–180). Mahwah, NJ: Lawrence Erlbaum Associates.

Freedman, H. (2009). *Our careers are our lives.* Retrieved August 1, 2013, from http://careers.theguardian.com/careers-blog/careers-are-our-life

French, L. (2011). The unspoken: The stresses of a novice nurse. *Nursing, 41*(12), 16–17. doi:10.1097/01.NURSE.0000407690.31430.ab

Gaylord, K. M. (2006). The psychosocial effects of combat: The frequently unseen injury. *Critical Care Nursing Clinics of North America, 18*(3), 349–357.

Geiger-Brown, J., & Lipscomb, J. (2010). The health care work environment and adverse health and safety consequences for nurses. *Annual Review of Nursing Research, 28,* 191–231.

Gkorezis, P., & Petridou, E. (2011). The impact of rewards on empowering public nurses. *Health Services Management Research, 24*(2), 5–59. doi:10.1258/hsmr.2010.010004

Globe News Wire. (2013). *Workplace stress on the rise with 83% of Americans frazzled by something at work.* Retrieved from http://globenewswire.com/news-release/2013/ 04/09/536945/10027728/en/Workplace-Stress-on-the-Rise-With-83-of-mericans-Frazzled-by-Something-at-Work.html

Gold, L., & Shuman, D. W. (2009). *Evaluating mental health disability in the workplace: Model, process, and analysis.* New York, NY: Springer.

Goldschmidt, K. J. (2011). "Techno-savvy" nurse or on the brink of "digital distress"? How to survive change in the delivery of pediatric nursing care. *Pediatric Nursing, 26*(5), 500–502. doi: 10.1016/j.pedn.2011.07.010

Government of Newfoundland Labrador. (2013). *The cost of conflict.* Retrieved from http:// www.psc.gov.nl.ca/psc/rwp/costofconflict.html

Greco, P., Laschinger, H., & Wong C. (2006). Leader empowering behaviours, staff nurse empowerment and work engagement/burnout. *Canadian Journal of Nursing Leadership, 19*(4), 41–56.

Gzorezis, P., & Petridou, E. (2011). The impact of rewards on empowering public nurses. *Health Services Management Research, 24*(2), 55–59.

Hansen, M., & Keltner, D. (2012). *Finding meaning at work even when your job is dull.* Retrieved June 4, 2013, from http://blogs.hbr.org/cs/2012/12/finding_meaning_at_work_even_w.html

Happell, B., Dwyer, T., Reid-Searl, K., Burke, K. J., Caperchione, C. M., & Gaskin, C. J. (2013). Nurses and stress: Recognizing causes and seeking solutions. *Journal of Nursing Management, 21*(4), 638–647. doi:10.1111/jonm.12037

Hasketh, K. L., Duncan, S. M., Estrabrooks, C.A., Reimer, M. A., Giovannetti, P., Hyndman, K., et al. (2003). Workplace violence in Alberta and British Columbia hospitals. *Health Policy, 63*, 311–321.

Hayes, L. J., Orchard, C. A., McGillis Hall, L., Nincic, V., O'Brien-Pallas, L., & Andrews, G. (2006). Career intentions of nursing students and new nurse graduates: A review of the literature. *International Journal of Nursing Education Scholarship, 3*, 1281.

Huston, J. L., & Brox, G. A. (2004). Professional ethics at the bottom line. *Health Care Manager, 23*(3), 267–272.

Institute of Medicine. (2004). *Keeping patients safe: Transforming the work environment of nurses.* Washington, DC: National Academies Press.

International Roundtable. (2009). *Impact of the recession on the mental health of workers and their families: Summary report.* Retrieved from http://www.google.ca/url?sa=t&rct= j&q=&esrc=s&frm=1&source=web&cd=1&ved=0CCs QFjAA &url=http%3A%2F% 2Fwww.mentalhealthcommission.ca%2FEnglish%2Fsystem%2Ffiles%2F private%2FWorkforce_International_Roundtable_ENG_0.pdf&ei=7LztUsKdE6S_sQTI-yoHwCQ &usg=AFQjCNEs7-0ARnhHKpKdB88qj5oGhGTEDA

Jasperse, M., Herst, P., & Dungey, G. (2014). Evaluating stress, burnout and job satisfaction in New Zealand radiation oncology departments. *European Journal of Cancer Care, 23*(1), 82–88. doi:10.1111/ecc.12098. Epub 2013 Jul 12.

Johnson, C. (2009). *Bad blood: Doctor-nurse behavior problems impact patient care.* Retrieved from https://www.ache.org/policy/doctornursebehavior.pdf

Johnson, M. (2012). *Workplace effect on attitude.* Retrieved from http://www.ehow.com/ facts_5921443_workplace-effect-attitude.html

Johnstone, M. J. (2012). Workplace ethics and respect for colleagues. *Australian Nursing Journal, 20*(2), 31.

Karanikola, M. N., & Papathanoasoglou, E. E. (2013). Exploration of the burnout syndrome occurrence among mental health nurses in Cyprus. *Archives of Psychiatric Nursing, 27*(6), 319–326. doi:10.1016/j.apnu.2013.08.004

Kashani, M., Eliasson, A., Chrosniak, L., & Vernalis, M. (2010). Taking aim at nurse stress: A call to action. *Military Medicine, 175*(2), 96–100.

Kath, L. M., Stichler, J. F., Ehrhart, M. G., & Schultze, T. A. (2013). Predictors and outcomes of nurse leader job stress experienced by AWHONN members. *Journal of Obstetric, Gynecological and Neonatal Nursing, 42*(1), E12–E25. doi:10.1111/j.1552-6909.2012.01430.x

Kelly, O. (2010). *Glossary: Coping.* Retrieved from http://ocd.about.com/od/glossary/g/Coping_Glossary.htm

Kennedy, D. M., Caselli, R. J., & Berry, L. L. (2011). A roadmap for improving healthcare service quality. *Journal of Healthcare Management, 56*(6), 400–402.

Kinoshita, Y., Furukawa, T. A., Kinoshita, K., Honyashiki, M., Omori, I. M., Marshall, M., et al. (2013). Supported employment for adults with severe mental illness. *The Cochrane Database of Systematic Reviews, 13*(9). doi:10.1002/14651858.CD008297.pub2

Kotter, J. (2014). *The 8-step process for leading change.* Retrieved from http://www.kotterinternational.com/our-principles/changesteps

Kovner, R., & Neuhauser, D. (Eds.). (2004). *Health services management* (8th ed.). Chicago, IL: Health Administration Press.

Laschinger, H. K. S., Leiter, M. P., Day, A., Gilin-Oore, D., & Mackinnon, S. P. (2012). Building empowering work environments that foster civility and organizational trust. *Nursing Research, 61*(5), 316–325.

Learner, E. E. (2008). *What's a recession anyway?* Retrieved from http://www.nber.org/papers/w14221

Lee, C., Scheunemann, J., Hall, R., & Payne, L. (2012). *Low staff morale & burnout: Causes & solutions.* Retrieved from https://illinois.edu/lb/files/2012/06/01/39974.pdf

MacBride-King, J. L., & Bachmann, K. (1999). *Solutions for the stressed-out worker. The Conference Board of Canada.* Retrieved from http://www.conferenceboard.ca/temp/6fb7209d-bd3c-40f1-8ddd-85a3bdd33cdf/worklife3.pdf

Maddalena, V., Kearney, A. J., & Adams, L. (2012). Quality of work life of novice nurses: A qualitative exploration. *Journal for Nurses in Staff Development, 28*(2), 74–79. doi:10.1097/NND.0b013e31824b41a1

Mahmood, A, Chaudhury, H., & Valente, M. (2011). Nurses' perceptions of how physical environment affects medication errors in acute care settings. *Applied Nursing Research, 24*(4), 229–237. doi:10.1016/j.apnr.2009.08.005

Mark, G., & Smith, A. P. (2012). Occupational stress, job characteristics, coping, and the mental health of nurses. *British Journal of Health Psychology, 17*(3), 505–521. doi:10.1111/j.2044-8287.2011.02051.x

Marshall, T., Goldberg, R. W., Braude, L., Dougherty, R. H., Daniels, A. S., Ghose, S. S., ... Delphin-Rittmon, M. E. (2013). Supported employment: Assessing the evidence. *Psychiatric Services, 11*(18). doi:10.1176/appi.ps.201300262.

Maslow, A. H. (1962). *Towards a psychology of being.* Princeton, NJ: D. Van Nostrand Company.

Matsumoto, M., Kamata, S., Naoe, H., Mutoh, F., & Chiba, S. (1996). [Investigation of the actual conditions of hospital nurses working on three rotating shifts: Questionnaire results of shift work schedules, feelings of sleep and fatigue, and depression]. *Seishin Shinkeigaku Zasshi, 98*(1), 11–26.

McDaid, D. (2008). *Countering the stigmatization and discrimination of people with mental health problems in Europe. Research paper produced for the European Commission Directorate-General for Employment, Social Affairs and Equal Opportunities.* Brussels, Belgium: European Commission. Retrieved from http://ec.europa.eu/health/ph_determinants/life_style/mental/docs/stigma_paper_en.pdf

McHugh, M. D., & Lake, E. T. (2010). Understanding clinical expertise: Nurse education, experience and the hospital context. *Research in Nursing Health, 33*(4), 276–287.

Milutinovic, D., Golubovic, B., Brkic, N., & Prokes, B. (2012). Professional stress and health among critical care nurses in Serbia. *Arhiv za Higijenu rada I toksikologiju, 63*(2), 171–180. doi:10.2478/10004-1254-63-2012-2140

Moneke, N., & Umeh, O. J. (2013). Factors influencing critical care nurses' perception of their overall job satisfaction: An empirical study. *Journal of Nursing Administration, 43*(4), 201–207.

Morelius, E., Gustafsson, P. A., Ekberg, K., & Nelson, N. (2013). Neonatal intensive care and child psychiatry inpatient care: Do different working conditions influence stress levels? *Nursing Research and Practice.* doi:10.1155/2013/761213

Moultry Belcher, L. (2013), eHow contributor. *How negativity in the workplace can affect you personally.* Retrieved from http://www.ehow.com/info_8608474_negativity-workplace-can-affect- personally.html#ixzz27U4ANJCp

National Institute for Occupational Safety and Health. (2008). *Exposure to stress: Occupational hazards in hospitals.* Retrieved March 15, 2013, from http://www.cdc.gov/niosh/docs/2008- 136/pdfs/2008-136.pdf

National Quality Institute. (2007). *Mental health at work.* Retrieved from http://www.nqi.ca/assets/files/P-R-C/MHatW-Flyer-17Jul2012.pdf

Neville, K., & Cole, D. A. (2013). The relationships among health promotion behaviors, compassion fatigue, burnout, and compassion satisfaction in nurses practicing in a community medical center. *Journal of Nursing Administration, 43*(6), 348–354. doi:10.1097/NNA.0b013e3182942c23.

Ni, C., Hua, Y., Shao, P., Wallen, G. R., Xu, S., & Li, L. (2013). Continuing education among Chinese nurses: A general hospital-based study. *Nurse Education Today, 8*(6). doi:10.1016/j.nedt.2013.07.013

Portela, L. F., Rotenberg, L., & Waissmann, W. (2004). Self-reported health and sleep complaints among nursing personnel working under 12 h night and day shifts. *Chronobiology International, 21*(6), 859–870.

Prosci. (2013). *The harder side of change.* Retrieved July 16, 2013, from http://www.change-management.com/tutorial-what-why-how.htm

Read, E. A. (2013). Workplace social capital in nursing: An evolutionary concept analysis. *Journal of Advanced Nursing, 15.* doi:10.1111/jan.12251

Reiersen Thompson, W. (2004). *The Psych Central report: Employment and mental illness.* Retrieved from http://psychcentral.com/newsletter/issue001/employment.htm

Rodwell, J., & Martin, A. (2013). The importance of the supervisor for the mental health and work attitudes of Australian aged care nurses. *International Psychogeriatrics, 25*(3), 382–389. doi: 10.1017/S1041610212001883

Ruggiero, J. S. (2005). Health, work variables and job satisfaction among nurses. *Journal of Nursing Administration, 35*(5), 254–263.

Ruokolainen, M., Mauno, S., & Cheng, T. (2013). Are the most dedicated nurses more vulnerable to job insecurity? Age-specific analyses on family-related outcomes. *Journal of Nursing Management.* doi:10.1111/jonm.12064

Salpeter, M. (2013). *10 signs that you're a 'problem' employee.* Retrieved from http://jobs.aol.com/articles/2013/05/15/signs-problem-employee

Scott, E. (2010). *Best types and sources of social support.* Retrieved from http://stress.about.com/u/ua/readerresponses/sources_of_social_support.htm

Scott-Clarke, E. (2011). *Today's workplace is changing and more focus is being put on the psychological health of employees.* Retrieved from http://www.benefitscanada.com/benefits/health-wellness/will-mental-health-standards-improve- workplaces-18018

Shirey, M. R., McDaniel, A. M., Ebright, P. R., Fisher, M. L., & Doebbeling, B. N. (2010). Understanding nurse manager stress and work complexity: Factors that make a difference. *Journal of Nursing Administration, 40*(2), 82–91. doi:10.1097/NNA.0b013e3181cb9f88

Smith, M., Segal, R., & Segal, J. (2013). *Stress symptoms, signs and causes.* Retrieved from www.helpguide.org/mental/stress_signs.htm

Spence Laschinger, H. K., Leiter, M., Day, A., & Gilin, D. (2009). Workplace empowerment, incivility, and burnout: Impact on staff nurse recruitment and retention outcomes. *Journal of Nursing Management, 17*(3), 302–311. doi:10.1111/j.1365-2834.2009.00999.x

Sveinsdóttir, H., & Blöndal, K. (2013). Surgical nurses' intention to leave a workplace in Iceland: A questionnaire study. *Journal of Nursing Management, 5.* doi:10.1111/jonm.12013

Tangri, R. (2003). *Stress costs stress-cures.* Victoria, BC: Trafford.

The Health Communication Unit, University of Toronto. (2004). *An introduction to comprehensive workplace health promotion.* Retrieved from http://www.thcu.ca/workplace/documents/intro_to_workplace_health_promotion_v1.1.fi nal.pdf

Tillott, S., Walsh, K., & Moxham, L. (2013). Encouraging engagement at work to improve retention. *Nursing Management (Harrow), 19*(10), 27–31.

Tomey, A. M. (2009). *Guide to nursing management and leadership* (8th ed.). St. Louis, MO: Elsevier-Mosby.

Trinkoff, A., Geiger-Brown, J., Brady, B., Lipscomb, J., & Muntaner, C. (2006). How long and how much are nurses working? *The American Journal of Nursing, 106*(4), 60–71.

Tschudin, V., & Schmitz, C. (2003). The impact of conflict and war on international nursing and ethics. *Nursing Ethics, 10*(4), 354–367.

Ulas, T., Buyukhatipoglu, H., Kirhan, I., Dal, M. S., Eren, M. A., Hazar, A., Demir, M. E., et al. (2012).The effect of day and night shifts on oxidative stress and anxiety symptoms of the nurses. *European Review for Medical and Pharmacological Sciences, 16*(5), 594–599.

Ulrich, C., O'Donnell, P., Taylor, C., Farrar, A., Danis, M., & Grady, C. (2007). Ethical climate, ethics stress, and the job satisfaction of nurses and social workers in the United States. *Social Science and Medicine, 65*(8), 1708–1719.

Van Bogaert, P., Wouters, K., Williems, R., Mondelaers, M., & Clarke, S. (2013). Work engagement supports nurse workforce stability and quality of care: Nursing team-level analysis in psychiatric hospitals. *Journal of Psychiatric and Mental Health Nursing, 20*(8), 679–686. doi:10.1111/jpm.12004

Violante, S., Benso, P. G., Gerbaudo, L., & Violante, B. (2009). Correlation between job satisfaction and stress factors, burn-out and psychosocial well-being among nurses working in different healthcare settings. *Giornale Italiano di Medicina del Lavoro ed Egonomia, 31*(1 Suppl A), A36–A44.

Walker, A., & Campbell, K. (2013). Work readiness of graduate nurses and the impact on job satisfaction, work engagement and intention to remain. *Nurse Education Today, 6917*(13). doi:10.1016/j.nedt.2013.05.008.

Wall, P. L. (2012). Posttraumatic stress disorder and traumatic brain injury in current military populations: A critical analysis. *Journal of the American Psychiatric Nurses' Association, 18*(5), 278–298. doi:10.1177/1078390312460578

Ward, L. (2011). Mental health nursing and stress: Maintaining balance. *International Journal of Mental Health Nursing, 20*(2), 77–85. doi:10.1111/j.1447-0349.2010.00715.x

Williams, D. B. (1996). Reward and recognition. *Nursing Case Management, 1*(5),199–200.

Williams, R. B. (2012). *The silent tsunami: Mental health in the workplace.* Retrieved April 1, 2013, from http://www.psychologytoday.com/blog/wired-success/201209/the-silent-tsunami-mental-health-in-the-workplace

Wolfe, M. (2013). *How negativity can affect employees.* Retrieved from http://www.ehow.com/info_8150602_negativity-can-affect-employees.html#ixzz27U3l8Nux

Wong, T. P. (2013). *Spirituality and meaning at work.* Retrieved from http://www.meaning.ca/archives/presidents_columns/pres_col_sep_2003_meaning-at- work.htm

World Health Organization. (2003). *Strengthening nursing and midwifery.* Retrieved from http://apps.who.int/gb/archive/pdf_files/WHA56/ea5619.pdf

World Health Organization. (2005). *Mental health policies and programmes in the workplace.* Retrieved from http://www.who.int/mental_health/policy/services/13_policies%20 programs%20in%20workplace_WEB_07.pdf?ua=1

World Health Organization. (2010). *Health impact of psychosocial hazards at work: An overview.* Retrieved from http://whqlibdoc.who.int/publications/2010/9789241500272_eng.pdf

World Health Organization. (2014a). *Mental health: Strengthening our response.* Retrieved from http://www.who.int/mediacentre/factsheets/fs220/en

World Health Organization. (2014b). *Stress at the workplace.* Retrieved from http://www.who. int/occupational_health/topics/stressatwp/en

Yamada, D. (2008). Workplace bullying and ethical leadership. *Journal of Values-Based Leadership, 1*(2), 49–62.

Yoder-Wise, P. S. (2011). *Leading and managing in nursing* (5th ed.). St. Louis, MO: Elsevier-Mosby.

Young, T. (2012). *Everything starts with attitude.* Retrieved from http://www.salestrainingplus. com/sales-marketing-information/sales-and-marketing-articles/57-everything-starts-with-attitude

3

The Perfect Storm

It's not the stress that kills us; it's our reaction to it.
—Hans Selye

LEARNING OBJECTIVES

By the end of this chapter, the learner will be able to:

1. Identify the elements of what creates a storm for the nurse at a personal and professional level.
2. Discuss what contributes to the development of a nurse leader's storm.
3. Discuss the impact on the organization as a result of nurses who are stressed.
4. Identify and discuss some of the core financial costs created as a result of nurses' mental health being jeopardized.
5. Highlight some of the physiological impacts of stress on the nurse as a person.

This chapter seeks to take you on a journey to illustrate why mental health in the workplace is a critical issue for nurses. On that journey, you will quickly come to realize that the Swiss cheese philosophy can apply to you as a person, you as a nursing professional, and you as a manager/leader, as well as your employing organization. Given all that nurses are responsible for, the acuity of their job, the legislation and environment under which they practice, and their own personal life endeavours, the holes in the Swiss cheese can indeed line up, and what can result is a perfect storm. The impact of poor workplace mental health is phenomenal and has far-reaching effects. Poor workplace mental health comes with a hefty price tag, not just for the organization that is providing the employment, but for the nurse as a person and human being and the nurse as a practicing professional as well. After having discussed the major contributing factors that can impact a nurse's workplace mental health in Chapter 2, we now endeavor to see exactly what damage can occur.

In the context of one's personal life and virtues, one's professional obligations, and organizational expectations, we investigate the numerous costs created when one's workplace mental health becomes jeopardized. When it comes to mental health, this perfect storm is brewing for each nurse as a person and a practicing professional, and for the health care organization. But let's not get discouraged, as we will later identify proactive and reactive measures that can be taken to prevent or address such stormy costs. The beauty of studying the topic of workplace mental health is that being aware of and recognizing the potential sources and outcomes of mental health is half the battle of overcoming any threats to one's mental health. And this is just the intention here—to at least recognize these costs.

In survey after survey, people are feeling more and more that their working environment is not psychologically safe (Williams, 2012). Nurses in particular are no exception. Research shows that a significant percentage of employees say they have coped with a mental disorder such as substance abuse, schizophrenia, depression, burnout, or addictions; the prevalence rate was as high as 44% in some cases (Williams, 2012). However, in spite of these costs, it is encouraging to see that some countries are making headway to address this growing concern. The Mental Health Commission of Canada, for example, recently become the first such commission in the world to release a workplace psychological standard calling for the presence of mentally healthy workplaces for all (Williams, 2012). As Sherman (2013) quotes Harvard University professor Dr. Amy Edmondson, "Psychological safety describes the individuals' perceptions about the consequences of interpersonal risk in their work environment. It consists of taken-for-granted beliefs about how others will respond when one puts oneself on the line, such as by asking a question, seeking feedback, reporting a mistake, or proposing a new idea. One weighs each potential action against a particular interpersonal climate, as in, 'If I do this here, will I be hurt, embarrassed or criticized?' An action that might be unthinkable in one work group can be readily taken in another, due to different beliefs about probable interpersonal consequences."

THE PERSONAL STORM

Most individuals enter the caring profession of nursing for various reasons; however, there is often much overlap in these reasons. Many often manifest a desire or compassion to help others. For various reasons, nurses seem to have an astute nurturance trait that they can use to identify with the suffering or the less fortunate. As a result, they often move their lives forward with an empathetic desire to help them overcome adversity or limitations of life. Nurses are also able to feed off the caring that they provide; they reap great self-satisfaction and rewards for the caring and altruistic work they do for others. The opportunity to help change lives and help others is often the motivation and drive behind wanting to become a nurse. As nursing was once a position filled by women only, it is anticipated that the maternal nurturing instinct played a pivotal role in the development of nurses and the roles that nurses were expected to perform (Donahue, 1996). A woman's own values, morals, ethics, and beliefs are often paralleled with those expected of a nurse. These same values, morals, ethics, and beliefs are often what characterizes the nurse who is perhaps also a mother, wife, sister, and daughter.

As much as individuals enter the nursing profession with hopes and wishes of doing good for others, all can become shattered once their own mental health becomes compromised. From an array of factors such as a nurse's coping skills, mental health, self-concept, work ethic, job satisfaction, pride, philosophy, supports, life experiences, and history, the potential for a perfect storm is stirring. So let's now explore the significance that workplace mental health has on the nurse as a person.

As a person as well, each nurse has his or her own response to stress and coping mechanisms that is used to survive troublesome and stressful ordeals in life. The health care organization for which nurses work is basically the bread and butter that support their livelihood, but it doesn't come without a price of its own. These pressures add to the already personal issues and professional expectations that go with being a nurse. No two individuals respond to stressful events in the exact same way. In Chapter 1, we saw how stress can physiologically impact the body and mind and predispose them to the development of physical and mental illnesses.

Given the intrinsic values and drives of most nurses, the addition of work as a source of negative stress can wreak havoc for the nurse as a person. The development and existence of a work environment that tests one's own mental health can not only predispose one to the development of a mental illness but also challenge one's already stretched coping resources. However, the potential for a perfect storm doesn't stop here.

The presence of negativity in the workplace creates stress for the nurse as a person. At times, it almost feels as though work is becoming a burden because of "other people's bad attitudes or because you know that you might be verbally or professionally attacked on any given day." This kind of stress can manifest physically with depression, increased fatigue, weight gain or loss, and a general lack of interest in your job (Moultry Belcher, 2013).

Nurses do not perform well at taking care of themselves (Nahm, Warren, Zhu, An, & Brown, 2012). They found that 72.2% of nurses lacked exercise and had an average body mass index (BMI) of 28.3; in addition, 53.8% had irregular meal patterns and 59.2% were either overweight or obese. The greater the perceived stress, the more irregular meal schedules and eating patterns became.

To best respond to stress, a nurse's self-care behaviors are critical to consider. Nurses know what it is they need to do to stay healthy; however, this knowledge does not translate well into their own daily self-care. This is particularly concerning in light of the fact that the population of nurses is one of the greatest aging workforces today.

For the nurse as a person, much damage can be created as a result of poor workplace mental health. Both physical and mental disorders can infectiously occur. Every aspect of the nurse's self-concept begins to fade; the self-esteem, self-value, and self-confidence that previously helped to define this nurse as a person all begin to slip away in both presence and strength. Nurses may begin to question themselves, their motives, their behaviors, their actions, and even their choice of words, regardless of the setting in which they find themselves. The threat to the nurse's own mental health and well-being is outstanding. The nurse begins to feel unappreciated, as a failure, and no longer as a valuable contributing member of society. When the stressfulness of various events accumulate, the nurse begins to feel overwhelmed, not sure where to turn or what to do next. Thoughts of self-doubt linger, feelings of hopelessness and helplessness set in, and stress levels skyrocket. Every aspect of the nurse's self-concept, self-worth, self-value, and self-esteem begins to erode, just as an ocean erodes the shoreline and the esthetic beauty it represents. As the cognitive processes of memory loss, confusion, and poor concentration grow, mental disorders such as anxiety disorders, mood disorders, and even psychological disturbances and somatoform disorders take root. Finally, one's altered mental health can precipitate physical health concerns and illnesses as well. In the absence of adequate coping resources and social supports and the presence of persistent and varied stressors, the seed is now set. The development of a mental illness for the nurse is perhaps the second most terrible outcome that can occur as a result of poor workplace mental health.

Physical

In Chapter 1, we got a close and personal view of the impact that stress can have on us as human beings. When you experience levels of bad and ugly stress that is repeated, consistent, and chronic in nature, your threshold of defenses and body functions become compromised. These health concerns focus primarily on our physical health—our cardiac and cardiovascular health, immunity, and gastrointestinal health. In other words, stress levels that cannot be returned to normal can result in heart disease (Scott, 2010; The Health Communication Unit, University of Toronto, 2004); hypertension and cardiovascular problems (National Institute for Occupational Safety and Health [NIOSH], 2008; The Health Communication Unit, University of Toronto, 2004); increased infections, particularly the common cold (Scott, 2010); autoimmune diseases (Scott, 2010); impaired gastrointestinal function (Geiger-Brown & Lipscomb, 2010; Johnson, 2012; NIOSH, 2008; The Health Communication Unit, University of Toronto, 2004); weight gain or loss (Moultry Belcher, 2013); and musculoskeletal problems (Geiger-Brown & Lipscomb, 2010; The Health Communication Unit, University of Toronto, 2004). Scott (2010) adds that when the stress is chronic, the concern is biggest. Other worries for concern for one's physical health as a result of chronic stress are obesity (Johnson, 2012), pain (Johnson, 2012), increased fatigue (Moultry Belcher, 2013), headaches (NIOSH, 2008), and sleep difficulties (NIOSH, 2008). This constellation of symptoms is what later became known as metabolic syndrome, in which the increased risk for the combination of high blood pressure, insulin resistance, and central obesity (excessive abdominal fat) has been linked to increased levels of cortisol in the bloodstream. Researchers have found that "greater levels of job stress increased people's chances of developing metabolic syndrome; the higher the stress level, the greater the chance of developing metabolic syndrome" (Scott, 2010).

Social

Successful social relations always help to control and buffer the stress we experience in life. However, the social relationships that people build, or should I say the lack thereof, are another fallout for how we face stress that can jeopardize our mental health. Experiencing stress and mental health concerns for prolonged periods of time can actually cause us to distance ourselves from some of our friends. We are spending so much of our time absorbed and worried about what is happening in our lives that our perceptions become significantly narrowed, and we cannot see the larger picture of how our friends can actually help us during these difficult, mentally challenging times. As suggested by Davis, Lind, and Sorensen (2013), nurses who rely on supportive social networks as a coping mechanism have lower levels of depersonalization.

Unequivocally, a lack of social support exacerbates our perception of stress and the onset of mental health concerns even more and is often positively correlated with emotional exhaustion, burnout, and depersonalization (Davis et al., 2013). One's stressed mental health can also result in work–family conflict (Geiger-Brown & Lipscomb, 2010).

Psychological/Mental

We would be remiss if we did not highlight here the impact that poor workplace mental health and unresolved stress have on our mental health. Just as we discussed in Chapter 2, there are many sources of stress of personal, professional, and organizational origin that can elevate our increased disposition to the development of mental health concerns. The impact that our poor and nonconducive workplaces has on our mental health is phenomenal and the very impetus for writing this book. High rates of stress are negatively correlated with low mental health; as stress levels increase, mental health decreases (Scott, 2010; The Health Communication Unit, University of Toronto, 2004). When we experience high and repeated levels of chronic stress, our self-concept can often change—that is, how we think about ourselves and how we fit into society, work, and other roles. Closely related to self-concept are our self-value and our self-esteem, which are crucial elements for how we view ourselves and how we feel others may view us.

Workplace mental health guru Shain suggests poor mental health can "result in a psychologically unsafe workplace possibly in the form of debilitating anxiety, depression, and burnout or even cardiovascular disease, higher consumption of alcohol and susceptibility to infectious diseases" (Williams, 2012). Stress affects nurses personally. It not only precipitates various mental disorders, such as different levels of anxiety and depression, but also generates fatigue (Kawano, 2008). Park (2005) adds that failure to manage change in the workplace "heightens stress, harassment and conflict" as it increases workers' vulnerability as a fertile target of bullying and violence (Johnson, 2012). Furthermore, nurses can suffer from emotional exhaustion (Canadian Mental Health Association [CMHA] Ontario, 2010a; Scott, 2010; Violante, Benso, Gerbaudo, & Violante, 2009), depersonalization (20%) (Violante et al., 2009), lack of interest in one's job (Moultry Belcher, 2013), irritability (NIOSH, 2008), and low levels of perceived personal accomplishment (43%; Violante et al., 2009).

The onset of depression for those experiencing prolonged levels of stress is a common occurrence (CMHA Ontario, 2010a; Johnson, 2012; Moultry Belcher, 2013; NIOSH, 2008; Scott, 2010), particularly when it is left unresolved (Johnson, 2012).

Mental health concerns can also develop from increased stress levels and result in illnesses such as anxiety (CMHA Ontario, 2010a), addictions (as will be discussed in Chapter 9), or psychosomatic disorders (CMHA Ontario, 2010a; Scott, 2010). If you recall from Chapter 1, we spoke about how stress ages and shrinks the brain; therefore, it of no surprise to us to hear that altered brain processes such as cognitive processing and memory difficulties can occur (Johnson, 2012).

An acute traumatic event can even cause posttraumatic stress disorder (PTSD) among nurses. However, it is important to recognize that not every traumatized person develops full-blown or even minor PTSD (NIOSH, 2008).

As a result of poor workplace mental health, tension and stress can disturb one's concentration (Cram & MacWilliams, 2014). Up to 80% find it difficult to concentrate as a result of stress and tension in the work environment (Advisory, Conciliation, and Arbitration Service, 2013).

Suicide

The very worst outcome that can occur as a result of a mentally unhealthy workplace, other than the development of a mental disorder, is of course suicide. Suicide is the ultimate damage that a workplace with poor mental health can create because it is irreversible.

A recent event that became globally well-known concerned the royal family, when Kate Middleton was pregnant and hospitalized and a radio show host tricked a nurse into giving him an update of Ms. Middleton's health status. This occurred in the spring of 2012. Jacintha Saldanha, 46 years old and mother of two, was on reception duty at the London hospital where the duchess was being treated when presenters Mel Greig and Michael Christian rang and pretended to be Queen Elizabeth and Prince Charles asking for a condition report (Smyth, 2013). Anxious, already dealing with a previously diagnosed depression, and distraught over the idea that she had wrongfully disclosed personal information about the Duchess of Cambridge, this nurse felt she had no other option but to take her own life.

While suicide rates among middle-aged nurses of the United States have declined in recent years (Anderson, Kochanek, & Murphy, 1995), the suicide rate among middle-aged female nurses has increased (Hawton & Vislisel, 1999). As found by Feskanich et al. (2002), a severe level of stress at home or at work was associated with an increased risk for suicide in female nurses. Forty-four percent of the women reported the same stress level at home and at work. Incidence rates for suicide were highest among those who reported severe (24.8 per 100,000) or minimal (13.3 per 100,000) levels of stress both at home and at work, with increased risks in the minimal and severe categories for both home and work stress. Even after adjusting for smoking, coffee consumption, alcohol intake, and marital status, risks remained high. This increase is believed to result from increased occupational stress levels and easier access to drugs. They further suspect that "the increased risk of suicide among the women who reported minimal stress at home or at work may reflect denial or it may be associated with other risks for suicide, such as social isolation and depression" (Feskanich et al., 2002). In a literature review by Hawton and Vislisel (1999), it was found that "there is evidence from several countries that female nurses are at increased risk of suicide." While there is very little information as to what are the specific causes, smoking and caffeine consumption are significantly related risk factors.

THE NURSE'S PROFESSIONAL STORM

Nurses are among the small number of professionals who are at increased risk for being vulnerable to the many different stressors they encounter daily. In many of the directions they turn, there is death, sickness, suffering, and pain. They deal with all of these saddening issues on a daily basis. They work in very emotionally charged positions where the caring and competencies they provide help generate wellness and recovery. However, this does not always occur, with a patient's deteriorating health status making a nurse's efforts to help the patient become well or better sometimes seem futile. Nurses at all ages and levels of experience come to understand that sometimes there are worse things for their patients than dying.

Nursing is one profession that is posited to experience a perfect storm, meaning that nurses often experience all the critical components to drain them physically, mentally, socially, spiritually, and emotionally of the energy needed to sustain their efforts and move them forward altruistically and competently to help others. Translated, the demands placed on nurses by their patients, colleagues, professional associations/unions, employing organization, government, and environment, accompanied by the demands they place on themselves, make for a possible tsunami of poor mental health in the workplace. Identifying and being aware of these issues will assist in the later development of strategies to help address and prevent the advent of the perfect storm.

For the nurse as a practicing professional, the impact of poor mental health at work remains phenomenal. All of the costs that impacted the nurse as a person now trickle into the realm of the nursing profession as well, only now the costs come to include the patients to whom the nurse is assigned and the nursing profession's status that currently exists. At the professional level, practicing nurses begin to experience such outcomes that their work ethic, levels of work satisfaction, pride, and even career trajectory becomes challenged. Similarly, from a clinical patient perspective, nurses begin to exhibit concerning behaviors such as poor clinical judgment, errors relating to medication and procedure, and an increase in questionable competent practice. The occurrence of many stressors can reach into the depths of professional practice. As on any other individuals, the impact of stress on nurses, as working professionals, is substantial at the least.

Compassion Fatigue

Nursing is a very giving and caring profession. Nurses, however, try to be everything to everyone and so can drain their own energies and resources quickly. Unfortunately, some nurses can also suffer from compassion fatigue. The occurrence of compassion fatigue further begins to play on the vulnerabilities of one's mental processes. Nursing is not as easy a job as many may think. However, nurses tend to endure more ingrained consequences of stress merely from the role they play in society with their caring, altruistic, and nurturing sense of self.

"Compassion fatigue is the combination of secondary traumatic stress and burnout experienced by helping professionals and other care providers" (Figley, 1995; Stamm, 1995). Its prevalence among nurses ranges from 16% to 39%, with burnout ranging from 8% to 38% (Hooper, Craig, Janvrin, Wetsel, & Reimels, 2010; Potter et al., 2010; Robins, Meltzer, & Zelikovsky, 2009; Yoder, 2010). Burnout, or cumulative stress, is the state of physical, emotional, and mental exhaustion caused by the depletion of a person's ability to cope with his or her environment (Maslach, 1982). In health care professionals, burnout is associated with increased turnover, employee absenteeism, poor coworker support, depersonalization, decreased performance, decreased patient satisfaction, and difficulty in recruiting and retaining staff (Garman, Corrigan, & Morris, 2002; Sundin, Hochwalder, & Lisspers, 2011; Vahey, Aiken, Sloane, Clarke, & Vargas, 2004).

Secondary traumatic stress has been defined as "the stress resulting from helping or wanting to help a traumatized or suffering person" (Figley, 1999, p. 10). Secondary traumatic stress is the trauma health care professionals experience as they provide care for others, and it correlates highly with burnout (Vahey et al., 2004; Yoder, 2010). The presence of secondary traumatic stress has been reported in forensic nurses and nurses who work in emergency departments, oncology, pediatrics, and hospice (Beck, 2011).

Compassion fatigue is a prevalent condition among health care providers. The development of resiliency to compassion fatigue may improve decision making, clarity of communication, and patient and nurse satisfaction (Potter et al., 2013).

Secondary traumatic stress arises from repeated exposure to traumatic events, as is the case in the ongoing care of patients with cancer. A caregiver's empathy level with traumatized individuals is hypothesized to play a significant role in the transmission of traumatic stress from patient to nurse (Figley, 1995). The more empathic a nurse, the greater the risk for developing compassion fatigue.

The typical nurse experiencing compassion fatigue often is nervous, cynical, and pessimistic; has low self-esteem; is angry toward coworkers; and dreads work. The stress of compassion fatigue is not restricted to work. At home, an affected nurse may be unable to sleep, have bad dreams, lose interest in social events or sexual activity, and experience changes in appetite (e.g., weight loss, weight gain) and relations with others (Potter et al., 2013). Health effects include potential mental and physical health issues and increased use of alcohol or drugs (Stamm, 2002). Nurses who have compassion fatigue may experience changes in job performance, negative effects in personal relationships, increased mistakes, noticeable personality changes, decline in health, and a desire to leave the profession or their specialty (Perry, Toffner, Merrick, & Dalton, 2011; Schwam, 1998). Compassion fatigue has significant implications for hospitals' efforts to maintain a competent and caring nursing staff, which is associated with patient satisfaction with nursing care and is a predictor of patients' overall satisfaction with hospital care (Vahey et al., 2004; Wolf, Colahan, & Costello, 1998).

Maiden, Georges, and Connelly (2011) reported that compassion fatigue correlated with nurses disagreeing with their institution's definition of medication error and fear as reasons for not reporting medication errors. The extent to which compassion fatigue affects clinical decision making and nurse judgment is yet to be thoroughly researched. Compassion fatigue can go beyond the impact on the well-being of individual nurses and can also impact larger organizational issues, such as staff turnover and patient satisfaction (Potter et al., 2013).

Job Burnout

Job burnout has become a global problem (Scott, 2010). Members of caring professions, such as nursing, are especially prone to burnout (Geiger-Brown & Lipscomb, 2010; Wright & Sayre-Adams, 2012). According to Smith, Segal, and Segal (2013), "job burnout is a state of physical, emotional and mental exhaustion caused by long-term exposure to demanding work situations. Burnout is the cumulative result of stress and can be hazardous to your health. Anyone can experience job burnout. However, professions with high job demands and few supports can increase the prevalence of burnout and reduce engagement. Helping professions, such as jobs in health care, teaching or counseling, often have high rates of burnout." Nursing has come to be known as a profession very demanding of one's physical and mental capacities and abilities, and job burnout is a well-recognized factor that impairs one's professional performance, judgment, and practice. As found by Mark and Smith (2012), increasing job demands are associated with higher levels of mental health problems such as anxiety and depression.

Job burnout is symbolized by three main characteristics (Smith et al., 2013):

1. Exhaustion (i.e., the depletion or draining of mental resources)
2. Cynicism (i.e., indifference or a distant attitude towards one's job)
3. Lack of professional efficacy (i.e., the tendency to evaluate one's work performance negatively, resulting in feelings of insufficiency and poor job-related self-esteem)

Burnout can stem from many and different negative conditions at work, most of which are also direct causes of stress and the eventual development of anxiety and other mood disorders. Many or some combination of the stressors identified in Chapter 2 can predispose one to the development of burnout and hence mental health concerns.

To set the record straight, just because burnout can occur among nurses does not mean you as a nurse will develop it. There are various factors that can predispose an individual to an increased risk for developing burnout. However, because burnout can sneak up on you unexpectedly, it is good to spot the cues before it goes too far. These cues are as follows (Mayo Clinic, 2013):

1. You literally dread Mondays (if you are an 8 to 4 worker) or the beginning of your series of shifts. You are using up a lot of energy worrying about this day.
2. You just cannot seem to get the energy or motivation to engage in some sort of social activity.
3. You often have a drink or two after you get home from work and fall asleep in front of the television.
4. You feel as if you are getting in a rut, all days begin to look alike, there is too much work to do in so little time, and you don't feel appreciated for what work you do.
5. You have become cynical, critical, impatient, and irritable.
6. You feel disillusioned and dissatisfied with your job.

If you're experiencing more than a few of these signs, it may be time to take a break, seek out support and career counselling, or talk to your manager about making some changes to your job. Seeking medical advice from your doctor or someone from the employee assistance program in your organization is highly encouraged. Because of the nature of burnout and the fact that it is often job-related and intense, it is best to recognize the warning signs before they occur.

Breach of Professional Nursing Standards of Practice or Nurse Practice Act

Nursing standards of practice are developed and designed as a guide for nurses on the knowledge, skills, judgment, and attitudes they need to provide quality, safe, and competent care to patients. They represent the rules of competent care and the benchmark of excellence and reflect the minimal level of care that should be provided to patients. The primary purpose of standards is to identify for nurses the public, government, and other stakeholders the desired and achievable level of performance expected of nurses in their practice, against which actual performance can be measured (College of Nurses of Ontario [CNO], 2002). The standards further act to promote, guide, and direct a nurse's professional practice, and failure to adhere to them will result in possible disciplinary action. Standards of practice in any profession are often developed at a higher political level of the nurses' governing body, association, or college and apply to all nurses within a province, state, county, or country, regardless of the practice setting in which they are employed.

The American Nurses Association (ANA) standards "are comprised of standards of care and standards of professional practice. The standards of care are based on the nursing process and describe a competent level of nursing care. Standards of professional performance cover quality of care, performance appraisal, education, collegiality, ethics, collaboration, research, and resource utilization" (Learning Express Editors, 2010). Regardless of the standards involved or how they are worded, prudently following the standards is something expected of all nurses, and any violation of the standards can be just cause for possible disciplinary action against the nurse. Having set the foundation, it should be easy to see now why the very presence of the standards can be stressful for nurses, and there are many legal and liability issues that can breach these standards of nursing practice.

The value of nursing standards and the importance of the expectation that they will be followed have been emphasized over and over again. However, when a nurse is stressed to the point that mental health and thought processes become compromised, standards of nursing practice can be violated. When nursing standards of practice are breached, patient care, quality, and safety become jeopardized, and any form of disciplinary action can occur, such as license suspension, adding yet another significant stressor.

Professional Misconduct

Yet another outcome closely linked to breaches of the standards of nursing practice that result from a nurse's response to a mentally unhealthy workplace is of professional misconduct. Nurse Practice Acts, Health Care Professions Acts, or whatever legislation exists in individual provinces and states help to guide nursing practice. Although these Nurse Practice Acts provide guidance and expectations of how a nurse is supposed to practice, it is still very much dependent on the nurse using his or her own clinical judgment as well to help determine what is and is not professional misconduct (CNO, 2002). Tasks that constitute a breach or abuse of the nurse–client relationship are considered professional misconduct and conduct that demonstrates a lack of integrity. In other words, a nurse's conduct that is harmful in any way, or that undermines or detracts from the professional caring relationship with and for the client, and is not consistent with expected professional standards defines professional misconduct (CNO, 2013). This act, which guides nursing practice and represents an important piece of legislation, can be quite stress-provoking for some. Nurses of all countries and states have a jurisdictional nursing practice act that should be followed, often referred to as a Nurse Practice Act. This act is legally binding in that it legally obligates all nurses to do what is best and most prudent to help ensure the delivery of safe, competent, and quality care to patients. Again, failure to do so can result in legal and disciplinary action against the nurse in question.

Professional misconduct in nursing comes in many different forms, incuding:

1. Failure to maintain the standards of practice: "Contravening a standard of practice of the profession or failing to meet the standard of practice of the profession."
2. Working while impaired: Actively providing care and intervention as a registered nurse while under the influence with impaired judgment as a result of using substances.
3. Abusive conduct: Any action or threat of action, verbal, physical, or emotional, from a nurse toward a client.
4. Theft: Misappropriation of property belonging to clients, visitors, or colleagues that results in a violation of trust by the nurse.
5. Failure to obtain informed consent and breach of confidentiality.
6. Failure to obtain client consent.
7. Breach of confidentiality: "Giving information about a client to a person other than the client or his or her authorized representative except with the consent of the client or his or her authorized representative or as required or allowed by law."
8. Failure to share information with a client: "Failing to reveal the exact nature of a secret remedy or treatment used by the member following a client's request to do so."
9. Inadequate documentation and record keeping.
10. Misrepresentation: "Inappropriately using a term, title, or designation in respect of the member's practice."
11. Failure to meet legal/professional obligations (contravention of statutory or College of Nurses of Ontario requirements): Nurses are committed to trust respect to help regulate the nursing profession and protect the public. Examples would include the following:
    a. Contravening a term, condition, or limitation on the member's Certificate of Registration.

    b. Contravening a provision of the Nursing Act, the Regulated Health Professions Act, or the regulations under either of those Acts.
12. Failure to comply with reporting obligations: "Failing to report an incident of unsafe practice or unethical conduct of a health care provider to the employer or other authority responsible for the health care provider or the College."
13. Conflict of interest: "Conflict of interest exists when a nurse's personal interests could improperly influence her/his professional judgment or conflict with her/his duty to act in the best interest of clients."
14. Inappropriate business practices if working as an independent business owner (e.g., fraud, excessive fee charges, etc.).
15. Disgraceful, dishonorable, and unprofessional conduct: "Engaging in conduct or performing an act relevant to the practice of nursing, that, having regard to all the circumstances, would reasonably be regarded by members as disgraceful, dishonourable or unprofessional."
16. Guilty of an offense: "An offence that is relevant to a nurse's suitability to practise nursing amounts to professional misconduct."
17. Finding of professional misconduct in another jurisdiction.
18. Sexual abuse: Sexual abuse of a client by a nurse.

Malpractice

Under the stressors of job demands, lack of control, stressed working relationships, and increasing workloads, one's thought processes, performance, and mental health can interfere and cause nurses to become victims of malpractice. Malpractice, often referred to as "professional negligence," is a more specific term that addresses a professional standard of care as well as the professional status of the caregiver and "any professional misconduct, unreasonable lack of skills or fidelity in professional or judiciary duties" (Wacker Guido, 2010, p. 93). To be liable for malpractice the "tortfeasor," or the person committing the wrong, must be a professional (p. 93). Malpractice is negligence as it pertains to a professional person. The only difference between malpractice and negligence is the status of the person committing the action or failing to act when legally required to do so (p. 94).

    This wrong or injudicious treatment results in injury, unnecessary suffering, or death to the injured party and proceeds from ignorance, carelessness, want of proper professional skills, disregard of established rules and principles, neglect, or a malicious or criminal intent (p. 93). In the case of a psychiatric/mental health nurse, the nurse has failed to act in a manner that was expected and in keeping with standards of practice, or failed to foresee the negative consequences that a professional person having the necessary skills and education should foresee (p. 93).

    There are six criteria needed to prove that malpractice has occurred. These include the following:

1. Injury is treatment-related or caused by a lack of or poor professional skill.
2. Expert evidence is required to determine whether the appropriate standard of care was breached.

3. The act or omission of an act involved an assessment of the client's condition.
4. The incident occurred in the context of the health care professional–client relationship or within the scope of activities the hospital is licensed to perform.
5. Injury occurred because the client sought treatment.
6. The act of omission was unintentional (p. 93).

Malpractice differs slightly from negligence. Negligence committed by a professional is malpractice, but not all malpractice is negligence. As highlighted above, *negligence* is defined as "failure to use such care as a reasonably prudent and careful person would use under similar circumstances" and *malpractice* as "improper or unethical conduct or unreasonable lack of skill by a holder of a professional or official position; often applied to physicians, dentists, lawyers, and public officers to denote negligent or unskillful performance of duties when professional skills are obligatory." The definition often further states, "Malpractice is a cause of action for which damages are allowed" (Stubenrauch, 2007).

When a nurse is assigned a patient, the nurse takes on the responsibility to provide for that person a high degree of care and due diligence. Fulfilling these responsibilities requires the nurse to follow the policies and procedures that define the basic standard of care as a professional. Unfortunately, nurses sometimes make errors, which can prove to be costly, if not fatal (Stubenrauch, 2007), such as the misuse of a medical product, failure to warn the doctor of changes in a client's condition, failure to properly assess vital signs, failure to monitor clients, chart documentation error, and medication errors.

Work Ethic

The area of the nurse's work ethic is concerning for the nurse, who is a practicing professional. When one's mental health becomes compromised as a result of stressors at work and elsewhere, the work ethic that was once characterized by vigor and ambition begins to dissipate. You no longer look forward to going to work, your energy level feels drained, and the altruistic motivation that once was is now beginning to fade. Furthermore, as a previously hard-working, eager, and dedicated nurse, you continue to see colleagues slacking off at work without any valid reason, so you too begin to slow down the pace and urgency. While other nurses stand around for prolonged periods of time gossiping and rumormongering, this begins to seem a more desirable and less energy-requiring task, so you too join in. This occurs particularly when workplace negativities predominate. Even if you are not participating, you may still have a compromised work ethic simply from taking the time to listen or from engaging in the negativity (Moultry Belcher, 2013).

Pride

A nurse's pride at work also begins to become compromised as a result of poor workplace mental health. The pride you once had in your job begins to dissipate. As the negativity of the organization begins to infiltrate the workplace environment, and workers continually slam the organization for its negativity and loss of respect for the worker, you begin to lose that sense of pride that first brought you to this career and organization initially.

Whereas you might have enjoyed your job and your particular responsibilities in the past, you can now find yourself with a general lack of enjoyment for what you do because you are working in a negative environment. You may have excelled at certain aspects of your job, but if the people you work with are constantly downing the company or your results and work, then you will feel a decreased level of pride in your job (Moultry Belcher, 2013).

Job Dissatisfaction

One's level of work satisfaction also becomes impacted as a result of a poor mental health workplace environment. If getting up to go to work begins to become a burden rather than something you once looked forward to and enjoyed, you are probably not satisfied with your job situation. Job dissatisfaction is one substantial cost that can result from increased stressors being experienced in the workplace and elsewhere (NIOSH, 2008; Scott, 2010). Researchers have found that many nurses are dissatisfied with their jobs (Ruggiero, 2005; Smith et al., 2013), in some nursing samples as many as 30% (Violante et al., 2009). In helping professions, such as nursing, work dissatisfaction positively correlates with strained interpersonal relationships, excessive workload and poor leadership (Moneke & Umeh, 2013), workplace incivility (Andersson & Pearson, 1999), and aggression and violence at work (Hasketh et al., 2003). It therefore stands to reason that one's work satisfaction will also suffer because of poor workplace mental health.

Job demand and job control have both been linked to job satisfaction in nurses (Rodwell & Martin, 2013). Other stressors impacting significantly on nurses' lack job satisfaction include work–family conflict (Farquharson et al., 2012), poor pay (Ernst, Messmer, Franco, & Gonzalez, 2004), insufficient time to do nursing care (Ernst et al., 2004), and lack of confidence in one's ability (Ernst et al., 2004). However, those nurses who were more senior with more years of experience were less concerned about time demands, pay, and task requirements than were younger nurses" (Ernst et al., 2004). Even among nursing faculty, a multiple regression result indicated that job satisfaction was significantly influenced ($p < 0.01$) by the presence of a mentoring relationship, salary, tenure status, psychological empowerment, and job stress (Chung & Kowalski, 2012).

Ambitions and Dreams

From a practicing professional perspective, one's career trajectory and ambitions may change direction as a result of poor workplace mental health. After you have worked 20 years on the same nursing unit and witnessed workplace mental health and staff morale deteriorate to the point you don't feel you can tolerate it any further, there may come a time for a long and perhaps overdue change.

The negative environment within which you currently work can be what motivates you to seek a change in pace. For nurses with significant seniority or at the end of the career, the prospect of having to search for another job brings with it a certain degree of stress and uncertainty as well. Your dreams and aspirations of climbing the corporate ladder do not seem feasibly inviting or important any longer, halted by the agonizing and even toxic environment your place of employment has become. Changing careers at any time is fraught with mental health challenges of its own.

Even novice nurses experience a significant degree of stress as a result of entering clinical practice on their own for the first time (Maddelena, Kearney, & Adams, 2013). Mark and Smith (2012) add that extrinsic effort and overcommitment are often associated with higher levels of mental health problems, such as anxiety and depression. Now that we have seen how the nurse as a practicing professional can potentially suffer and incur mental health challenges because of the mentally unhealthy workplace, we will now turn our attention to the impact of a negative attitude.

The Fallout of a Negative Attitude

The health effects of a negative attitude are phenomenal. A negative attitude compromises not only your physical health but your mental health as well. In fact, many of the most common causes of sudden death in the United States (Young, 2012), Canada, and elsewhere are stress-related diseases, such as heart disease, cardiovascular disease, and cancer. Therefore, the negative emotions of fear and anxiety not only paralyze our bodies and motivate us to "use hurtful and dangerous behaviors" (Williams, 2007) but also precipitate the development of physical disease and illness. Williams explains that this increased susceptibility to illnesses develops as a result of a negative attitude and other bad mental habits, which occur when we "fail to discipline our minds." The body's response to stress, which may be one of fear, anxiety, worry, and anger, produces increased levels of circulating catecholamines such as adrenalin (as we pointed out in Chapter 1), alters the body's chemistry, rapidly uses up available nutrients, and therefore weakens our immune systems, thus making the human body vulnerable to the development of disease and illness (Williams, 2007). Because the body cannot differentiate between true emergency situations and everyday sources of stress, the same stress response will occur. Therefore, in the presence of a negative attitude that occurs on a regular basis, the body repeatedly experiences the stress response, which continues to pump unhealthy amounts of adrenalin into our bodies every day. The bottom line message here is, "Don't let simple unimportant items bother you, it is best to invest your energies into positive and productive thoughts." This is a skill that can be learned, but you need to be persistent to achieve it. Williams suggests that we can control our attitude.

Just as your attitude can influence your workplace, so too can your workplace influence your attitude. As highlighted previously, we spend roughly 30% of our life working; this is a significant amount of time to allow the events and atmosphere of a workplace to mold and add to the development of our attitudes, whether they be good or bad. Although you are able to control your own attitude and are free to pick and choose how it develops, sometimes external influences, such as those experienced at work, can exert insidious effects. For example, you work on a neurosurgery unit, and every day when you go to work, you are faced with colleagues from all disciplines who are typically ignorant, disrespectful, and just downright nasty to one another. You remain a neutral participant who focuses only on doing what it is you have to do to get the job done and your patients cared for. A workplace atmosphere such as this is definitely not a healthy one. Although many people suggest that what happens at work stays at work, this is actually a myth (Johnson, 2012).

"Imagine going to work daily with people who are rude and disrespectful. Even though people believe what is done at work stays at work, that is not true. Work carries over into the private lives of employees, and negative attitudes can lead to a negative effect not only on the company but also on the employee as well" (Johnson, 2012). A negative work attitude can actually cost an employee his or her job. Most employers terminate and let go employees who do not have team spirit because that lack of unity can become a pattern for other employees (Johnson, 2012).

Whether your bad attitude created a snowball effect to compromise your own mental health or the toxic workplace environment negatively impacted your attitude, it remains a professional cost for you. Either way, you struggle internally to say focused, confident, and aware to ride out the storm.

THE LEADER'S STORM

As a nurse leader, you can be in the midst of stormy waters trying to keep good morale on your unit, satisfied and engaged nurses, and quality patient care while also trying to meet organizational expectations, values, missions, and strategic goals. These numerous responsibilities and accountabilities can insidiously create for you a storm all its own.

Complacency

Over time, compliance and poor work ethic turn into uncaring complacency as employees see no purpose to their efforts. In this stage, they come to work and go through the motions just to collect a paycheck every week. As trust is a critical part of being committed to an organization and a job, it is important that employees trust one another. Trust in the other employees and performing work that matters are the two things that must be accomplished to gain employees who are committed to the cause. In the absence of trust, there is high turnover of staff, increased numbers of employee problems, poor teamwork and cooperation, higher operating and labor costs, lower levels of customer satisfaction, and decreased ability to attract and retain the best and brightest talent available.

According to human resources expert Bob McKenzie (2014), when complacency at work occurs, "the human mind that wants to be urgent, becomes urgent about the rules of what CANNOT be done." In other words, the employee decides when and what she or he will be urgent in addressing. The "human mind thinks: I can't, so I'll be urgent about NOT doing," and this occurs in two forms: complacency and false urgency. With complacency, individuals rationalize that they cannot complete the tasks required of them. These people are very passive and do little or nothing to improve themselves and develop and have themselves convinced that they just cannot do what is being asked of them (McKenzie, 2014). If you are a patient, the mere thought of your nurse being complacent should sound scary, not to mention it being poor professional practice.

False urgency, on the other hand, occurs when people act and look busy, but in fact they aren't. Even though they look busy, they are in fact fulfilling no valuable role or task. These individuals are very busy at trying to "look" busy. You may in fact perceive that your colleagues are too busy to help you because they are rushing around the unit, at an unusually quiet time for some unknown reason, so therefore you do not ask them to help you. Instead, you decide to take on an onerous task yourself and, yes, more added stress.

Poor Organization

As a result of poor workplace mental health, 57% find it harder to juggle multiple tasks (Advisory, Conciliation, and Arbitration Service, 2013). Kuan (2013) suggests that being organized is one of the greatest keys to a successful and rewarding career. She states that doing simple things like managing your time efficiently and effectively is vital to avoid disorganization. She adds that you need to become organized, and to do so you must stay on top of things and stop procrastinating. If not, you can and will easily become buried under the stress of everyday events. As nursing managers and leaders often deal with multiple ongoing issues and hassles throughout their workday, it is easy to comprehend how a manager's or leader's stress can culminate in a tidal wave for the perfect storm.

Staffing Difficulties

When tension is running high, workload is elevated, patients are acute and complex, and poor leadership exists, staffing problems of nurses on any unit are often commonplace. The lack of enough staff to adequately cover the unit is the most stressful event perceived by staff nurses (Alnems, Aboads, Al-Yousef, Al-Yateem, & Abotabar, 2005). According to the ANA (2014), "Registered nurses have long acknowledged and continue to emphasize that staffing issues are an ongoing concern, one that influences the safety of both the patient and the nurse. There is a strong relationship between adequate nurse-to-patient ratios and safe patient outcomes. Rising patient acuity and shortened hospital stays have contributed to challenges."

Poor Motivation

For the practicing nurse, a workplace that drains one's mental energies can also inadvertently reduce motivation (Cram & MacWilliams, 2014). As found by Dana (2001), "Over 65% of performance problems result from strained relationships between employees, not from deficits in [an] individual employee's skill or motivation." Furthermore, job satisfaction (Kath, Stickler, Ehrhart, & Schultze, 2013), intent to quit, and mental health symptoms were the most significant outcomes of stress (Kath et al., 2013). Autonomy, for example, moderated relationships between perceptions of stress and outcomes, with low autonomy showing greater negative outcomes when levels of stress were higher (Kath et al., 2013).

Low Morale

Morale can be the fuel that drives an organization forward or the fuel that feeds the fires of employee discontent, poor performance, and absenteeism (Vitt, 2014). When morale is low in health care settings, nurses are most often the professionals to feel the pinch. Nurses are present in the organization 24/7 and are most often on the front line when dealing with patients after other staff and physicians have left for the day. Low morale for nurses is a costly liability for many reasons. Low morale can result in increased levels of absenteeism, poor performance, complacent attitudes, and general discontent.

From a professional practice perspective, another cost associated with nurses' poor workplace mental health is that of decreased staff morale. If one nurse is feeling overwhelmed, frustrated, and discouraged, then in all likelihood other nurses may be feeling this way as well. Therefore, what occurs is a nursing unit that is just existing and doing only what it has to, to ensure safe and quality patient care, but even here, there are no guarantees.

Workplace Negativism

Workplace negativism can be not only a source of mental health strain but also a cost. A prevailing negative atmosphere where employees can feel demoralized, belittled, harassed, and demeaned at work can create serious adverse and unwanted effects. This is not just about whether people are able to get along with one another, smile, and be friendly; it is also about the lives of vulnerable patients who seek our help and an organization's bottom line. This insidious negativity can affect employees in a number of different ways inclusive of communication, productivity, consumer/patient relations, and recruitment and retention (Wolfe, 2013).

A negative and even hostile environment can significantly diminish *communication*. For example, nurses may be hesitant to speak for fear of ramifications, or because of strife and conflict they actively choose not to speak to each other. Poor communication infringes on critical, timely, and accurate information getting relayed through the proper channels. Work becomes less efficient and more difficult, and policies and procedures often take the backseat and are deemed as not important, thus creating a dangerous, poor-quality, and substandard basis of nursing (Wolfe, 2013).

Productivity also suffers when a negative atmosphere dominates the workplace. Because morale is often low, employees become less motivated, they lose interest and faith in the organization's mission and values, and they generally spend less time at work and not accomplishing tasks as well as they should (Wolfe, 2013). Furthermore, 62% often take longer to do tasks (Advisory, Conciliation, and Arbitration Service, 2013).

Patient and consumer relations also feel the pinch of a negative work environment. Nurses can choose to be less informative, less supportive, and less helpful toward patients and families when they are engulfed by a negative work atmosphere (Wolfe, 2013). This typically leads to increased patient complaints, increased legal suits, jeopardized patient health and life, increased risk for making mistakes, and increased negative media attention, and can even cause patients to turn away and seek a competitor's services.

Recruitment and retention also suffer because of a negative workplace atmosphere. Often, a reputation precedes itself, and at a time when nursing shortages are commonplace, a negative work environment can drive skilled employees away, make it difficult to recruit experts or necessary to spend a great deal of money and use up resources in efforts to recruit, hire, and orient that new employee into the workplace (Wolfe, 2013).

The Cost of Conflict

In Chapter 2, we learned a great deal about how conflict can be a significant source of stress and tension in the workplace, so much so as to negatively impact a nurse's mental health. The impact of conflict in the workplace can be devastating—to the individuals involved, to colleagues and teams, to clients, and to the business as a whole and the organization as a whole. "Unresolved conflict represents the largest reducible cost in many businesses, yet it remains largely unrecognized" (Dana, 1999). The number of employees seeking help for work-related conflict has increased from 23% in 1999 to close to 30% in 2001 (Warren Shepell, 2002). In one U.K. study, a 46% increase in conflict at work has been identified (Park, 2005). Some of the results of unresolved conflict in the workplace include the following (Center for Conflict Resolution International, 2013): stress, frustration, anxiety, loss of sleep, strained relationships, presenteeism, employee turnover, decreased productivity, increased patient complaints, absenteeism, sabotage of efforts, injury, accidents, and a rise in disability claims. Furthermore, in the presence of unresolved conflict, a team member's commitment to the team and the team mission can decrease, and team members are likely to leave the company or use valuable time searching for career alternatives (Barnes-Slater & Ford, 2002). Other consequences of increased conflict-related stresses include a greater incidence of substance abuse, heart problems, back problems, cancers, mental health problems, workplace injury, and interpersonal conflict (Health Canada, 2000).

As a result of poor workplace mental health, 37% of sufferers are more likely to get into conflict with colleagues (Advisory, Conciliation, and Arbitration Service, 2013). Unresolved conflict instills worry, fear, and trepidation among nurses, decreases patient satisfaction, and even compromises patient care quality and creates further conflict (Fink, 2007). Conflict among colleagues can have an indirect influence on the therapeutic nurse–client relationship. Poor relationships among members of the health care team negatively affect the delivery of care. For example, workplace bullying can erode a nurse's confidence and compromise her or his ability to foster therapeutic relationships with clients. Conflict among colleagues can further lead to antagonistic and passive–aggressive behaviors (such as bullying and horizontal violence) that compromise the therapeutic nurse–client relationship and jeopardize every aspect of patient care. If not managed well, conflict can hinder a nurse's ability to provide quality client care and can escalate into violence and abuse (CNO, 2002).

Failure in Achieving Organizational Goals

Escalating levels of stress and nurses' mental illness can jeopardize the achievement of the operational and strategic goals of an organization. For a nurse manager in particular, whose key tasks are to serve as a decision maker; inspire staff; and engage, educate, execute, and evaluate actions, projects, and progress, the cumulative stressors that she or he may face at work can potentially interfere with the success of such goals.

Dysfunctional Team Dynamics

In an environment where teamwork is not just desired but required, it is critical for nurses to make teamwork a priority and help ensure that it remains functional at best. When teamwork becomes dysfunctional and one would prefer not to have to be part of a team to achieve patient care and organizational goals, the fallout can be detrimental for the nurse, the nurse leader, the patient, and the organization. For example, a lack of interest in critical teamwork and collegial relations can result in errors, poor clinical judgment, treatment delays, poor morale, increased work dissatisfaction, poor coordination of priorities and tasks, loss of motivation, standard and rule complacency, and loss of interest in the workplace (Dale Carnegie, 2013).

AN ORGANIZATION'S STORM

In the midst of the changing landscape of health care organizations, there is a potential for the perfect storm from many a perspective. This landscape and its accompanying paradigm shift have created a health care delivery system in most countries that sees a more educated patient population, an aging demographic, an aging workforce, an increased use of advanced technology, and many patients who require complex care. All of these factors together amount to one significant threat: enormous health care costs that seem to keep climbing with each fiscal year. How can any country be expected to sustain such exponential increases in its health care spending? Are we all not oblivious to the obvious? If health care spending continues to climb significantly, as we have witnessed thus far up to 2013, how will we be able to ensure the health and safety of our patients and our health care professionals, such that quality, competent care is delivered and received?

Within the larger health care organization, an even bigger perfect storm is brewing, that being the magnitude of an organizational storm. As the mental health of a workplace becomes altered and deteriorates, many organizational factors contribute to fueling this event, some of which may or may not be under the control of the organization itself. Unknown to many front-line nurses and other employees, organizations are often engaged in a regular balancing act to maintain the equilibrium of health and safety for all. Under the watchful eye of the accrediting bodies, their board of directors/ trustees, their chief sponsors and owners, and the public, they work within the confines of their available resources and fiscal restraints to ensure safe, quality, efficient, and competent patient care and an occupationally safe and healthy work environment for their employees. However, given the significant costs to organizations that poor mental health can produce, it would be most prudent for them to work to bring these concerns within their span of control. It is the purpose of this section to highlight the various costs an organization can incur as a result of a mentally unhealthy work environment.

Large hospitals and health care organizations are challenged daily to provide a healthy workplace environment. Many of today's health care organizations are quite large and even monstrous in size and geographical dispersion. However, the mere size of them poses a challenge to keep a pulse on every single aspect of function. Often, it is not until something goes wrong, such as an adverse event, that organizations realize there is trouble in the operational platform and then respond. In essence, an organization's response is usually reactive, not proactive.

Although health care organizations strategically aim to function optimally, efficiently, and effectively, the health and well-being of the employees do not often surface as a priority. What often occurs is that the health and welfare of the employees, such as nurses, become lost in the midst of other priorities, such as budget planning, quality assurance, and fiscal responsibilities. Nurses, for example, are the most abundant health care professionals who keep health care organizations afloat. They work 24/7, whereas most other health care professionals work the regular day shift from 8 a.m. to 4 p.m. The nurse is there every step of the way, during all hours of operation of the organization or hospital, and is often that "middle man" who relays information and initiates the reporting hierarchy to reach executive teams when things go wrong, no matter what time of the day, night, week, month, or year. As suggested by Williams (2012), "Maintaining a psychologically healthy workplace is cost-effective through higher employee commitment and motivation, reduced absenteeism, and reduced health care costs."

Regardless of the critical role that nurses play in health care organizations, the response of the organizations and the work environment in which they provide care can be fraught with issues that impact nurses' functionality and desire to optimize service and care delivery. These issues may or may not be within the control of the organization as a whole and may include organizational challenges from above, but in any event they still represent a key source of stress and pressure on nurses in their day-to-day professional activities.

Nurses are one key group of professionals who support the operational platform of health care organizations. As a health care organization works to address and meet its operational goals, fiscal responsibilities, and mandate for the people it serves, it is frequently challenged by external and internal sources. These external and internal sources that truly test the organization's ability to achieve its goals, mandates, and strategic directions often arise from societal, employee, and patient issues. Regardless of the sources, the organization attempts to meet its goals, mandates, and strategic directions, but in a manner that may impact the workplace environment of the nurse. Organizational issues tend to have a trickle-down effect. Once it arrives under the umbrella of nursing and how a nurse is expected to do his or her work with whatever resources are available, it is then in a place to potentially impact on the nurses' stress level and hence mental health. Therefore, whatever occurs at the organizational level and all the challenges faced at that level can impact significantly on the already bombarded and stressed nurse. In this respect, the very goal of an organization to promote safe and quality patient care has much potential to become jeopardized as a result of the many organizational pressures and expectations placed upon the nurses keeping the organization together.

Core Financial Costs

Around the world, poor mental health in the workplace is costing countries staggering billions of dollars each year. For example, in Australia in 2012, it came with the price tag of 6.5 billion dollars in business losses (Hamilton, 2013). A similar trend occurs in Canada as well, costing that country $33 billion annually (Mood Disorders Society of Canada, 2009).

Significant financial costs associated with job stress are continuously absorbed by the U.S. economy. Health care expenditures have increased nearly 50% for workers who perceive their jobs as stressful and nearly 200% for those who report high levels of job stress and depression (Alves, 2005). According to national estimates, the total cost of job stress incurred by the U.S. economy ranges from $250 to $300 billion annually (Jones, Tanigawa, & Weisse, 2003).

In Canada, 82% of organizations rank mental health conditions as one of their top three causes of short-term disability and 72% as top three causes of long-term disability. It was estimated that up to $51 billion annually in Canada could be saved if mental health problems could be prevented. A Wilson Banwell study in 2008 stated, "Research strongly supports the need for employers to make workplace mental health a high priority business issue. It is not simply the right thing to do; it makes a company more competitive and profitable" (Williams, 2012).

According to a *USA Today* report, based on research by Harvard University Medical School, untreated mental illness costs the United States a minimum of $105 billion in lost productivity each year. Most organizations' health coverage plans show that physical ailments are covered, while mental health problems lag far behind. Serious mental illnesses cost society almost $200 billion in lost earnings per year (Williams, 2012). For an average company of 500 employees, untreated depression alone costs $1.4 million in lost work days and lost productivity per annum, and this does not include the costs related to bipolar disorder and anxiety disorders (Williams, 2012). Furthermore, mental health problems cost employers in the United Kingdom £30 billion a year through lost production, recruitment, and absence—so why aren't we doing more about it (Advisory, Conciliation, and Arbitration Service, 2013)?

Organizational Costs

The costs to a health care organization as the result of a workplace environment gone bad where nurses do not feel a sense of valued mental health are phenomenal. These costs manifest themselves in the form of recruitment and retention issues, decreased productivity, absenteeism, increased disability claims, increased injury and accidents, increased sick leave, strained relationships, presenteeism, increased liability, damaged reputations, increased grievances and litigation, sabotage of the organization's efforts, societal and family harm, increased incidence of bullying and violence, and increased incidence of employee loss and turnover. As identified here, there are many mitigating factors that can help define the organizational costs associated with poor workplace mental health.

Decreased Productivity

When an employee's mental health is maximally challenged as a result of a difficult workplace, productivity declines (Fink, 2007). This occurs particularly when morale is low and nurses are preoccupied with worry and stress, which results in low motivation, creativity, and inspiration and suboptimal levels of focus and concentration. Furthermore, nurses can lose faith in the mission and values of the organization and tend to spend fewer hours at work with less work getting done (Wolfe, 2013). Brun, Biron, Martel, and Ivers (2003) have found that while "3% of people are absent from work due to psychological disorders, 40% of those who remain at work show signs of heightened psychological stress, and are unable to work at full capacity." Those with depression in particular have been found to work at only 62% of their full capacity (Mood Disorders Society of Canada, 2009). Cornell University Professor Phyllis Gabriel states, "The burden of mental disorders on health and productivity throughout the world has long been profoundly underestimated. ... Mental health problems strongly influence employee performance, rates of illness, absenteeism, accidents and staff turnover" (Williams, 2012). Further, a simple loss of productivity of 25% (doing things other than work-related activities, such as discussing a dispute, playing computer games, finding reasons to get out of the area) reduces an average work week to fewer than 20 hours (Cram & McWilliams, 2009).

For managers and health care leaders as well, a great amount of time is lost attending to workplace mental health issues. Their attendance to conflict is one such example. Managers can spend as much as 30% (Thomas & Schmidt, 1976) to 42% (Watson & Hoffman, 1996) of their time addressing conflict in the workplace. Chief executive officers as well have spent "up to 70% of their time on conflict" (Taylor, 2003) and 20% on litigation-related activities (Levine, 1998).

A recent Gallup Organization poll found that "there are 22 million actively disengaged employees costing the American economy as much as $350 billion per year in lost productivity including absenteeism, illness, and other problems that result when employees are unhappy at work." (Fink, 2007).

In the absence of rewards or recognition for nurses, many negative ripple effects occur, all of which can be potentially damaging to the organization as a whole (me). What often occurs as a result is a decrease in nurse confidence, esteem, and value of self; a decreased sense of trust in the organization; retention and recruitment challenges; increased turnover of staff; increased risk for emotional exhaustion and burnout; and therefore an increased risk for the development of a mental illness and increased feelings of disrespect, demoralization, and discontent (Guarding Minds @ Work [GM@W], 2012).

When opportunities for involvement and influence are absent, both nurses and the organization suffer. Nurses can be left feeling voiceless, helpless, alienated, and indifferent to the organization. As a result, they feel frustrated, dissatisfied, discontent, cynical, and even critical or the organization's efforts (GM@W, 2012). Hence, nurses can become distressed and experience burnout as a result. On the other hand, the organization will typically experience increased staff turnover, decreased productivity, increased operational costs, and a missed valuable opportunity for it to do better by drawing on nurses' expertise, rich backgrounds, and seasoned experiences. Furthermore, low engagement can cause reduced productivity and a lower level of work quality, whereas high engagement can raise your productivity and quality levels and also help your business to attract and retain talented new members of staff (Culture Consultancy, 2013).

Absenteeism

Absenteeism is an age-old issue related to increasing organizational costs. Workers who have higher levels of job stress call in sick more often and so have a higher rate of absenteeism (Advisory, Conciliation, and Arbitration Service, 2013; Fink, 2007; NIOSH, 2008; Scott, 2010), particularly when those employees are nurses (Kawano,

2008). In a national study of 50,000 employees, it was found that "the greater the number of sources of stress reported in the social environment at work, the greater the likelihood of reporting more than 10 days off as a result of ill health" (Health Canada, 1998). Stressors of interpersonal relations, job control, and management practices, in particular, cause employees to be absent for 6 or more days (Health Canada, 1998) and a yearly total of 35 million workdays to be lost each year (Williams, 2012). Bullied employees, in particular, take on average 7 more sick leave days per year than do other employees (Knight, 2004).

The actual cost of employee absence alone can range from $1.7 billion (Warren Shepell, 2005) to $8.6 billion (Canadian dollars) in Canada (The Health Communication Unit, University of Toronto, 2004). Even though unscheduled absenteeism related to workplace stress and mental health concerns take billions of dollars off the bottom line for U.S. businesses, organizations have failed to make significant headway against the costs of workplace mental health (Fink, 2007). With climbing workplace expenses, only 31% of employers had plans to address mental health and mental illness in the workplace, 64% had no structured process for supervisors to support employees returning to work after any illness or disability, 84% had no process to address significant changes in employee productivity or behavior, and only 20% had any plans to address stigma associated with mental illness (Mood Disorders Society of Canada, 2009). Yet, employers could save billions in the form of $5,000 to $10,000 per employee per year for those receiving treatment in terms of average wage replacement, sick leave, and prescription drug costs alone (Mood Disorders Society of Canada, 2009). Even a positive workplace attitude can help lower absentee rates because employees are more likely to go to work when the working environment is positive. Among nurses, a multiple regression revealed that work–family conflict was identified as a significant predictor of absence due to sickness (Farquharson et al., 2012).

Disability Claims

The rising trend of disability claims and associated expenses also represents a significant portion of organizational costs as a result of poor workplace mental health. According to Corbitt Clark (2005), "job stress is a key driver of health care costs," which are 50% higher than those for those employees not experiencing high levels of stress.

"Depression and high stress were found to have the greatest impact on worker health care costs, increasing these costs more than obesity, smoking or high blood pressure," which in some cases were 46% higher for workers who felt they were under a lot of stress (The Health Communication Unit, University of Toronto, 2004). In one investigation, 56% of employers stated that the rising cost of mental health claims is a concern, as they account for 72% of short-term disability claims, 82% of long-term disability claims, and a 27% increase in long-term disability costs, with depression the fastest-growing category of claims for each of short-term, long-term, and permanent leave from work (Mood Disorders Society of Canada, 2009). Similarly, as found by Warren Shepell, "Workplace stress and work-related conflict are among the top eight reasons why employees request counseling assistance" (Warren Shepell, 2002).

In spite of these rising costs, only 28% of employers even track disability claims (Mood Disorders Society of Canada, 2009). Given acts such as harassment, "absenteeism, employee theft, sabotage, not to mention the cost of employee turnover (estimated to be as much as 75% to 150% of base salary), it is understandable why companies are beginning to pay attention" (Taylor, 2003). Mental illness seems to be the fastest-growing reason for short- and long-term disability claims, accounting for about 30% in Canada and costing business $6 billion in lost productivity and absenteeism in 2011, according to the Mental Health Commission. In its national strategy last May, the Mental Health Commission listed new health and safety standards among its key recommendations (Gordon, 2013).

Physical Injury and Accidents

When workplace stress and mental health concerns rise, so too does worry about increased risk for worker injury and accidents. There is increasing evidence that stress leads to errors and errors lead to accidents (Nguyen, Lieu, Bibbings, & Roger, 2002). As reported by the National Institute for Occupational Safety and Health (1992), "Psychosocial factors relating to the job and work environment play a role in the development of work-related musculoskeletal disorder of the upper extremity and back." Furthermore, when the physical environment of an organization is lacking safety, it can result in a more dangerous workplace and hence employees feeling less engaged and secure (GM@W, 2012).

Damaged Reputation

An organization has a lot more than just money on the line when it comes to failure to provide a psychologically safe workplace. Its reputation can become tarnished as a result. A hospital or health care organization that fails to look after its nurses, create a positive work culture, and address poor patient care issues is one that most people will try to avoid. When employee mental health suffers, effects trickle down to impact patient care and safety, and the reputation of the organization is at risk for being damaged or destroyed. The costs of the damaged reputation include lost revenue, loss of inspiration and motivation of staff, poor perceptions by people in society, and damaged marketing strategies because the organization is no longer enthusiastically perceived by others (Lickerman, 2010).

Critical Incidents and Adverse Events

In the presence of mental health challenges exhibited by nurses, critical incidents, adverse events, and sentinel events may all occur at a significant cost to the organization. Given the role that nurses play in all sectors of health care delivery, no nursing setting would be exempt from such potential. What is crucial to understand here is that nurses care for vulnerable patients and are given the responsibility and accountability to meet their needs while they are in an altered state of health. However, when a nurse's mental health becomes impaired, errors in clinical judgment and provided treatments can occur and result in critical incidents and adverse events. These incidents and events can result in the death, disability, or illness of patients, colleagues, and families and visitors. At the end of the day, in a toxic work environment that stretches nurses' stress and mental health to the maximum, an organization's priority of providing continuous quality improvement can easily get lost among the stormy waves, resulting in critical and adverse events.

Grievances and Litigation

From a labor and legal perspective, an organization can also bear the brunt of housing a poor psychological workplace environment. Failure to provide a psychologically safe workplace can lead employees to engage lawyers in pursuit of court settlements (Williams, 2012).

The rise in harassment complaints has gained increased momentum in recent years. As found by Taylor (2003), "The number of employees seeking help for harassment has almost tripled from 1999 to 2001," reaching 52% in some areas of the United Kingdom (Park, 2005). Further, as added by Kleiman, Kass, Wackerfuss, and Benek-Rivera (2007), "Sexual harassment is associated with more conflict in work teams, less cohesion, and less success in meeting financial goals."

Court costs and delays add to these rising figures. For example, "in the United States an average of 2 years is required for the Equal Employment Opportunity Commission to investigate most claims" (Busch, 1997). As suggested by Taylor (2003), "The math isn't complicated. A complaint that escalates to a lawsuit can easily cost $50,000 to $100,000 and take 3 to 5 years to settle. It doesn't stop there."

Organizations should also recognize that when there is a possible infringement of an employee's workplace rights, payout of liability and litigation claims increases. In 64% of cases involving wrongful termination, the organization pays upward of $600,000 (Bureau of National Affairs, 1998). The Mood Disorders Society of Canada (2009) reports that the percentage of court-awarded settlements due to mental injury in the workplace has risen by 700% in the last 5 years.

Shain, Arnold, and GermAnn (2012), add that the growing number of case law precedents, legislative changes, and tribunal deliberations supports a trend toward envisioning the duty to provide a psychologically safe workplace as being included in an employment contract. As such, "a political legal storm is brewing in the area of mental health protection at work. This storm brings with it a rising tide of liability for employers" (Williams, 2012).

Sabotage of the Organization's Efforts

We have previously discussed how unresolved conflict can jeopardize one's workplace mental health. As another fallout of that unresolved conflict, the organization can also experience some underhanded hidden costs. According to Dana (2001), there has been found "a direct correlation between prevalence of employee conflict and the amount of damage and theft of inventory and equipment. Also, "covert sabotage of work processes and of management's efforts usually occurs when employees are angry at their employer."

Community and Family Harm

When the mental health of employees at work becomes jeopardized, it can spill over into people's families and communities alike. The stress and threatened mental health that unresolved conflict causes is one such example of how this can happen. This can often occur in the form of "inner-directed harm (suicidal behavior, recklessness, agitated depression and abuse of alcohol, drugs) and outer-directed expressions (threatening behaviour, emotional and/or verbal abuse, bullying, harassment, assault, domestic violence, road rage)" (Health Canada, 2000), all of which impact loved ones, friends, spouses, and families and alter the various roles individuals play in society, such as being a nurse, mother, aunt, neighbor, or volunteer. These are the very communities and families that health care organizations are there to serve and protect.

Poor Consumer/Patient Relations

An organization has to remain cognizant of its core purpose as well, that being the concern of its patients and consumers and the care they receive. Poor workplace mental health among nurses can negatively impact patient/consumer relations. For example, when workplace negativity flourishes, employees are stressed, and mental health is at risk, relations with patients/consumers suffer and up to 50% are less patient with patients/consumers (Advisory, Conciliation, and Arbitration Service, 2013). As an end result, employees may choose to be less helpful and less reactive to customer needs, so patients/consumers defect to competitors (Wolfe, 2013).

Recruitment and Retention

Directly related to an organization's damaged reputation as being a "not so nice place to work," challenges concerning recruitment and retention can rear their ugly heads. In times of great stress and strained mental health, employees can create a great turnover of staff and retention and recruitment difficulties, costing millions along the way (Fink, 2007). When a program or facility is known for its poor leadership, lack of interest in continuing education opportunities, substandard salary scales, and rigid micromanagement techniques, the nurses whom it wishes to retain and recruit will in all likelihood experience difficulties of performance, increased costs of overtime, and a decrease in the quality of care they wish to provide.

A negative work environment, in particular, can send you looking for the nearest job classified section faster than anything else. Even if you have put in a certain amount of time with the company and are seeking to move up its corporate ladder, too much negativity may negate these goals and instead cause you to seek opportunities elsewhere. This, in turn, adds more stress to you because you are now faced with the prospect of finding a new employer and the change that can entail (Moultry Belcher, 2013). For the organization, it translates into additional expenses in terms of time and money devoted to the recruitment and hiring of a new employee, integrating the new employee into the workforce with training, and getting him or her in sync with the business (Wolfe, 2013).

"High staff turnover not only means the added costs of losing an experienced worker, recruiting and retraining a successor (at an estimated cost of 1.5 times the employee's annual salary), but it also causes lower productivity of a new worker, and low morale effects on managers, peers and subordinates" (Duxbury & Higgins, 2003). "The turnover costs for an employee are anywhere between 75% and 150% of the annual salary" (Phillips, 1990). Further, unresolved conflict, for example, represents "the decisive factor in at least 50% of departures, and up to 90% of involuntary departures" (Dana, 2001).

The cause of the event determines whether an employee is more likely to contribute to absenteeism or presenteeism. Individuals who have undergone treatment for a physical illness, such as a heart condition, have a higher correlation with absenteeism than presenteeism, whereas individuals who have sought psychological help or undergone counselling have a higher correlation with presenteeism than absenteeism (CMHA Ontario, 2010b).

Compassion fatigue can go beyond the impact on the well-being of individual nurses and can also impact larger organizational issues, such as staff turnover (Potter et al., 2013). Among nurses, a multiple regression revealed that work–family conflict is a significant predictor of intention to leave (Farquharson et al., 2012).

Presenteeism

Presenteeism is another negative outcome of poor workplace mental health. Presenteeism is the "action of employees coming to work despite having a sickness that justifies an absence, therefore they are performing their work under suboptimal conditions because they did not give themselves enough time to get well. This absence of days from work when one is feeling unwell can actually be a healthy coping strategy for some" (CMHA Ontario, 2010b). "When employees come to work not mentally present because of an illness, extreme family or life pressures, or stress, they are not giving themselves adequate time to get better" (Canadian Centre for Occupational Health and Safety, 2012). In addition, their performance at work can deteriorate even further (Warren Shepell, 2005). This is estimated to be three times more common than absenteeism (Warren Shepell, 2005), to be more costly than absenteeism (CMHA Ontario, 2010b), and impact an organization just as sickness or absence in terms of productivity and performance. "Presenteeism is most common in people with children, lower waged workers, employees with poor health status, and those who have difficulties setting limits when confronted with excessive demands" (CMHA Ontario, 2010b).

This can also occur when employees intend to leave the organization and fail to do so. As suggested by Duxbury and Higgins (2003), these "employees tend to have lower commitment, be more dissatisfied with their jobs, and reduce morale in the area in which they work." What seems to happen is that they "retire on the job" and hence do not pull their own weight, leading to heavier workloads in other areas (Duxbury & Higgins, 2003).

Any host of stress sources identified in Chapter 2 can precipitate the development of presenteeism. These can include not being able to afford to take the day off, not having a backup plan to take the day off, having even more to do after returning to work, being committed to personally attending meetings or events, and being concerned about job insecurity related to downsizing or restructuring. Heavy workload was found to be the most important predictor of increased presenteeism, followed closely by higher skill discretion, harmonious relationships with colleagues, role conflict, precarious job status, and higher self-efficacy (CMHA Ontario, 2010b). Unequivocally, presenteeism occurs less often when there is a good deal of trust, social support, and decision-making authority present (CMHA Ontario, 2010b).

Costs to the Patient

The very impetus and existence of hospitals and health care organizations is to provide safe, quality, and competent health care to the citizens of society as they face actual or threatened disease, illness, and injury. The international guidelines for nurses developed by the International Council of Nurses outlines that patient safety is fundamental for quality care (International Council of Nurses, 2002). When nurses' stress reaches dangerously high threshold levels and mental health becomes jeopardized, patient care can suffer. For example, a nurse's stress level in the emergency department is considered quite high, and very often it is correlated with decreasing patient safety (Carayon & Gurses, 2005; Elfering, Semmer, & Grebner, 2006; Meurier, Vincent, & Parmer, 1997). Furthermore, nursing working conditions that are characterized by a shortage of nursing staff to complete the work are inextricably linked to poor quality of care, unsafe patient care, and increased stress levels among other nurses (Geiger-Brown & Lipscomb, 2010; Moneke & Umeh, 2013). In various other settings as well, the correlation of rising stress with declining patient safety and care has been anecdotally noted.

Workplace mental health appears to an outcome involving two key players, the nurses and the employer. However, let's not forget the most important person in this shuffle, the vulnerable patient for whom your care is being sought. Unequivocally, at the patient level, concerns of abundant stressors impacting on the professional nurse also become apparent. The cost here is the patients and patient care that can be compromised (Adriaenssens, de Gucht, & Maes, 2012; Kawano, 2008). From a patient safety perspective, medication errors, errors in clinical judgment, patient harm, and professional misconduct can all occur. Further, patient satisfaction suffers (Kawano, 2008), and there are often increased complaints of the care received (Fink, 2007).

Medication errors in particular have been proved to be correlated with the poor mental health of nurses (Deans, 2005; Health Canada, 2008; Rassin, Kanti, & Silner, 2005). As suggested by the Massachusetts Nurses Association (2011), "In today's complex patient care environments, medication errors can occur in the practice of even the most diligent nurses." In one study from Ohio, the stress scores of various nursing units were strongly correlated with the occurrence of medication errors ($R = 0.40$). As found by Fogarty and McKeon (2006), "Deficiencies at the organizational level affect the psychological well-being of hospital employees, and distressed employees are more likely to engage in substandard work practices that ultimately endanger the patients under their care." Mahmood, Chaudhury, and Valente (2011) add that even the stress caused by the physical work environment can increase the risk for making medication errors.

Errors in clinical judgment have been found repeatedly in the literature as an outcome when nurses experience high stress levels and threats to their own mental health because of events occurring in the workplace. As Dugan et al. (1996) found, a relatively strong relationship exists between a hospital unit's stress continuum scale and the occurrence of patient incidents that include patient falls and medication errors.

Shirey, Ebright, and McDaniel (2013) found that nurse managers' chronic exposure to stress and work complexity negatively affects their heath, concentration, and decision-making processes, potentially threatening individual, patient, and organizational outcomes. Further, the nurse manager's role, organizational context, and situation factors also influence their cognitive decision-making processes.

Mahmood et al. (2011), in their study to assess nurses' views of how the physical work environment impacted the occurrence of medication errors, found that several physical environmental factors, particularly in the area of the nursing station, lead to medication, documentation, and other types of nursing errors. Hence, the layout of the physical workplace increased stress levels of nurses and potentially affected patient outcomes.

Patient Satisfaction

Patient dissatisfaction is also a fallout from a workplace that is stressful for nurses. The majority of research linking patient satisfaction to nursing stress levels suggests a negative correlation, and that as a nurse's stress level increases, patient satisfaction decreases. Compassion fatigue, for example, can go beyond the impact on the well-being of individual nurses and impact patient satisfaction as well (Potter et al., 2013). However, as much as patient satisfaction has been used as an indicator of the quality of care received from nurses, Johansen (2012) found that while emergency department nurses acknowledge that patient satisfaction is important to consider, it does not necessarily represent the quality of patient care provided.

SUMMARY

As we have seen, nurses are integral players in the operational fulfillment of their own needs, those of the profession, and those of the organization. Cumulatively, when the personal, professional, and organizational goals experience challenges and threats to their integrity, not only the nurse and professional but also the organization and society and, most importantly, the patient are ultimately impacted. The impact of stress for nurses has no boundaries, and stress can literally create illness for the nurse, jeopardize patient care, and prevent an organization's fulfillment of its mandate.

DISCUSSION QUESTIONS

1. Identify and discuss the impact that stress can have on you physically, psychologically, and socially.
2. What are the various outcomes that can occur for the leader as the result of increased stress levels?
3. What are the organizational costs incurred as a result of stressed nurses?

REFERENCES

Adriaenssens, J., de Gucht, V., & Maes, S. (2012). The impact of traumatic events on emergency room nurses: Findings from a questionnaire survey. *International Journal of Nursing Studies, 49*(11), 1411–1422. doi:10.1016/j.ijnurstu.2012.07.003

Advisory, Conciliation, and Arbitration Service. (2013). *Promoting positive mental health at work.* Retrieved from http://www.acas.org.uk/index.aspx?articleid=1900

Alnems, A., Aboads, F., Al-Yousef, M., AL-Yateem, A., & Abotabar, N. (2005). *Nurses' perceived job related stress and job satisfaction in Amman private hospitals.* Retrieved from http://www.google.ca/url?sa=t&rct=j&q=&esrc=s&source=web&cd=1&cad=rja&ved=0CC4Q FjA A&url=http%3A%2F%2Ffaculty.ksu.edu.sa%2Fmsawalha%2FDocuments%2FMy% 2520public ation.pdf&ei=r3QqUoXIH5Tb4AP9k4DgBg&usg=AFQjCNGc5QDBdGt99ix 5STHP2EuXIa1J9w &bvm=bv.51773540,d.dmg

Alves, S. L. (2005). A study of occupational stress, scope of practice and collaboration in nurse anesthetists practicing in anesthesia care settings. *AANA Journal, 73*, 443–452.

American Nurses Association. (2014). *Nurse staffing.* Retrieved from http://www. nursingworld.org/MainMenuCategories/ThePracticeofProfessionalNursing/ NurseStaffing

Anderson, R. N., Kochanek, K. D., & Murphy, S. L. (1995). Report of final mortality statistics. *National Center for Health Statistics Monthly Vital Statistics Report, 45*(11), Suppl. 2.

Andersson, L. M., & Pearson, C. M. (1999). Tit for tat? The spiraling effect of incivility in the workplace. *The Academy of Management Review, 24*(3), 452–471.

Barnes-Slater, S., & Ford, J. (2002). *Measuring conflict: Both the hidden costs and the benefits of conflict management interventions.* Retrieved from http://www.mediate.com/articles/ fordSlater.cfm

Beck, C. T. (2011). Secondary traumatic stress in nurses: A systematic review. *Archives of Psychiatric Nursing, 25*(1), 1–10. doi:10.1016/j.apnu.2010.05.005

Brun, J.-P., Biron, C., Martel, J., & Ivers, H. (2003). *Evaluation of workplace mental health: An analysis of human resources management practices* (Études et Recherches Report No. R-342). Quebec, Canada: Institut de Recherche Robert-Sauvé en Santé et en Sécurité du travail.

Busch, R. F. II. (1997). The conundrum: Conflict—the solution: Designing effective conflict management systems. *Preventive Law Reporter, 12*(1997–1998). Retrieved from http://heinonline.org/HOL/LandingPage?handle=hein.journals/prevlr16&div= 8&id=&page=

Bureau of National Affairs. (1998). *Without just cause: An employer's practical guide on wrongful discharge.* Washington, DC: Author.

Canadian Centre for Occupational Health and Safety. (2012). *Workplace stress.* Retrieved from http://www.ccohs.ca/oshanswers/psychosocial/stress.html

Canadian Mental Health Association Ontario. (2010a). *Job burnout.* Retrieved from http://wmhp.cmhaontario.ca/workplace-mental-health-core-concepts-issues/ issues-in-the- workplace-that-affect-employee-mental-health/job-burnout

Canadian Mental Health Association Ontario. (2010b). *Presenteeism.* Retrieved from http://wmhp.cmhaontario.ca/workplace-mental-health-core-concepts-issues/ issues-in-the- workplace-that-affect-employee-mental-health/presenteeism#_ftn3

Carayon, P., & Gurses, A. P. (2005). A human factors engineering conceptual framework of nursing workload and patient safety in intensive care units. *Intensive Critical Care Nursing, 21*(5), 284–301.

Center for Conflict Resolution International. (2013). *About workplace conflict.* Retrieved from http://www.conflictatwork.com/conflict/cost_e.cfm

Chung, C. E., & Kowalski, S. (2012). Job stress, mentoring, psychological empowerment, and job satisfaction among nursing faculty. *The Journal of Nursing Education, 51*(7), 381–388. doi: 10.3928/01484834-20120509-03

College of Nurses of Ontario. (2002). *Professional standards revised.* Retrieved from http://www.cno.org/Global/docs/prac/41006_ProfStds.pdf

Corbitt Clark, M. (2005). *The cost of job stress.* Retrieved from http://www.mediate.com/articles/clarkM1.cfm

Cram, J. A. & McWilliams, R. K., (2009). *From conflict to opportunity: A guide to understanding and managing workplace conflict.* Medford, MA: Cramby River Consultants.

Cram, J. A., & MacWilliams, R. K. (2014). *The cost of conflict in the workplace.* Cramby River Consultants. Retrieved from http://www.crambyriver.com/coc.html

Culture Consultancy. (2013). *What is employee engagement?* Retrieved from http://www.cultureconsultancy.com/links/should-i-worry-about-employee-engagement

Dale Carnegie. (2013). *After effects of poor employee relationship management.* Retrieved March 30, 2013, from http://www.managementstudyguide.com/effects-of-poor-employee-relationship- management.htm

Dana, D. (1999). *Measuring the financial cost of organizational conflict.* Prairie Village, KS: MTI Publications.

Dana, D. (2001). *The Dana measure of financial cost of organizational conflict.* Prairie Village, KS: MTI Publications.

Davis, S., Lind, B. K., & Sorensen, C. (2013). A comparison of burnout among oncology nurses working in adult and pediatric inpatient and outpatient settings. *Oncology Nursing Forum, 40*(4), E303–E311. doi:10.1188/13.ONF.E303-E311

Deans, C. (2005). Medication errors and professional practice of registered nurses. *Collegian, 12*(1), 29–33.

Donahue, P. (1996). *Nursing, the finest art: An illustrated history.* St. Louis, MO: Mosby.

Dugan, J., Lauer, E., Bouquot, Z., Dutro, B. K., Smith, M., & Widmeyer, G. (1996). Stressful nurses: The effect on patient outcomes. *Journal of Nursing Care Quality, 10*(3), 46–58.

Duxbury, L., & Higgins, D. (2003). *Work-life conflict in Canada in the new millennium: A status report.* Retrieved from http://publications.gc.ca/collections/Collection/H72-21-186-2003E.pdf

Elfering, N. K., Semmer, S., & Grebner, D. (2006). Work stress and patient safety: Observer-rated work stressors as predictors of characteristics of safety-related events reported by young nurses. *Ergonomics, 49,* 457–469.

Ernst, M. E., Messmer, P. R., Franco, M., & Gonzalez, J. L. (2004). Nurses' job satisfaction, stress, and recognition in a pediatric setting. *Pediatric Nursing, 30*(3), 219–227.

Farquharson, B., Allan, J., Johnston, D., Johnston, M., Choudhary, C., & Jones, M. (2012). Stress amongst nurses working in a healthcare telephone-advice service: Relationship with job satisfaction, intention to leave, sickness absence, and performance. *Journal of Advanced Nursing, 68*(7), 1624–1635. doi:10.1111/ j.1365-2648.2012.06006.x

Feskanich, D., Hastrup, J. L., Marshall, J. R., Colditz, G. A., Stampfer, M. J., Willett, W. C. et al. (2002). Stress and suicide in the nurses' health study. *Journal of Epidemiology and Community Health, 56*(2), 95–98.

Figley, C. F. (1995). Compassion fatigue as secondary traumatic stress disorder: An overview. In C. F. Figley (Ed.), *Compassion fatigue: Coping with secondary traumatic stress disorder in those who treat the traumatized* (pp. 1–20). New York, NY: Brunner/Mazel.

Fink, N. (2007). *The high cost of low morale: How to address low morale in the workplace through servant leadership.* Retrieved from http://www.roberts.edu/Academics/AcademicDivisions/BusinessManagement/msl/Community/Journal/TheHighCostofLowMorale.htm

Fogarty, G. J., & McKeon, C. M. (2006). Patient safety during medication administration: The influence of organizational and individual variables on unsafe work practices and medication errors. *Ergonomics, 49*(5–6), 444–456.

Garman, A. N., Corrigan, P. W., & Morris, S. (2002). Staff burnout and patient satisfaction: Evidence of relationships at the care unit level. *Journal of Occupational Health Psychology, 7,* 235–241. doi:10.1037/j.1076-8998.7.3.235

Geiger-Brown, J., & Lipscomb, J. (2010). The health care work environment and adverse health and safety consequences for nurses. *Annual Review of Nursing Research, 28,* 191–231.

Gordon, A. (2013). *Canada launches workplace standards for mental health and safety.* Retrieved from http://www.thestar.com/news/world/2013/01/16/canada_launches_workplace_standards_for_mental_health_and_safety.html

Guarding Minds at Work. (2012). *A workplace guide to psychological health and safety.* Retrieved from http://www.guardingmindsatwork.ca/info/index

Hamilton, C. (2013). *Work mental health issues cost billions.* Retrieved January 29, 2013, from http://www.theherald.com.au/story/1244549/opinion-work-mental-health-issues-cost-billions

Hasketh, K. L., Duncan, S. M., Estrabrooks, C. A., Reimer, M. A., Giovannetti, P., Hyndman, K., et al. (2003). Workplace violence in Alberta and British Columbia hospitals. *Health Policy, 63,* 311–321.

Hawton, K., & Vislisel, L. (1999). Suicide in nurses. *Suicide Life Threat Behaviors, 29,* 86–95.

Health Canada. (1998). *Health Reports, 10*(3), 47–62.

Health Canada. (2000). *Best advice on stress risk management in the workplace, 15–16.* Retrieved from http://www.mentalhealthworks.ca/sites/default/files/stress-part-1_e.pdf

Health Canada. (2008). *Correlates of medication error in hospitals.* Retrieved from http://www.statcan.gc.ca/daily-quotidien/080514/dq080514b-eng.htm

Hooper, C., Craig, J., Janvrin, D. R., Wetsel, M. A., & Reimels, E. (2010). Compassion satisfaction, burnout, and compassion fatigue among emergency nurses compared with nurses in other selected inpatient specialties. *Journal of Emergency Nursing, 36,* 420–427. doi:10.1016/j.jen.2009.11.02

International Council of Nurses. (2002). *ICN position statement on patient safety.* Retrieved from http://www.icn.ch/pspatientsafe.htm.

Johansen, M. L. (2014). Conflicting priorities: Emergency nurses' perceived disconnect between patient satisfaction and the delivery of quality patient care. *Journal of Emergency Nursing, 40*(1):13–19. doi:10.1016/j.jen.2012.04.013

Johnson, M. (2012). *Workplace effect on attitude.* Retrieved from http://www.ehow.com/facts_5921443_workplace-effect-attitude.html#ixzz27TzxKpeK

Jones, D., Tanigawa, T., & Weisse, S. (2003). Stress management and workplace disability in the US, Europe and Japan. *Journal of Occupational Health, 45,* 1–7.

Kath, L. M., Stichler, J. F., Ehrhart, M. G., & Schultze, T. A. (2010). Predictors and outcomes of nurse leader job stress experienced by AWHONN members. *Journal of Obstetric, Gynecological and Neonatal Nursing, 42*(1), E12–E25. doi:10.1111/j.1552-6909.2012.01430.x

Kawano, Y. (2008). Association of job-related stress factors with psychological and somatic symptoms among Japanese hospital nurses: Effect of departmental environment in acute care hospitals. *Journal of Occupational Health, 50*(1), 79–85.

Kleiman, L. S., Kass, D. S., Wackerfuss, A., & Benek-Rivera, J. (2007). Fighting back: Legal options for same-sex harassment vctims. *Journal of Individual Employment Rights, 12*(4), 303–312.

Knight, J. (2004, August 17). *Bullied workers suffer 'battle stress.'* BBC News Online. Retrieved from http://news.bbc.co.uk/2/hi/business/3563450.stm

Kuan, K. (2013). *12 secrets to a rewarding nursing career.* Retrieved from http://www.nursetogether.com/twelve-tips-for-a-rewarding-nursing-career#sthash.QF1jLE5t.dpuf

Learning Express Editors. (2010). *Standards of nursing practice.* Retrieved from http://www.education.com/reference/article/standards-nursing-practice/?page=3

Levine, S. (1998). *The many costs of conflict*. Retrieved from Mediate.com

Lickerman, D. (2010). *The value of a good reputation*. Retrieved from http://www. psychologytoday.com/blog/happiness-in-world/201004/the-value-good-reputation

Maddalena, V., Kearney, A. J., & Adams, L. (2012). Quality of work life of novice nurses: A qualitative exploration. *Journal for Nurses in Staff Development, 28*(2), 74–79. doi:10.1097/ NND.0b013e31824b41a1

Mahmood, A., Chaudhury, H., & Valente, M. (2011). Nurses' perceptions of how physical environment affects medication errors in acute care settings. *Applied Nursing Research, 24*(4), 229–237. doi:10.1016/j.apnr.2009.08.005

Maiden, J., Georges, J. M., & Connelly, C. D. (2011). Moral distress, compassion fatigue, and perceptions about medication errors in certified critical care nurses. *Dimensions of Critical Care Nursing, 30*, 339–345. doi:10.1097/DCC.0b013e31822fab2a

Mark, G., & Smith, A. P. (2012). Occupational stress, job characteristics, coping, and the mental health of nurses. *British Journal of Health Psychology, 17*(3), 505–521. doi:10.1111/j.2044- 8287.2011.02051.x.

Maslach, C. (1982). *Burnout—The cost of caring*. Englewood Cliffs, NJ: Spectrum.

Mayo Clinic. (2013). *Job burnout: How to spot it and take action*. Retrieved August 5, 2013, from http://www.mayoclinic.com/health/burnout/WL00062

McKenzie, B. (2014). *Are your employees committed, compliant or complacent?* Retrieved from http://www.hrcsuite.com/productivity/committed

Meurier, C. E., Vincent, C. A., & Parmer, D. G. (1997). Learning from errors in nursing practice. *Journal of Advanced Nursing, 26*, 111–119.

Moneke, N., & Umeh, O. J. (2013). Factors influencing critical care nurses' perception of their overall job satisfaction: An empirical study. *Journal of Nursing Administration, 43*(4), 201–207. doi:10.1097/NNA.0b013e31828958af

Mood Disorders Society of Canada. (2009). *Quick facts: Mental illness and addictions in Canada*. Retrieved from http://www.mooddisorderscanada.ca/page/quick-facts

Moultry Belcher, L. (2013). *How negativity in the workplace can affect you personally*. Retrieved from http://www.ehow.com/info_8608474_negativity-workplace-can- affect- personally.html#ixzz27U4ANJCp

Nahm, E. S., Warren, J., Zhu, S., An, M., & Brown, J. (2012). Nurses' self-care behaviors related to weight and stress. *Nursing Outlook, 60*(5), e23–e31.

National Institute for Occupational Safety and Health. (1997). *Musculoskeletal disorders and workplace factors: A critical review of epidemiologic evidence for work-related musculoskeletal disorders of the neck, upper extremity, and low back*. Retrieved from http://www.cdc.gov/ niosh/docs/97-141/pdfs/97-141.pdf

National Institute for Occupational Safety and Health. (2008). *What are the potential adverse health effects of occupational stress?* Retrieved from http://www.cdc.gov/niosh/ docs/2008- 136/pdfs/2008-136.pdf

Nguyen, L., & Bibbings, R. (2002). Exploring the links between stress and accidents in the workplace: A literature review. *Journal of the Institution of Occupational Safety and Health, 6*(2), 9–20.

Park, R. (2005). *Failure to manage change heightens stress, harassment and conflict at work, survey claims*. Retrieved from http://www.trainingreference.co.uk/news/bp050128.htm

Perry, B., Toffner, G., Merrick, T., & Dalton, J. (2011). An exploration of the experience of compassion fatigue in clinical oncology nurses. *Canadian Oncology Nursing Journal, 21*, 91– 105.

Phillips, D. T. (1990). The price tag of turnover. *Personnel Journal, 12*, 58.

Potter, P., Deshields, T., Berger, J. A., Clarke, M., Olsen, S., & Chen, L. (2013). Evaluation of a compassion fatigue resiliency program for oncology nurses. *Oncology Nursing Forum, 40*(2), 180–187. doi:10.1188/13.ONF.180-187

Rassin, M., Kanti, T., & Silner, D. (2005). Chronology of medication errors by nurses: Accumulation of stresses and PTSD symptoms. *Issues in Mental Health Nursing, 26*(8), 873–886.

Robins, P. M., Meltzer, L., & Zelikovsky, N. (2009). The experience of secondary traumatic stress upon care providers working within a children's hospital. *Journal of Pediatric Nursing, 24*, 270– 279.

Rodwell, J., & Martin, A. (2013). The importance of the supervisor for the mental health and work attitudes of Australian aged care nurses. *International Psychogeriatrics, 25*(3), 382–389. doi:10.1017/S1041610212001883.

Ruggiero, J. S. (2005). Health, work variables and job satisfaction among nurses. *Journal of Nursing Administration, 35*(5), 254–263.

Schwam, K. (1998). The phenomenon of compassion fatigue in perioperative nursing. *Association of Perioperative Registered Nurses Journal, 68*, 642–645, 647–648. doi:10.1016/S0001- 2092(06)62569-6

Scott, E. (2010). *Chronic job stress is a risk factor for heart disease.* Retrieved from http://stress.about.com/od/stresshealth/a/jobstress.htm

Shain, M., Arnold, I., & GermAnn, K. (2012). The road to psychological safety: Legal, scientific, and social foundations for a Canadian national standard on psychological safety in the workplace. *Bulletin of Science Technology Society, 32*(2), 142–162.

Sherman, R. O. (2013). *Creating psychological safety in our workplaces.* Retrieved from http://www.emergingrnleader.com/emergingnurseleader-8/

Shirey, M. R., Ebright, P. R., & McDaniel, A. M. (2013). Nurse manager cognitive decision-making amidst stress and work complexity. *Journal of Nursing Management, 21*(1), 17–30. doi: 10.1111/j.1365-2834.2012.01380.x

Smith, M., Segal, J., & Segal, R. (2013). *Preventing burnout.* Retrieved from http://www.helpguide.org/mental/burnout_signs_symptoms.htm

Smyth, S. (2013). *'I hold radio DJs responsible, make them pay for my mortgage': The suicide note left by nurse who hanged herself over Kate Middleton hospital prank call.* Retrieved June 2, 2013, from http://www.dailymail.co.uk/news/article-2316055/Jacintha-Saldanha-suicide-note-Kate-Middleton-hospital-prank-holds-radio-DJs-responsible.html#ixzz2cWrkfmfB

Stamm, B. H. (2002). Measuring compassion satisfaction as well as fatigue: Developmental history of the compassion satisfaction and fatigue test. In C. R. Figley (Ed.), *Treating compassion fatigue* (pp. 107–119). New York, NY: Brunner-Routledge.

Stubenrauch, J. M. (2007). Malpractice vs. negligence. *American Journal of Nursing, 107*(7), 63.

Sundin, L., Hochwalder, J., & Lisspers, J. (2011). A longitudinal examination of generic and occupational specific job demands and work-related social support associated with burnout among nurses in Sweden. *Work, 38*, 389–400. doi:10.3233/WOR-2011-1142

Taylor, R. (2003). Workplace tiffs boosting demand for mediators. (2003, March 17). *National Post.*

The Health Communication Unit, University of Toronto. (2004). *The psychosocial work environment, the organization of work and the management culture of the workplace have the most dramatic impact on employee stress and health outcomes.* Retrieved from http://www.thcu.ca/workplace/documents/intro_to_workplace_health_promotion_v1.1.final.pdf

Thomas, K., & Schmidt, W. (1976, June). A survey of managerial interests with respect to conflict. *Academy of Management Journal, 19*(2), 315–318.

Vahey, D. C., Aiken, L. H., Sloane, D. M., Clarke, S. P., & Vargas, D. (2004). Nurse burnout and patient satisfaction. *Medical Care, 42*(2, Suppl.), II57–II66. doi:10.1097/01.mlr.0000109126.50398.5a

Violante, S., Benso, P. G., Gerbaudo, L., & Violante, B. (2009). Correlation between job satisfaction and stress factors, burn-out and psychosocial well-being among nurses working in different healthcare settings. *Giornale Italiano di Medicina del Lavoro ed Ergonomia, 31*(1, Suppl. A), A36–A44.

Vitt, L. A. (2014). Raising employee engagement through workplace financial education. *New Directions for Adult and Continuing Education, 2014*(141), 67–77.

Wacker Guido, G. W. (2010). *Legal and ethical issues in nursing* (5th ed.). Toronto, Ontario: Pearson.

Warren Shepell. (2002). *Workplace trends linked to mental health crisis in Canada.* Retrieved from http://www.warrenshepell.com/newsroom/pr-nov152002.asp

Watson, C., & Hoffman, R, (1996). Managers as negotiators. *Leadership Quarterly, 7*(1).

Williams, G. D. (2007). *Attitude and stress, effects on the body.* Retrieved from http://EzineArticles.com/702403

Williams, R. B. (2012). *The silent tsunami: Mental health in the workplace.* Retrieved from http://www.psychologytoday.com/blog/wired-success/201209/the-silent-tsunami-mental-health-in-the-workplace

Wolf, Z. R., Colahan, M., & Costello, A. (1998). Relationship between nurse caring and patient satisfaction. *Medsurg Nursing, 7,* 99–105.

Wolfe, M. (2013). *How negativity can affect employees.* Retrieved from http://www.ehow.com/info_8150602_negativity-can-affect-employees.html#ixzz27U3l8Nux

Wright, S., & Sayre-Adams, J. (2012). Reassess the stress. *Nursing Standard, 26*(42),18–19.

Yoder, E. A. (2010). Compassion fatigue in nurses. *Applied Nursing Research, 23,* 191–197. doi:10.1016/j.apnr.2008.09.003

Young, T. (2012). *Everything starts with attitude.* Retrieved from http://www.salestrainingplus.com/sales-marketing-information/sales-and-marketing-articles/57-everything-starts-with-attitude

4

The Role of the Organization in Creating and Fostering Positive Workplace Mental Health

*Employees who believe that management is concerned about them as
a whole person—not just an employee—are more productive, more
satisfied, more fulfilled. Satisfied employees mean satisfied customers,
which leads to profitability.*
—*Anne Mulcahy*

LEARNING OBJECTIVES

By the end of this chapter, the learner will be able to:

1. Better understand and articulate some of the different strategies that organizations can complete to help foster a mentally healthy workplace
2. Discuss the value of workplace mental health champions and the roles you feel they can play in helping nurses at work
3. Identify active or new and arising legislation in your state, province, and country that you feel would help to steer organizations toward building and maintaining positive workplace mental health
4. Understand how some of the internal workings of an organization, such as communication, morale, recruitment and retention, and recognition and reward, help to foster positive workplace mental health
5. Identify the value of culture, psychological job fit, staff engagement, shared governance, and respect in a workplace
6. Discuss how organizations can motivate and engage nurses to create higher retention and recruitment rates
7. Identify and discuss some health promotion strategies an organization can offer to its nurses to help build and strengthen workplace mental health
8. Discuss the value that leaders have in helping to build an organization that has positive mental health

An organization functions only as well as the people who help to run it. Nurses are most often the backbone of what keeps large health care organizations operating functionally and efficiently. Nurses are the body, mind, and spirit of most health care facilities/hospitals, are visible 24/7, and have the most contact with clients on a daily and ongoing basis.

As employers, accredited bodies, and sources of health care services, be they public or private health care organizations, hold a significant responsibility to the shareholders, boards, governing bodies, governments, and society at large for creating and fostering a positive environment of workplace mental health. They are also held to stringent levels of accountability, transparency, and obligation in accordance with various legislative acts and public policy and standards.

Organizations are under much pressure and high expectations to ensure that the workplaces they provide are in synchrony with government legislation and accreditation standards, and as such are healthy ones. There are many measures and efforts that organizations can work toward and support to help ensure that the workplace for nurses is safe and healthy, and that it posesses no threat to anyone's mental health. As suggested by Williams (2012), "protecting psychological well-being is a basic and key element of being a responsible employer."

Quite often, we witness most government and other health care dollars being dedicated to acute surgical and medical programs. This leaves only a small fraction of total health care dollars invested into other programs, such as mental health. Unknown to many, mental health is just as, if not more, important than the physical health that you see supported by surgical and/or medical programs and services. By the time you finish this chapter, you will quickly learn why.

Although society is seeing some money diverted by organizations to help build a mentally healthy workplace, with British Columbia's spending increasing by 52% over the past 10 years (Williams, 2012), it has yet only scratched the surface.

GOOD BUSINESS SENSE

Health care facilities and/or organizations that strive to create, offer, and maintain mentally healthy workplace environments are a win–win situation for everyone involved and make good business sense. Although organizations strive to keep staff healthy, engaged, effective, and productive, doing so is one of the most challenging aspects of business operations. In essence, good health means good business. To achieve such a goal makes good business sense not only for the organizations but also for the nurses, other staff, and patients/families. As the business of the day for health care organizations/facilities is promoting good health for all, then it would be in the best interest of any health care organization to do so in a manner that promotes and fosters productivity, clinical efficiency, positive collegial relations, good public relations, and fiscal responsibility. When the organization or corporation is a health authority, hospital, and/or some other health care service facility, the impact is even more substantial because the positive effects not only impact the employees of the health care facility but also enhance the delivery of services that patients seek at the health care facility.

To any health care organization/facility, the value of good workplace mental health is substantial. The operational cost savings that result from good mental health, in the form of decreased absenteeism, increased productivity, decreased use of sick leave, increased staff recruitment and retention, and decreased workers' compensation claims, reflect good business operations. Furthermore, good mental health adds significantly to levels of nurse satisfaction and contentment, which in turn help to build on the provision of safe and quality patient care and hence patient satisfaction, optimal recovery, and a greater chance of decreasing the use of hospitals.

Good workplace mental health for nurses is an all-around crucial need for organizations to maintain. The integral role that nurses play in the successful operation of any health care organization needs to be recognized and addressed. Furthermore, monitoring nurses' mental health is a valuable policy for organizations to maintain, for without emotionally stable nurses, patient care becomes compromised, operational costs skyrocket, the potential for liability increases, and every aspect of a health care organization's business suffers.

Operationally, the existence of a workplace that is mentally unhealthy presents many issues of concern and liability. These can potentially jeopardize the success of the business by increasing operating costs and decreasing its revenue phenomenally. Such costs become evident through employees' increased rates of absenteeism, sick leave, workers' compensation, and staff turnover, as well as decreased efficiency, productivity, and output. In an environment where there is inconsistency of staff and increased workloads because of fewer and/or absent staff, there is also bound to be significantly less turnaround of patients, longer patient stays, poorer quality of patient outcomes, concerns about patient safety, and a greater risk for liability. Furthermore, the poorer care outcomes of patients during their initial hospital stay will result in a higher readmission rate for them after discharge. Yet again, this equates to another costly venture by having to hospitalize individuals repeatedly.

Because nurses are often the main front-line practicing professionals providing many of the services of these health care facilities and/or organizations, the mental health of nurses is crucial to ensure the success of the health care business from every perspective. It would be most prudent for health care organizations to recognize the possibility of mental health concerns among their employees now, and to invest proactively today instead of incurring unnecessary costs later. The Partnership for Workplace Mental Health, a program of the American Psychiatric Foundation (APF; 2014), offers similar advice. In essence, health promotion ventures are often easy and cost-effective, and they can often be undertaken without any disruption to the operations of the health facility/business.

Nurses who have mental illnesses, impending mental illnesses, and/or mental health concerns and who are not treated adequately or provided a healthy environment in which to work end up costing the health care organization significantly. Such costs often take the form of expenses incurred for the provision of health and mental health care and services, pharmaceutical products and services, and short- and long-term disability claims. Furthermore, the expenses and rising premiums that result can be easily mitigated or avoided entirely when health promotion measures are many and implemented, problems are detected, and treatment is timely. Failure to intervene for mental illnesses and maintain mental health can result in higher assessment and treatment costs. These measures help to ensure a higher-quality standard of care, support a better quality of life for individuals, and avoid unnecessary suffering and costs incurred as a result (APF, 2014).

The costs of doing nothing to address the mental health concerns and issues of nurses are astronomical. The continued presence of mentally drained and stressed nurses can lead not only to unwell and ineffective nurses and increased replacement costs, but also to increased patient liabilities and possibly the delivery of a compromised quality of care to the patient, as we have seen in Chapter 3.

RESPECT, COURTESY, CONSIDERATION, AND CIVILITY

What many of us consider the basics of human communication are not always used or employed as best practices. While we learned much about communication in Chapter 1, the parameters of respect, courtesy, consideration, and civility should not be taken for granted. Each requires a conscious effort to be used, practiced, and relayed accurately to others with whom we engage and interact with daily. Many organizations and their administrative leaders often need reminders about the value that respect, courtesy, consideration, and civility should have, and the influence they can exert on the workplace environment.

First, to enhance our understanding of these valuable characteristics, they need to be defined. Respect "essentially refers to a moral attitude that, when translated into action, is manifest as showing regard, esteem, admiration, and kindly consideration for another" (Johnstone, 2009). In other words, respect "manifests as the 'good' treatment of people and invariably results in their being humanised" (Johnstone, 2012), while courtesy represents consideration, cooperation, and/or generosity or "behavior that is marked by polished manners or respect for others" (*Merriam-Webster's Collegiate Dictionary*, 2014). Believe it or not, I could not find one nursing reference that identifies and defines "courtesy." One nursing reference speaks to courtesy as a very positive trait for nurses to value as being what you "display towards your colleagues in front of patients" and by doing so it further "strengthens their trust in your professionalism" (Davies, 2012). Equally, courtesy means "polite behavior that shows respect for other people, something you do to be kind to others" (*Merriam-Webster's Collegiate Dictionary*, 2014). In addition, consideration means being "thoughtful of the rights and feelings of others" in a manner that displays respect, kindness, and thoughtfulness (*Merriam-Webster's Collegiate Dictionary*, 2014), and civility symbolizes civilized conduct or a polite act or expression demonstrated by an individual and one that represents courtesy and politeness (*Merriam-Webster's Collegiate Dictionary*, 2014). Disseminated as a frequent tweet recently was that "politeness has become so rare, that some people today mistake it for flirtation" (Hudspeth, 2013).

An organization has the power, authority, and skilled human resources to develop policies and procedures around the values of disrespect, lack of courtesy and consideration, and incivility in the workplace. While we will be elaborating further on incivility and respect in Chapter 7, when we discuss workplace bullying among nurses, they are included here as issues that organizations can address in promoting and fostering mentally healthy workplace environments for their nurses.

An organization should help to ensure that nurses in the workplace are respectful, civil, courteous, and considerate to one another as well as to colleagues, patients, families, and visitors. The use of respect, courtesy, consideration, and civility by nurses when interacting with others illustrates much genuineness, concern, empathy, and dignity toward others, and is easily identified and perceived by those who bear witness to it. Furthermore, it helps to support the very premise of nursing—that of being a caring profession.

A positive workplace environment where respect, courtesy, consideration, and civility are encouraged provides a spin-off of multiple benefits for an organization. A nurse's workplace environment that is rich in respect, courtesy, consideration, and civility also strengthens other operational indicators (Guarding Minds @ Work [GM@W], 2012). Other beneficial spin-offs from a positive workplace environment include:

1. Greater job satisfaction
2. Positive perceptions of fairness
3. Increased cooperation and collaboration
4. Increased positive attitude
5. Increased morale
6. Increased teamwork
7. Increased interest in one's own personal and professional development
8. Increased engagement in problem resolution and conflict management
9. Enhanced nurse–manager relations
10. Decreased use of sick leave
11. Increased retention and decreased turnover of nurses

In identifying all of these benefits, we are not oblivious to the reality that workplace environments are often challenged with ongoing operational issues and restraints, patient complexities, family complaints, and interpersonal dynamics. A perfect work environment does not exist, and not everyone is going to be happy and content "all" of the time at their place of work. However, what can realistically be achieved is a workplace environment that does all it can, that has supportive leaders and a strong supportive organization whose executives take much pride in its values of respect, courtesy, consideration, and civility. To help further enforce such favorable workplace characteristics, it is up to health care organizations to develop zero-tolerance policies against anything that would oppose or compromise a collegial, respectful work environment.

The absence of respect, courtesy, consideration, and civility breeds an environment of emotional exhaustion, increased conflict, decreased productivity, withdrawal of self, animosity, and discontent. For an organization, it further increases costs, risk for legal liabilities, and grievances; compromises patient care; and can even damage the public reputation of the organization.

STRESS MANAGEMENT INTERVENTION

Stress management is not new to health care organizations. "Health care occupations have long been known to be highly stressful and associated with higher rates of psychological distress than many other occupations. Working with people and the health and lives of other people as nurses do is one of the highest psychologically distressing occupations around" (NIOSH, 2008). As identified in Chapter 2, nurses have numerous sources of stress that can be experienced, as well as associated costs (Chapter 3); however, we need to find ways to ameliorate this stress.

Nurses are exposed to a number of stressors, ranging from work overload, time pressures, and lack of role clarity to dealing with infectious diseases and difficult, ill, helpless patients. Such stressors can lead to physical and psychological symptoms, absenteeism, turnover, and medical errors. However, the literature points to both organizational and worker-focused interventions that can successfully reduce stress among health care workers. Although organizational interventions (because they address the sources of stress) are preferred, interventions that combine worker and organizational components may have the broadest appeal as they provide both long-term prevention and short-term treatment components.

"Occupational stress interventions can focus either on organizational change or the worker. Worker-focused interventions often consist of stress management techniques such as training in coping strategies, progressive relaxation, biofeedback, cognitive-behavioral techniques, time management, and interpersonal skills" (NIOSH, 2008). "Another type of intervention that has shown promise for reducing stress among health care workers is innovative coping, or the development and application by workers of strategies like changes in work methods or skill development to reduce excessive demands. The goal of these techniques is to help the worker deal more effectively with occupational stress. Worker-focused interventions have been the most common form of stress reduction in U.S. workplaces. Although worker interventions can help workers deal with stress more effectively, they do not remove the sources of workplace stress, and thus may lose effectiveness over time. Mental health support intervention may be needed in the event of a significant event at a health care organization" (NIOSH, 2008).

PSYCHOLOGICAL PROTECTION

We have just discussed psychological support and its value in promoting a mentally healthy workplace for nurses. Closely related to psychological support is psychological protection. Psychological protection is yet another technique that organizations can use to their advantage to build and support good mental health for nurses in the workplace. Psychological protection can be defined as the measures that an organization puts in place so nurses feel secure, safe, and protected from psychological harm and/or injury. In the nursing profession, this sense of safety is demonstrated when nurses feel it is safe to go that extra mile to that next step forward and put themselves on the line to voice their opinion, lobby government, seek input from others, report nursing errors, or present new and innovative ideas to courageously introduce a change in practice or policy (GM@W, 2012). However, many nurses are often apprehensive about taking such actions or voicing such concerns for fear that they may be reprimanded or ostracized, or that they may experience negative ramifications from others—colleagues and/or leaders. Hence, they can often unknowingly turn a blind eye rather than identify and report risks and challenge the status quo.

The psychological protection that an organization offers enables nurses to demonstrate and maintain esteem, confidence, and autonomy by letting them know that they can take steps to do what they believe or know is right and so experience emotional well-being, and that the organization will do its best to eliminate any threats to the nurses' mental health and overall well-being. Without any measure of psychological protection, nurses will begin to feel demoralized, threatened, stressed, pressured, and disengaged in their work and professional relations because they feel they are working in an environment of unpredictability, ambiguity, and uncertainty (GM@W, 2012).

For an organization, psychological protection will often come in the form of policies or government-imposed legislation. Such examples include whistle-blower legislation and policies of protective disclosure. Under whistle-blower legislation or a protected disclosure policy, for example, an organization commits itself to maintaining the highest ethical standards in its activities by protecting any employee who acts to expose wrongdoing to the organization and further to act immediately on this reported wrongdoing. The specific purposes of such legislation and policy are the following (Athabasca University, 2012; New South Wales Government, 2009):

1. To protect persons who, in good faith, make such disclosures by prohibiting subsequent reprisals against them
2. To provide a mechanism through which nurses can confidentially disclose wrongdoing, unethical conduct, fraud, or abuse of public trust that they observe in the context of performing their duties or activities
3. To prescribe procedures for making such disclosures
4. To provide a mechanism for appropriate investigation of and response to such disclosures
5. To protect against the serious and substantial waste of public money

The mere presence of whistle-blower legislation and/or protected disclosure policies, which health care organizations are advised to develop and enforce, should symbolize the extent to which an organization will go to offer its nurses/employees a significant degree of psychological protection.

ORGANIZATIONAL CULTURE

Health care organizations have a tremendous responsibility for providing safe, quality, and competent care to the people they serve. At the same time, they also have to monitor and guide the work of thousands of employees, meet expected standards of practice and strategic directions for accreditation, and fulfill the organizational mandate and vision under the watchful eye of their board of trustees/directors—all while maintaining an acute sense of responsibility, fiscal stewardship, transparency, and accountability to the public. One is left to wonder then how they can possibly even notice the culture that is being created and growing within the confines of their facilities. If and when they finally do, it is often too late or in response to an adverse event that occurred because of their unawareness.

In many respects, health care organizations are so caught up with their own agendas that they tend to forget about the front-line workers, particularly the nurses, who form much of the backbone that supports and fulfills the main goals of the organizations. From an organizational perspective, the human factor often goes unnoticed and underutilized. As technological advances skyrocket and engineered robotics become integrated into the mainstream of society, they may come with a human price tag within an organization, at least from a consumer perspective. When was the last time you called a hospital and got a human voice? One that was not prerecorded, of course. When was the last time you received a personally signed letter from a hospital chief executive officer (CEO)? For the employees, as well, the same applies: When was the last time a senior vice president visited your nursing unit? You have been working on this unit as a nurse for 20 years and have yet to see any one of the four CEOs who passed through the organization during that time. If you are a nursing manager trying to get in touch with someone from human resources, good luck with that; you probably need to push three or four recorded options to get the one you need, and then if you are lucky you "may" get a real person who can help answer your questions, but don't get your hopes up because this person has a recorded voice mailbox, too.

But wait; let's move this philosophy to the bedside, where care is given to patients who are in their weakest and most vulnerable state. The electronic blood pressure cuff that is frequently used has removed the need for this nurse–patient contact. Use of the pulse oximeter and iPad as assessment and documentation tools creates a similar outcome of decreasing interpersonal contact. The point is that when you take the human factor out of the provision of patient care at all levels, a cold, impersonal automation is left to flourish. The organization is so preoccupied with fulfilling its mandate and organizational goals in the most financially responsible manner possible that the people within the organization and therefore patient care ultimately suffer. For any health care organization, a balancing act is truly needed to find equilibrium.

The effects of technology are far-reaching, both positively and negatively. On the downside, they can help to create an impersonal culture (Bailey, 2011). Instead of freeing the nurse for more patient contact time, a paradigm shift in society has now produced more patients with more complex needs and demands, nursing shortages, and increased workloads because of fiscal cutbacks. This only serves to decrease nurse–patient human contact even more.

Culture is an important element of an organization that represents the set of values, assumptions, attitudes, conventions, and behaviors of the group of people who work there (Yoder-Wise & Kowalski, 2006). It symbolizes the "signature" of the organization, which is unique because it sets the tone, meaning, atmosphere, and expectations of those new to the organization. Within an organization, many norms, practices, and beliefs are held; however, they do not all necessarily reflect what is right or even moral. These cues and innuendos represent what is considered acceptable behavior and/or practices in an organization (GM@W, 2012). Organizational culture is something that is learned, and it means connecting behavior and gestures with consequences (Kramer, Schmalenberg, & Maguire, 2004).

It would be most prudent for health care organizations to realize, even more so today, that it is the employees who are the most valued asset to the functioning of an organization. A realization is needed by every health care organization, if it wishes to succeed, that the human beings or people connected to it are a valuable resource. Person-to-person contact works best and helps to illustrate the genuine interest and desire of an organization to meet the needs of all people; therefore, it is one of the best investments that an organization can make.

Because an organizational culture helps to set the tone and even the level of comfort of an organization, a culture that is characterized by caring, trust, learning, honesty, fairness, and integrity is a model and the most desirable organizational culture any nurses could wish for (GM@W, 2012). For most organizations, the key person who has much influence on the culture of an organization regarding nurses is the chief nursing officer. This person is positioned to help fulfill many valuable, culturally focused goals of an organization, such as (Yoder-Wise & Kowalski, 2006, p. 145):

1. Create an environment where nurses can flourish
2. Support nurses and convey a sense of genuine caring about them as individuals
3. Provide sufficient learning opportunities for nurses to feel nurtured and supported intellectually
4. Engender enthusiasm

An organization that has a positive, open, and uplifting culture creates a positive influence on maintaining nurses' good workplace mental health. An environment fostered by cooperation, open collaboration, honest interpersonal peer interactions, and employee commitment and loyalty would in all likelihood produce increases nurse engagement, job satisfaction, and retention and recruitment rates, and therefore decreased organization costs and increased productivity.

A negative organizational culture, on the other hand, can easily challenge nurses' mental health and be detrimental to the function of the organization, morale, and patient care delivery. What often occurs when a negative organizational culture exists is that nurses' stress levels, absenteeism, and staff turnover increase; their engagement, satisfaction, and well-being decrease; and a financially challenged and struggling organization occurs (GM@W, 2012). A hospital or health care organization that is competitive and profit-driven under private ownership would harvest an organizational culture of chaos and division in which extreme levels of stress and burnout are the norm.

In recent years, the development of strategies to build and promote positive work cultures has been emerging. The FISH (so-called because the philosophy was founded in a fish market) culture is one such example. When an organization adopts a FISH culture, it has been proven that there are many positive spin-offs. The following FISH philosophy, from Charthouse Learning (2013), is one to embrace. CEO John Christensen states, "Whatever the subject, how we **talk** about our work shapes the way we **think** and **act** at work. In other words, our conversations **are** our culture." The recognized trademark of the FISH! philosophy—Be There, Play, Make Their Day and Choose Your Attitude™—helps us talk honestly, safely, and optimistically about the kind of workplace culture we want to create … together. This philosophy is based on the premise that our conversation and dialogue are critically important and reflect an openness and transparency, so people are living, doing, and talking about issues and things openly and honestly. It is about working together in harmony, being supportive of others, and making their day. Furthermore, it helps to make work playful, creative, innovative, and just plain fun, yet achieves productivity, optimal outputs, better patient care (in the case of nurses), and a more respectful workplace. (For further information on the FISH philosophy, please visit their website at http://www.charthouse.com/productdetail.aspx?nodeid=11986.)

Nursing or Employee Culture

In the increased pace of many acute care settings, in particular with risky workloads and a lack of manager presence and input, what fosters is a culture of "who cares?" Furthermore, some of the busiest acute units are also the units that experience a higher turnover of staff (Berry & Curry, 2012; Colosi, 2013). Colosi (2013) adds that the turnover rate for nurses in the United States working in medicine and surgery and even emergency areas have consistently exceeded the national average; in 2013 they were 16.8% and 16.5%, respectively. Here, novice nurses and new hires, who are perhaps reluctant to oppose current bad practices of a unit, can easily slide into and fall prey to the very same behaviors that were modeled before them.

SHARED GOVERNANCE

Shared governance is one example of how organizations can help to ensure that their organizational culture will grow to become a positive one and hence create a mentally healthy workplace. Shared governance can be defined as "a process for empowering nurses in the practice setting" (Sullivan, 2012). The nurse leader plays a key role in and can influence the culture of effective governance by building trust and respect and by challenging the behaviors that have led to poor quality care (Bassett & Westmore, 2012). Even in Magnet hospital settings, shared governance has furthered the development of a positive nursing practice environment (Clavelle, O'Grady, & Drenkard, 2013).

Shared governance is a framework that can be operationalized within a health care organization/facility to help nurses maintain a strong voice and provide input into their practices and feedback on changes needed. It also allows them to maintain a strong sense of autonomy and integrity and feel like valued partners in shared decision making because they are involved actively in the decision-making processes of nursing and in patient care delivery (Porter O'Grady, 2004). Other benefits of shared governance for nurses are that it helps to promote their sense of value and self-concept. As a result, nurses begin to feel valued by the organization and productive in clinical settings, and they have some measure of control over their practices, efficiency, and accountability (Sullivan, 2012).

Most hospitals and/or health care organizations have generated their own models of shared governance. As a result, there are several models in circulation; however, no one model seems to fit the bill for everyone. Figure 4.1 is a generic overview of the critical components of a shared governance model that captures each of the important elements in which nurses can and should play a vital role.

A person's mental health is an integral component of his or her total well-being. However, it can be challenged by numerous and different personal, professional, and organizational factors. The promotion of good mental health along life's continuum is something everyone strives to be prepared for. Throughout life we all face many of life's different challenges, but we endeavor to develop strategies and coping mechanisms to minimize the impact these destructive forces can have on us.

An organization that employs hundreds of nurses is in a very positive strategic position to help support and influence the health practices, mental health practices, and awareness of its nurses. Given the very hectic and busy life that most nurses

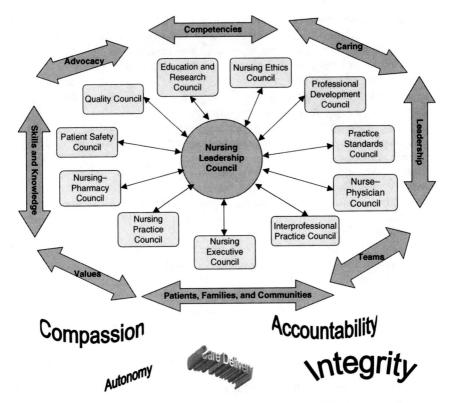

FIGURE 4.1   Employee wellness: Mental health promotion and illness prevention.

lead, they often forget to look after themselves, particularly when it comes to health promotion and illness prevention decisions. An organization that is interested in maintaining the good mental health of its nurses will do much for its operational success because an organization is only as good as the people who work there.

In terms of mental health promotion and mental illness prevention, the following are different strategies an organization can offer and maintain to support the optimal mental health of its nurses. An employer should:

1. Educate its nurses on all available resources that are in existence to help support nurses. This would include resources both internal and external to the organization.
2. Offer regular in-house services to nurse leaders and managers so that they are aware of these resources and can reinforce their use with their frontline nurses.
3. Identify mental health champions in key areas of the organization so that they can provide a supportive internal networking system to help out in mental health crisis events that may arise.
4. Provide structured, up-to-date, and focused mental health training for these champions that will cover such areas as verbal de-escalation, supportive counseling, advocacy and guidance, therapeutic crisis intervention, and suicide intervention.

5. Implement and support educational and public relations initiatives that are visible and transparent to nurses on such topics as smoking, drugs, alcohol, exercise, gambling, nutrition, sleep, and stress management.
6. Ensure that the organization's employee assistance program (EAP) is a top priority for the organization and that it is there as an open door policy, can be used freely and appropriately, and is highly accessible and visibly marketed throughout the organization for everyone to see.
7. Develop a comprehensive plan or strategy that includes the four key work factors of physical environment, organization, employee resources, and professionalism (me).
8. Identify, develop, and enforce zero-tolerance policies that challenge an organization's values, such as respect and integrity.
9. Use all organizational communication media/avenues to disseminate the message that employee mental health is a top priority for the organization and that you are there to talk openly about it.
10. Delegate the human resources department to hold regular or at least annual employee health conferences/workshops on selected key issues, such as stress management, the value of exercise, and the impact of sleep, diet, and other factors on mental health.
11. Recognize the value of the employee health and wellness department and optimize every opportunity to illustrate how valuable a resource it is.

The whole concept of mental health promotion takes us back to the old saying that "an ounce of prevention is worth a pound of cure." When the mental health of nurses is involved, the same theory applies to what organizations can do to promote prevention.

Health promotion policies in particular are one key mechanism that can help build a mentally healthy workplace. Health promotion policies can provide a user-friendly framework for the planning, development, implementation, and evaluation of healthy public policies (The Health Communication Unit, University of Toronto, 2004). A policy manual that focuses on the health of your employees will go far with respect to how you view and support your employees when it comes to their health, mental health, and overall well-being. Including real-life examples and issues that most employees typically face, such as workplace stress and work–life conflict, can help build an allegiance on the part of your employees.

The development of brochures and signage that focus on issues such as the value of communication, dealing with stress, and working through conflict is also a valuable strategy that organizations can undertake. Again, it lets your employees know that you take these issues very seriously and are willing to engage with and be supportive of them in such areas.

However, these policies are of no benefit if they are just sitting on the shelf covered in dust. Make them public, use your printing room/shop to develop and highlight some of the key messages of those policies, and post them in highly visible areas for all nurses and other staff to see. Use a high-gloss print and rich, eye-catching colors.

RECOGNITION AND REWARD

An organization that values its employees is an organization that will succeed in today's ever-changing and complex society. Recognition and reward of staff is simply acknowledging, respecting, and appreciating the efforts, accomplishments, and endeavors of nurses that often take them beyond the call of duty, and letting them and others know that these nurses excel in whatever they do. However, this is something that must be done in a timely, fair, appropriate, and consistent manner (GM@W, 2012).

There are various forums in which an organization can recognize nurses for their good efforts, admirable accomplishments, and a performance well done. Such forums and/or events can include the following:

1. Offer competitive salaries and/or bonuses (such as signing bonuses) if and when appropriate and possible.
2. Recognize years of service worked with a small memento or gift certificate.
3. Recognize accomplishments such as completion of educational programs through continuing education incentives, bursaries, and scholarships.
4. Offer small monetary incentives/bonuses for not having used any sick leave days during any fiscal or calendar year.
5. Host nursing gala award events. These should be annual events where nurses and their peers are recognized and nominated for various admirable attributes and efforts in their everyday work. Some categories would include most outstanding nurse on any unit, most caring nurse, best student mentor, and greatest nurse leader, manager, or educator; to name just a few.

The recognition and reward of nurses who are outstanding in their performance and efforts for one reason or another is of immense benefit for an organization. Some fringe benefits include increased nurse motivation; increased sense of job pride and commitment; increased rates of retention and recruitment; increased self-esteem, self-value, and self-concept; enhanced nursing unit and/or team success; increased nurse interest and participation in work issues and projects; encouragement of excellence; and increased positive output and work environment, one characterized by courtesy, respect, and understanding in relations with colleagues, clients/families, and/or other professionals (GM@W, 2012).

As suggested by human resource specialist Derek Irvine (2011), sometimes all employees need to know is that someone is paying attention to what they are doing and/or what they are achieving in the workplace, and that it has meaning and importance. He has blogged on several other aspects of promoting recognition and reward and the benefits they bring. Previously, he has also suggested such employer strategies as hosting annual awards dinners, recognizing successes and accomplishments in a timely manner (not months or years later), making the recognition or reward specific to the task at hand (not just a quick "thanks" as you pass through the hallway or stairwell), and making it personal by communicating how the success, event, and/or action impacted you as a member of the same organization. Finally, he suggests that this be done in a spontaneous or surprising manner, such that it is not expected and not contingent on an action that needs to be performed. As suggested by Irvine, "Engaging in a coaching or feedback conversation to acknowledge the employee's efforts and redirect to more important paths is also a powerful form of recognition" (Irvine, 2011). Furthermore, you need to walk the talk, not just talk the talk. "When providing people with the direction and expected behaviors, you need to be alert to the fact that they will hold you accountable. People want to know if you are walking the talk. They will be watching your every move and you need to be one in the same . . . every minute of every day."

In his work and research on employee recognition and reward, Irvine's (2011) review of the Ascent Group's annual report revealed many highlights of making recognition and reward a success. Some quotes follow:

1. **"Reinforce behaviors and reward results.** Recognize the right behaviors and communicate such that the employee's behavior becomes a model within the work group." When you define the behaviors that reflect your values, your employees begin to see the values come alive in their daily work.
2. **"Be timely, specific, and communicate!** Make sure you recognize behavior and reward results in a timely manner so employees know exactly why they are being recognized." Recognition given at the annual banquet or performance review does nothing to reinforce in the moment precisely what it is you need them to repeat. Make sure messages of recognition are specific and reference the value demonstrated.
3. **"Match the reward to the person and the achievement."** Every person is different. A BBQ isn't motivating for a person who lives in a high-rise apartment building. A gift card to a steakhouse isn't rewarding for a vegetarian. Let your employees choose what's personally memorable and culturally relevant for them.
4. **"Involve employees in the design and refinement of your reward and recognition programs."** Turn employees into program evangelists, ensuring rapid program adoption.
5. **"Don't just offer rewards and recognition for frontline employees."** Extend the program to cover all employees in the department so the entire group is working toward the same goals.
6. **"Look to technology to facilitate program administration and tracking."** Doing any of this strategically—especially on a global scale—is far beyond the capabilities of an Excel spreadsheet.
7. **"Measure the effectiveness and impact of your reward and recognition programs."** Without a strong technology solution, it is impossible to measure results.

IDENTIFYING A MENTALLY HEALTHY WORKPLACE CHAMPION

An organization can take into consideration many different aspects when it is deciding who can best fill the shoes of a workplace champion for mental health (Mental Health Commission of Canada [MHCC], 2013):

- Identify an individual with the organizational competencies and influence to be successful.

■ These aptitudes should be balanced with a personal connection to the issue and with passion and energy for the work.
■ Ensure that the person has sufficient corporate support and commitment.

The champion of workplace mental health is one who can provide passionate leadership, liaise effectively with all stakeholders to ensure successful implementation, communicate with employees, consider how recognition and reward for contributing to a mentally healthy workplace can be incorporated into the strategy, support and encourage all stakeholders to walk the talk, and promote and maintain engagement at all levels so that workplace mental health remains a valued priority (MHCC, 2013).

STAFF ENGAGEMENT

The engagement of nurses in the workplace is an integral component for both nurses and corporations. Staff engagement can be defined in many ways. Williams (2010) identifies some core definitions of employee engagement as follows:

1. "Commitment, work ethic, and loyalty."
2. "A combination of perceptions—including satisfaction, commitment, pride, loyalty, sense of personal responsibility, and willingness to be an advocate for the organization—that have an impact on behavior."
3. "An individual sense of purpose and focused energy, evident to others in their display of personal initiative, effort, and persistence, that is directed toward organizational goals."

Many opportunities arise within corporations for nurses to become more and better engaged in the operational mandate of the organization. Some such opportunities may include workplace policies and procedures, projects, and new initiatives. Staff engagement is recognized as one of the most significant investments that organizations can make for themselves, their business, and their clientele (Irvine, 2013a).

Employee engagement presents many benefits for the organization. Openly involving and inviting nurses to participate in organization, planning, goals, and program, can be a win–win policy for the organization. Good employee engagement for an organization often translates into increases in profitability; productivity and reputation; attendance; earnings where applicable; nurse morale, job satisfaction, and motivation; quality of patient care and service delivery; innovation; organizational citizenship behaviors; and nurses' personal behaviors and choices that are of hidden benefit to an organization. Engagement also results in decreased turnover (GM@W, 2012; Williams, 2010).

With engagement, nurses feel more valued, motivated to exceed, and emotionally passionate about their jobs. Furthermore, nurses feel more energized, enthusiastic, empowered, and satisfied when they feel that they are engaged and even valued by their employing organization (GM@W, 2012). Engagement supports nurses so that they come to enjoy, look forward to, and feel more connected and committed to their work and the organization as a whole.

Unfortunately, the lack of engagement of nurses in the workplace has been a long-standing issue and concern. A lack of engagement is what is often found and reported. When nurse engagement is lacking, a nurse's personal life and professional quality of work life decrease, as do an organization's bottom line. In the absence of engagement, nurses can often feel emotionally exhausted, not interested, and not valued, and so they are not productive. Organizationally, productivity decreases, staff turnover increases, and workplace deviance flourishes as nurses exert minimal effort to complete tasks and absenteeism increases (GM@W, 2012).

Leaders can create staff engagement through many avenues. Dale Carnegie (2012) suggests that "employee engagement and loyalty are more vital than ever to an organization's success and competitive advantage" and that "the biggest hurdle facing today's leaders is how to interact with and create an engaged workforce."

As a leader, you have a sense about who knows what and who does not when it comes to the organization's mission, values, and purpose. However, as recently found, "the average person in the trenches does not know what game they are supposed to be playing or how to play it" (Lee, 2012). In a survey of employees conducted by Leadership IQ, only 34% of employees said they could articulate their employer's strategic goals. Even worse, when asked to explain their understanding of those goals, only 51% of the people who said they could were able to do so. Thus, only about one in six employees actually knew what their employer was trying to achieve. Only one in six knew what game they were supposed to be playing and how the game was played. "If you don't know or know very little about what it is your organization is trying to achieve and how to get there, you will not be able to engage in the overall excitement" (Lee, 2012).

David Lee (2012), founder of Human Nature at Work, states that if you suspect that the nurses of your organization do not feel engaged, you need to do something about it. You need to make sure they know what it is the organization values, and staff engagement is one such priority for many organizations. Make it a point at a town hall meeting or provide some graphic poster highlighting the value of engagement to say these things:

1. Your mission and vision in non–business-speaking terms
2. Your strategic goals
3. Key initiatives
4. What other departments or divisions are doing
5. Current marketplace realities and how your marketplace works
6. Business financials and how their work impacts these
7. How their job contributes to the big picture
8. How specifically they can maximize their contribution

Better yet, make the most of the time you spend with your employees. Tap into your staff meetings, place the topic of engagement and respectful workplace on your agenda, bring it up at performance appraisals, and ensure that the following are mentioned at some point in time:

1. Share this story with your employees and fellow managers.
2. Ask your employees how "in the loop" they feel.
3. Ask them to articulate your mission, vision, and strategic goal.

4. Ask them to identify their key result areas—how they provide the most value and maximally contribute to your strategic goals.
5. Find out what information they feel they are lacking and what they want to know more about. You can use the aforementioned list to facilitate this conversation:
   a. Your mission and vision in simple lay terms
   b. Your strategic goals
   c. Your key initiatives
   d. What other departments or divisions are doing
   e. Current marketplace realities and how your marketplace works
   f. Business financials and how their work impacts these
   g. How their job contributes to the big picture
   h. How specifically they can maximize their contribution
6. Collect and continually share stories that illustrate and dramatize the following:
   a. What your organization is striving to achieve and why
   b. The difference your organization makes and the value you provide
   c. The challenges you face and how you are overcoming them
   d. Employee contributions

It is important for organizations to realize that a happy nurse is an engaged nurse. Irvine (2013a, 2013b) writes about four ways to create a happy and engaged workforce. The following are vital for organizations to recognize if they wish to attract and maintain their workforce:

1. **Build a strong social fabric.** The Gallup Q12 assessment of employee engagement includes the question "I have a best friend at work" for a reason. Building close relationships with others at work changes the focus of projects from simply "work that must get done" to "work that we accomplish together." It's an important twist to happiness in the workplace.
2. **Promote activities that fit their strengths, values, and lifestyle.** Don't we all work much more efficiently, effectively, and—yes—happily when we're doing what we know we do well and what we agree with morally and ethically? When our company's values align with our own, it's easier to be happy at work.
3. **Practice gratitude.** Practicing gratitude is much more than just being thankful. Truly "practicing gratitude" means we also step outside ourselves and our own priorities to notice what others around us are doing and the great work they are delivering (whether it's directly helpful to us or just generally good). That ability to look beyond the personal gives us all greater perspective on what the group as a whole is doing to achieve the mission.
4. **Give them direction.** Of course, having that greater perspective requires that we first understand what the greater mission is and how we as individuals can contribute to achieving it. Companies of all stripes and colors have these missions, visions, strategic objectives, and 5-year plans. The challenge lies in translating that for employees into personal, meaningful work, which has been identified through rigorous research as the primary motivator in the workplace, by far.
5. **Recognize people.** With respect to building a supportive culture at work, a culture must be created that is owned by every employee. And the most solid

culture to build that can feed all of these elements is a true culture of recognition. A culture of recognition is supported by a strategic and social employee recognition program that encourages everyone to notice, appreciate, and recognize others for living the company values and contributing to the strategic objectives. Detailed messages of praise from peers and managers give us the perspective we need on the importance, value, and meaningfulness of what we do every day, and that leads to happy and engaged employees.

6. **Offer challenges.**
7. **Spotlight the deeper meaning in the work.**
8. **Remember that employees are humans, not robots.**
9. **Make space for employees' lives.**

Dishman (2013) suggests the following five rules for happy employees:

1. Happy employees don't stay in one role for too long. Movement and the perception of improvement create satisfaction. Status quo, on the other hand, creates burnout.
2. There is a strong correlation between happiness and meaning; having a meaningful impact on the world around you is actually a better predictor of happiness than many other things you think will make you happy.
3. A workplace is far likelier to be a happy place when policies are in place to ensure that people regularly receive acknowledgement and praise for a job well done.
4. Recognize that employees are people first and workers second, and create policies that focus on their well-being as individuals.
5. Emphasize that work–life integration as a balance may be hard to achieve. The glass always has to be perceived as half full, not half empty.

Unequivocally going hand in hand with a lack of workforce engagement, there are other known reasons why people quit their jobs. According to a study reviewed by Toth (2012), the following are the top 10 reasons why people often quit their jobs: limited career opportunities (16%), lack of respect/support from supervisor (13%), money (12%), lack of interesting/challenging job duties (11%), lack of leadership from supervisor (9%), bad work hours (6%), unavoidable reasons (5%), bad employee relations by supervisor (4%), favoritism by supervisor (4%), and lack of recognition for contributions (4%).

Toth (2012) has found that 88% of employees leave their job and/or organization because of things other than money. This contradicts widespread beliefs and myths that 89% of employers believe employees leave because of money. From one of the many webinars by Toth (2012) in the area of staff engagement, he shares the following facts and figures:

1. Only 29% of employees are truly engaged.
2. Disengaged employees are five times more likely to leave than engaged employees.
3. Despite all the investment in and attention paid to engagement in recent years, engagement is actually decreasing.
4. Pay doesn't rank among the top four engagement drivers.

The golden rule applies to organizations, as well; you treat your employees the way you'd like to be treated yourself. According to the experts, the number-one thing managers can do to make employees stay is to "value" them (Right Management), "care" about them (Monster/Unum), and be "genuinely interested in their well-being" (Towers Watson, 2012).

HOW TO KEEP EMPLOYEES HAPPY AND ENGAGED

Figure 4.2 is the Magical Wheel of Engagement as designed by Toth (2012).
   In accordance with Toth's model, employees desperately want their leaders to:

- **Envision** a bold, clear, and inspirational future
- **Empathize** with them to understand their motivations and strengths
- **Enhance** their skills through education, exposure, and experience
- **Empower** them to do meaningful work
- **Evaluate** them on a truthful and timely basis
- **Encourage** them as much as is humanly possible

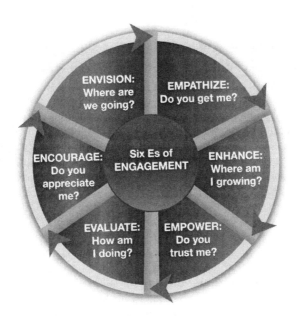

FIGURE 4.2   Toth's Magical Wheel of Engagement.

Toth (2013) says, "If you do those six things, your employees will feel the LOVE and will stay with you forever. If you don't, they won't."

Human capital and expanding on efforts to increase staff engagement are truly a win–win situation for everyone. All too often in today's industrialized countries do we hear about the rapid growth and expansion of satellite service sites in health care organizations. Haydon (2013a) suggests that the rapid growth of organizations can lead to "damaged human capital," and no one benefits when your human resources are playing second fiddle to operational success. First off the mark, disengaged employees can cost organizations upwards of $3,400 for every $10,000 worth of salary (Haydon, 2013b). If an organization is driven by productivity, cutbacks, and a polished reputation where employees are left feeling stressed, overworked, and disrespected, then yes, they will become disengaged.

As found by Decision-Wise (2013) and highlighted by Haydon (2013b), "Employee engagement and customer satisfaction are strongly correlated (as are customer satisfaction and financial performance, but that's a different study). When comparing individual locations across the client company, the locations with the highest proportions of *fully engaged* employees had nearly 3 times higher growth in customer satisfaction ratings than the locations with the highest proportion of *disengaged* employees. So, as your company experiences exponential growth, don't let it be at the expense of your most influential employees. How your customers are treated directly affects how they spend their money—and how they spend their money determines whether or not your company will be open tomorrow."

Involvement and Influence From the Top

Beyond the engagement of nurses in the workplace is the motion of getting them involved. Where there is an opportunity to exert influence in the day-to-day decision-making process of an organization, nurses' good mental health is encouraged and promoted. Collectively, nurses feel they have much to contribute to what work is done, when it is done, and who should be involved for the best potential outcome for all.

Numerous aspects of nurses' work can invite them to have a greater say, and such opportunities can relate to their specific role/job, unit/departmental activities, program or team activities, patient relations, family meetings, and issues involving the organization as a whole (GM@W, 2012). The advent of nurses being able to become intricately involved in organizations supports many short- and long-term benefits for both. Nurses who feel they are contributing positively to the work of an organization, or who feel they are at least being given the opportunity to do so, feel more engaged in their work, have greater job satisfaction and pride, have an enhanced sense of self and value, and are more willing to go that extra mile to ensure that the job gets done and done right. In addition, they are provided the opportunity to showcase their knowledge and skill set, enhance organizational commitment, and increase creativity and innovation for successful options. For the organization, the benefits are significant, often in the form of increased output and productivity, decreased operational costs, and hence greater recruitment and retention success.

The involvement and visible interaction of senior leaders and executives of an organization are highly motivational (MHCC, 2013). According to the MHCC, there is a significant role to be played by many departments in an organization toward building a healthy workforce and environment. At all levels of an organization, much can be done to build on and enhance workplace mental health. For senior leaders, in particular, the following are recommended:

1. Developing a concise statement of principle on the workplace mental health strategy
2. Setting the measurement framework by identifying tool(s) and data to assess the current state of workplace mental health
3. Leading the collaborative development of a full workplace mental health policy along with employees, unions, and other stakeholders
4. Ensuring that policies and strategic direction are implemented

Even the board of directors has a valuable role to play (MHCC, 2013):

1. Setting strategic direction to include workplace mental health
2. Approving mental health policy, providing direction, and reviewing outcomes
3. Keeping workplace mental health on the board agenda by reporting on progress

Other levels and departments of an organization can also be active in creating and fostering a mentally healthy workplace environment. As we have previously discussed throughout this book, communication is everything when you are trying to build and sustain a healthy workplace environment. The communication department can therefore contribute, as stated by the MHCC (2013):

1. Raised awareness of the mental health strategy, policy statements, and interventions among internal and external stakeholders.
2. Development of the brand to promote and market the organization as a mentally healthy workplace.

The finance department or the holders of the pocketbook of an organization's funds can also contribute to such efforts by (MHCC, 2013):

1. Reviewing the chief financial operating framework or strategic plan to consider how to record and measure workplace mental health impacts
2. Partnering with benefits providers, the EAP, human resources, and occupational health, outside consultants, or an insurer to obtain utilization data
3. Benchmarking with existing published financial data
4. Picking relevant key indicators that can be followed forward to assess the impact on workplace mental health
5. Considering ways to measure the risk abatement and return on investment of the organizational mental health strategy

Health care professionals should not be left to find their own way to cope with the complexities of patient care. Internal work processes need redesigning (Elmqvist, Fridlund, & Ekebergh, 2012).

Clear Leadership and Expectations

In order to run a ship, the captain must provide clear direction and expectations to all seamen and shipmates on board, such that a smooth journey is traveled. In health care organizations there is no immunity against rippled waters of order, tidal waves of errors, or the tsunami of crises and adverse and sentinel events. However, as on a ship, the CEO, executive teams, and all employees of an organization are not guaranteed a smooth journey.

The provision of clear and understandable directions is a sure factor of success in any organization. It is critical for all employees of any organization to have effective leadership and support, so that nurses know what they need to do when an unexpected event occurs. Furthermore, it is very important for nurses to know how they can contribute or are contributing to the goals of the organization and any changes in the planned strategic directions needed (GM@W, 2012). Directions and expectations that are provided in a timely, organized, easy-to-understand, clear, and concise manner are the ones that get heard and that are supported and adhered to by nurses/employees. As long as these directions and expectations are clearly articulated, relevant, and understood, then there should be very little reason or opportunity for the mental health of the nurses of an organization to become compromised because of misinterpreted, misleading, or confounding leadership directions and expectations.

When effective leadership and clear direction are provided, nurses will most often experience increased morale, resiliency, and trust. This openness and understanding that everyone is on the same page and moving forward with the same plan serves to decrease levels of nurse frustration, animosity, and conflict. However, at the same time, nurses become more content in their workplace and less likely to call in sick or seek workers' compensation for lost time (GM@W, 2012).

The Safety of the Workplace Environment

The physical safety of a workplace environment is perhaps one of the main issues that organizations can help to ensure so that effort and energies are not wasted on worry about something so fundamental to all human beings and even animals. According to Maslow's hierarchy of needs, physical safety is the first and foremost fundamental need for everyone's healthy development (Maslow, 1962), and the physical environment of the workplace is no different. An organization that does all it can to help ensure a safe workplace, is one that is taken seriously and respected by its employees.

A safe physical environment for employees is one that will help them feel more secure, protected, and engaged. Guarding Minds @ Work (2012) suggests that "higher levels in the confidence of the safety protection at work results in lower rates of psychological distress and mental health issues" and that "safety is enhanced through minimizing hazards, training, response to incidents, and the opportunity to have meaningful input into the workplace policies and practices. The concept of 'safety climate' is linked to this factor as they both relate to the larger culture or climate of the organization." Measures that can help organizations achieve such a goal can include the development of policies and crisis intervention training (such as a code white team in your health care facility) and a demonstrated concern for employees' physical safety. In today's climate, most health care organizations also have in place an occupational health and safety committee, an occupational health department, or a human resources department of health and wellness, all of which can help orchestrate interventions to promote and maintain a physically safe workplace environment.

Policy and Program Development

The development of policies within an organization is an effective, evidence-informed manner to promote positive mental health for the nurses employed there. Policies serve many purposes within an organization (Finkelman, 2006, p.173).

Policies and procedures should be the mainstay of what an organization expects of all staff and nurses. Policies and procedures are standard across an organization, evidence-informed, consistently enforced for everyone, and representative of acceptable practices. They are the most called-upon resource that guides the practices and expectations of an organization. As a result, the establishment of policies and procedures should prove beneficial not only for organizations but also for individual nurses. The mere existence of standardized policies and procedures can act as a significant support to nurses in their daily job. Generally, policies and procedures give nurses an increased sense of assuredness and confidence that their performance is up to standard and organizational expectations. Furthermore, they can help give nurses a greater sense of self-esteem, satisfaction, and well-being because they know they are doing exactly as is expected, needed, and supported by research.

For the organization, the benefits come in the form of increased standards and quality of care, consistency of practices and expectations, an increased sense of fairness for all nurses, and a smoother operational and functional organization. In addition, inadequacies, violations of the organization's values and mandate, and patient safety issues resulting from nurses' incompetence, poor performance, poor judgment, and unsafe or unacceptable patient care can be addressed in a sophisticated manner.

The absence of standardized policies and procedures can be detrimental to both nurses and the organization. Without policies and procedures, workplace conflict would escalate, tensions would rise, and self-doubt and poor esteem would increase; also, nurses would begin to feel uncertain, unsupported, and alienated. Organizationally, chaos would foster a culture of disrespect and discontent, in which liabilities would increase and standards of patient care would be repeatedly jeopardized.

Protective Disclosure Policies

The development of protective disclosure policies and/or whistleblower policies is yet another measure that organizations can complete to help enhance nurses' workplace mental health.

Workload Management

The topic of workload management is one that seems to always receive a great deal of attention in the nursing profession. In Chapter 3, we saw firsthand how increased workload can lead to increased stress and even burnout. In a climate of nursing shortages, work overload, complex patient care, and budget restraint, the topic of workload management should be critical for any organization to recognize and address.

An organization that can help achieve a balanced workplace for nurses should elicit great admiration and envy. A nursing environment where workload management is monitored and well maintained produces many benefits for both the nurses and the organization. A balanced workload decreases levels of stress, increases fulfillment and job satisfaction, and has a positive organizational ripple effect in the form of greater productivity, increased commitment, and enhanced recruitment and retention. To address and monitor workload balances for nurses, organizations can adopt many strategies.

However, in the absence of close monitoring and maintenance of workload management, nurses feel physically and psychologically drained, without control, overwhelmed, and stressed, and they experience a decreased sense of self-adequacy, value, and personal achievement. For the organization, the quality of patient care suffers, liabilities increase, and human resource replacement costs escalate.

Psychological Job Fit

A disconnect between nurses' skill mix, knowledge, competencies, and experience and the actual job they are hired to fulfill can wreak havoc with their mental health at work. Nurses' competencies and practices are forever changing and evolving, and it is important for organizations to be cognizant of this. An organization's department of human resources can help determine if the psychological job fit is optimal, and that the hired nurse has the knowledge, skills, and expertise to complete all the requirements of the job. Furthermore, an organization's professional practice department and chief nurse officer can be consulted on these matters. As found by Spence-Laschinger, Wong, and Greco (2006), when job fit or perceived job fit is poor, it can negatively impact nurse empowerment, energy, and motivation and so result in burnout and emotional exhaustion. Furthermore, what a nurse feels she or he can and cannot do (subjective job fit) may conflict with what the organization determines the nurse can and cannot do (objective job fit; GM@W, 2012).

A psychological job fit that matches the needs and skills of the nurse with the mandate and requirements of the job helps to build and support a mentally healthier workplace. The benefits arising from an appropriate psychological job fit are many and include the following:

1. Decreased health complaints
2. Decreased absenteeism rates
3. Increased self-esteem, value, and self-concept
4. Increased job satisfaction, performance, and commitment
5. Decreased turnover and increased retention
6. Decreased risk for the development of mental illness

A poor psychological job fit that goes unrecognized and unchecked has negative ramifications for both the nurse and the organization. The nurse experiences emotional exhaustion; increased stress levels, uncertainty, and frustration; and decreased energy and motivation. From an organizational perspective, there is decreased productivity, increased liability, decreased morale, and increased conflict (GM@W, 2012).

Recruitment and Retention Challenges

It is no secret that nursing shortages loom in all sectors of health care. Any country, state, or province that is not experiencing a nursing shortage is a rarity. Given that a nursing shortage dominates many countries globally, it should be all the more important for health care organizations to perform prudently and competitively, but to do so in a manner that is supportive, inviting, and admirable for nurses seeking employment opportunities. Hidden discrimination, with the screening out of employees who have a diagnosed mental illness, is no longer acceptable practice, although in some cases it may still go undetected. However, health care organizations need to move past this policy as nurses with mental illnesses are just as, if not more, competent than their mentally healthy counterparts.

PROMOTING GOOD MENTAL HEALTH AND PREVENTING ILLNESS IN THE WORKPLACE

Promoting and strengthening the mental health of employees and creating a mentally healthy and friendly workplace environment are important undertakings for organizations. The promotion of good mental health in the workplace helps to achieve several goals, such as increased productivity, engagement, and commitment. Sturgeon (2012) suggests that it is an essential component of health in general; however, it is unfortunately often overlooked.

There are many different strategies a health care organization can utilize to help promote and foster positive mental health in the workplace. These include strategies such as the following:

1. Inviting a guest speaker who is a dietician (I could just as easily have said a diabetes educator) to talk about good nutrition and "eating on the run";
2. Developing and offering a mini-gym for employees, free of charge, to promote exercise and increased activity;
3. Scheduling small retreats for the staff; and
4. Developing a schedule for weekly or monthly activities, such as a staff BBQ, a staff walk, and so on.

Organizations need to be aware of the amount of stress their employees are experiencing. Changes to the organization can make for a more mentally healthy workplace, especially when employees feel appropriately rewarded for their effort and in control of their work (CMHA, 2010). Employment and work conditions are important determinants of health for adults, so employers and employees must work together to identify areas where improvements and changes are needed at both a managerial and an individual level. The participation of employees at all levels must be supported through programs that allow them to be involved in making decisions about issues that affect mental well-being in the workplace (Keleher & Armstrong, 2005). In addition to participation, programs that focus on enhancing employees' sense of control, initiative, appreciation, self-esteem and self-worth, sense of belonging, and social support result in improvements in both the mental health and productivity of an organization (Lahtinen, Joubert, Raeburn, & Jenkins, 2005).

Effective interventions by organizations should help to reduce the strain of deteriorating workplace mental health, and some of these can easily be achieved through such supports as counseling to improve coping skills, increasing an employer's awareness of mental health issues, identifying common goals and positive aspects of the work process, creating a balance between job demands and occupational skills, providing training in social skills, developing the psychosocial climate of the workplace, providing counseling, enhancing work capacity, implementing early rehabilitation strategies, assessing workload, enhancing job control and decision-making latitude, and enhancing social support (Funk, Gale, Grigg, Minoletti, & Yasamy, 2005; World Health Organization [WHO], 2001).

Once employers know what is available to them, it is critical to pass this knowledge on to employees. Other strategies organizations can employ include the following (Scott-Clarke, 2011):

1. Better educate employees on the resources that are available, both inside the organization and in the community
2. Ensure that front-line managers are aware of the resources and have received proper training in how to help employees in the workplace who may be struggling with a mental health issue
3. Utilize your benefits plan and EAP providers to ensure you are getting as much as you can out of your programs.

The Global Business and Economic Roundtable on Addiction and Mental Health has also produced a comprehensive plan to help employers, employees, and unions deal with mental health issues in the workplace. The plan contains comprehensive guidelines to promote mental health as a workplace asset and to reduce the rates of disability due to mental disorders. Bill Wilkerson (2013), chairman of both the U.S.–Canada Forum on Mental Health and Productivity and the Great-West Life Centre for Mental Health in the Workforce, advises the following:

1. Champion mental health personally and create opportunities for open discussion and dialogue on the topic.
2. Audit the organization's disability experience, tackle trouble spots in work environments, and fight negative management practices reflected in higher rates of employee absence.
3. Develop specific policy objectives and concrete targets to reduce mental disabilities to 10% from 30% to 40% of the total disability experience, and decrease long-term disability claims (due to mental health conditions) to virtually zero over 5 years.
4. Equip managers with the tools and training needed to assume accountability for mental health standards in the workplace.
5. Alert managers to one particularly jarring fact: The longer an employee is off work, the less likely it is that that employee will ever return.

6. Disability leave policies should allow for the time it takes for treatments to work, for recovery to occur, and for a gradual return to work based on sound medical and management grounds.
7. An employee's reduced symptoms and recovery of functional capabilities should be matched with accommodations at work to help the employee ease back into the job.

Work–Life Balance

Organizations can also help employees achieve better work–life balance. The following strategies have been recommended (Workplace Mental Health Promotion, 2013):

1. Identify ways of reducing employee workloads. Special attention needs to be given to reducing the workloads of managers and professionals in all sectors. Employees should be asked for suggestions; they are often in the best position to identify ways of streamlining work.
2. Reduce reliance on both paid and unpaid overtime by employees.
3. Recognize and reward overtime work.
4. Reduce job-related travel time for employees.
5. Make alternative work arrangements more widely available within the organization. These might include flextime or the opportunity to work at home for part of the work week.
6. Give employees the opportunity to say no when asked to work overtime. Saying no should not be a career-limiting move. Employees should not have to choose between having a family and career advancement.
7. Examine work expectations, rewards, and benefits through a "life cycle" lens (i.e., what employees are able to do and motivated to do and what rewards and benefits they hope will change with each life cycle stage).

Address Stigma

We will talk in depth about stigma in Chapter 11, but the value of organizations recognizing that it exists is important. For an organization, the presence of stigma among colleagues, particularly when it is directed against those who have known mental health and/or addiction concerns, can be highly debilitating.

Because stigma can create just as much, if not more, stress than other matters, it can acutely impact the goals an organization sets out to achieve, such as safe, competent patient care and a safe, healthy workplace environment. The absence of these can cripple productivity, jeopardize service delivery and patient care, and so increase liability. There is much that organizations can do to help address and/or minimize the existence and impact of stigma.

TRANSPARENCY AND ACCOUNTABILITY

Transparency and accountability are the order of the day for all health care organizations. In an era when people are more educated and nurses race against the clock of technology and deal with advanced care practices and complex clients, it should be an issue of urgent concern for organizations to accept and communicate information regarding adverse events, mistakes, and inefficiencies. Gone are the days of hiding errors, brushing mishaps under the rug, and turning a blind eye to poor or substandard practice. Today, focus and value are placed on organizations accepting responsibility for what they do and what they can offer, on their being transparent to society regarding what information is available and what realistically occurs, and on using honesty as the best policy to disseminate any vital information needed to reach those involved. All nurses, and leaders in particular, should strive to demonstrate integrity and good clinical judgment when making decisions, engaging in teamwork, implementing care, and orchestrating change.

Accountability and transparency are two important elements of good governance. They are not easily separated because they encompass the same goals and use the same actions to achieve those goals. Transparency is a powerful force that, when consistently applied, can help fight corruption, improve governance, and promote accountability. While the concept of *accountability* refers to the legal and reporting framework, organizational structure, strategy, procedures, and actions, *transparency* refers to timely, reliable, clear, and relevant public reporting on an organization's status, mandate, strategic directions, activities, financial management, operations, and performance. In any event, both accountability and transparency serve to help ensure the following (Kanwit, 2008):

1. Individuals are held responsible for their actions and decisions.
2. Quality control and assurance obligations are met.
3. Standards of patient care are upheld.
4. Identified areas of risk are identified, addressed, and followed up.
5. Legal obligations, audit processes, and performance measures are met.
6. Financial statements and public funds are clearly identifiable with supporting rationale.
7. High standards of integrity, morals, values, and ethics are being practiced.
8. Policies, procedures, and practices are aligned with evidence-based research that is current, safe, validated, and effective.
9. Open and/or public reporting is expected and will include any peer reviews, audit findings, and external reviews.
10. Report cards, scorecards, and/or collated data findings are maintained and shared publicly.

Contrary to popular findings about the positive aspects of accountability, Harber and Ball (2003) have determined otherwise. They suggest that "accountability" has come to mean something much more and much worse than initially thought. It seems to carry a meaning of "who is to blame?" In other words, if there is accountability, then someone is behind the error in judgment or practice, someone is to blame, and "how should they be punished?" They add that this approach can lead to blame avoidance, blame shifting, cover-ups, infighting, defensive behaviors, and anti-learning dynamics and be the cause of even further dysfunction in a health system that has already been diagnosed as being among the least healthy work environments in the country.

This could drive nurses into hiding their errors, covering up their mistakes, pointing fingers, scapegoating, and denying responsibility. Although this suggests yet another irony of trying to govern and create a healthy and respectful workplace, the research to support such a stance is very limited.

PROMOTING HUMAN RIGHTS AT WORK

It is safe to say that most, if not all, countries have some form of declaration of human rights. These human rights dictate and expect that a society support the concept that all individuals should have an opportunity equal with that of other individuals to make for themselves the lives that they are able and wish to lead and to have their needs accommodated, consistent with their duties and obligations as members of society, without being hindered or prevented from doing so by discriminatory practices based on race, national or ethnic origin, color, religion, age, sex, sexual orientation, marital status, family status, disability, or conviction for an offense for which a pardon has been granted or in respect of which a record suspension has been ordered (Government of Canada, 2013b).

Extending human rights to the workplace, the Equality and Human Rights Commission of Britain (2010) suggests that such a workplace is "an environment where everyone is treated with dignity and respect, where the talents and skills of different groups are valued, and where productivity and customer service improve because the workforce is happier, more motivated, and more aware of the benefits that inclusion can bring."

Building an inclusive workplace has many benefits for the people and the organization. The Equality and Human Rights Commission suggests that these benefits include promoting equality, human rights and increased productivity, improved motivation and retention, and the creation of an inclusive and adaptable service for employees and patients. An inclusive workplace can be created in the following steps, with more detail available at the website of the Equality and Human Rights Commission of Britain (2010):

1. Consider what you want to achieve and what the benefits will be.
2. Undertake an inclusion review of your workplace.
3. Decide where work is needed and create an action plan.
4. Communicate the plan with staff and put the plan into action.
5. Review, monitor, and evaluate the plan's impact and use what you find to plan future action.

In achieving an inclusive workplace, the benefits are multifold and include such things as attracting new talent and creative and innovative employees; increasing retention rates of productive and committed employees; creating a culture change that permeates all programs, departments, and even the community at large; creating a larger appeal to patients and businesses; and optimizing the organization's reputation as a leader in health care delivery and services (Equality and Human Rights Commission of Britain, 2010).

STANDARDS OF WORKPLACE MENTAL HEALTH

The creation of standards of workplace mental health is not something that has yet caught on among businesses and large organizations. Just as the professional and governing body of a discipline has standards and expected practices, workplaces can do the same. In very recent years, there has been a noticeable movement on this paradigm shift in workplaces. In January 2013, Canada was the first country in the world to release such a precedent-setting standards document with its creation of the National Standard for Psychological Health and Safety in the Workplace (Goar, 2013; Gordon, 2013; MHCC, 2013). This document was developed in response to rising concerns about the effect that mental health was having on the workplace, productivity, safety, and risk as well as rising disability claims—all very common threads found in many other countries (Gordon, 2013). This standardized tool will help organizations to "tackle the issue by creating workplaces that promote mental health, reduce stress, and support employees dealing with mental illness." This 61-page "code of good practices is endorsed by business, labour, the federal government, the nonprofit sector, and the aboriginal community. It reflects a societal recognition that mental illness can no longer be neglected or treated as a personal weakness. It is the culmination of 14 years of research, advocacy, consciousness-raising, and consensus building." Although the standard is voluntary and not legislated or mandated, in brief, mental illness is an issue that no business can afford to ignore. It is free and can be downloaded from http://shop.csa.ca/en/canada/occupational-health-and-safety-management/cancsa-z1003-13bnq-9700-8032013/invt/z10032013/?utm_source=redirect&utm_medium=vanity&utm_content=folder&utm_campaign=z1003.

The purposes of the standard are the following (Morneau Shepell, 2013):

1. Reduce people and cost risks related to mental health.
2. Promote productivity and engagement.
3. Reduce potential liabilities related to the workplace legislation and employee mental illness.
4. Develop and continuously improve work environments.

Furthermore, it can"help companies identify potential hazards to mental health and where they can improve policies and practices. The new standard will allow organizations to analyze their own workplaces to assess and control risks associated with organizational changes and job demands, introduce practices to support psychological well-being, and review how well policies and approaches are working" (Gordon, 2013).

FORMS OF LEAVE

Organizations can become very creative with their benefits packages in trying to address the impact that poor mental health has on their organization and on the backbone of employees who enable it to function. One such idea is the creation and/or use of what we will call "mental health days." The development and implementation of mental health days as part of an employee's pay and benefits package is one way that organizations can demonstrate their support for a mentally healthy workplace. These should not be meant to be included in their number of sick leave days, but instead should be separate days in their own right. London states,"Wouldn't it be great if America's workers could take time off to rest, manage their stress, or even see a mental health professional? I am proposing that businesses should institute two or three paid 'mental health days' a year as part of their employee benefits package" (London, 2011). What London proposes is that "people need a mental break from the anxieties and stresses inherent in daily living." Given this, he would like to see "mental health days" become part of an organization's benefit package. He adds that "taking such a step would finally put us on the way toward establishing at least intellectual parity for mental health problems. This, in turn, would lessen the stigma associated with emotional disorders" (London, 2011).

A WHO Health and Work Performance Questionnaire that assesses sick days recently found that the number one reason for absenteeism on the job is depression. Furthermore, a February 2010 issue of the *Harvard Mental Health Letter* found that depression and anxiety are among the top five reasons for absenteeism (London, 2011).

While employees realize they get only so many sick leave days per year, they often feel hesitant about using them for reasons other than sickness, such as just needing a break from work. However, as London (2011) points out,"The ability to take a sick day because of extreme anxiety or stress is just as important as being able to do so because of a severe upper respiratory infection." London advocates and calls to formalize such a benefit; as society grows and evolves, the acceptance of mental health days will also grow and perhaps even minimize the effects of stigma, fear, shame, embarrassment, and discrimination that often accompany leave for stress and mental health reasons. This would put the long-tucked-away issue of mental health at work on the table for open discussion and awareness and optimistically would enhance much needed dialogue about it.

Staff Morale

If an organization wishes to succeed in its operational efficiency, commitment, and mandate with good public relations, the delivery of good quality of care, and engaged employees, the morale of nurses is an absolute necessity. Generally, the morale of staff is defined as the "psychological state of a person as expressed in [his or her] self-confidence, enthusiasm, and loyalty to a cause or organization." Morale is also reflective of the interest, commitment, optimism, and intended conviction about the rightfulness and worth that their actions will exert on the cause in the hope they may be recognized and/or rewarded for such efforts in the future.

Morale serves many purposes for nurses as well as the organization. Most positive efforts and initiatives that an organization introduces and implements will ultimately have a positive effect on the morale of nurses. Sadly, many of these organizational efforts are only common sense items for organizations/businesses that wishes to exceed. Some such actions include, but are not limited to, the following:

1. Be respectful of nurses.
2. Empower nurses. Invite them to participate in the development of a policy and let them chair the policy working group to share their expertise and concerns.

3. Provide feedback and coaching. When opportunities arise, feedback and coaching can be done during a performance appraisal and more immediately through a simple e-mail to just say "thank you for your continued support and efforts."
4. Provide organizational perks and activities. Orchestrate a summer staff BBQ or outing/retreat, or for long hours and days of hard work during a very busy time, offer them some unexpected time off. Take advantage of the different celebrations in society, such as during Christmas; offer the nurses who are working a hot Christmas dinner with all the trimmings.
5. Offer competitive pay, compensation, and benefits packages.
6. Keep the lines of communication open, regular, and consistent.
7. Make regular staff meetings a must, where all nurses can add items of concern to the meeting agenda. Offer regularly held town hall meetings to keep all staff up to date on organizational challenges and positive result/outcomes, and what's important for staff to know.
8. Offer educational initiatives and support them with such things as scholarships, awards, and internal research moneys for nurses who would be interested.
9. Make the organization's operational plan, framework, and goals visible, and be clear as to what the expectations are. This should be done in a manner that promotes fairness and responsibility, respects diversity, and supports any and all efforts.

In most cases, opportunities to promote the morale of nurses do not have to be extensive; as much can be done merely by recognizing a nurse's ongoing commitment and dedication. A mechanism such as boosting staff morale gives much credence to the old adage "An ounce of prevention is worth a pound of cure." A little effort and energy to acknowledge nurses for their hard work and accomplishments will go far in preventing such things as compromised quality of patient care, poor job satisfaction, and decreased commitment and dedication. An organization needs to show it has the desire, interest, commitment, and attention to maintain and boost the morale of its nurses. The use and dissemination of work satisfaction and employee engagement surveys are one simple yet effective means by which organizations can gauge the existing levels of nurse morale.

Poor morale at work impacts significantly on nurses' workplace mental health. Many researchers have found that in today's health care climate, boosting the morale of nurses is a never-ending effort (Callaghan, 2003). Fraught with nursing shortages, increased workloads, and budget spending constraints, the morale of nurses continues to be jeopardized (Callaghan, 2003; Montoro-Rodriguez & Small, 2006). Low morale among nurses often translates into questionable self-competence and self-confidence, increased absenteeism, and again, organizationally, increased costs, increased liabilities, and compromised output, such as in the form of questionable patient safety and quality of care, poor patient satisfaction, and increased costs because of increased nurse absenteeism rates, much of what we highlighted as a cost in Chapter 3.

As found by Montoro-Rodriguez and Small (2006), "Staffing issues such as morale and turnover are thought to have a direct bearing on the quality of the resident experience." Morale and job satisfaction were shown to depend more on variables that can be controlled by managers—such as shift scheduling and allocation and adequate resources—than on individual characteristics that are beyond managers' control. Furthermore, they found that "morale was weak among staff preferring confrontational or avoidance styles of conflict resolution."

Staff morale, satisfaction, and burnout were significantly affected by all aspects of work demand. All were found to exhibit a relationship to the following (Montoro-Rodriguez & Small, 2006):

1. Frequency of shift rotation—decreased satisfaction;
2. Available resources;
3. Conflict resolution styles—in particular, the cooperative style of conflict resolution had a more significant effect on job satisfaction;
4. Adequacy of facility supplies and frequency of team care planning meetings were associated with improved satisfaction;
5. Adequacy of facility supplies;
6. Number of assigned residents per shift; and
7. Frequency of change in assigned residents; each reduced morale and reduced the degree to which respondents considered their work a positive experience.

Responsible and Effective Communication

As we explored in Chapters 1 and 2, the topic of communication underpins not only many mental health issues and concerns in the workplace but also various strategies that can help address such issues. For many employees, it is critical to receive responsible and effective communication from organizations as well as from colleagues and others. There are several things executive and senior leaders of organizations can engage in to make this happen. Employees want and expect to know what is happening within an organization, what their priorities should be, if they change, and all information required for them to do their job efficiently and effectively.

Motivating Employees

Motivating employees is one of the best practices an organization can perform. The following are some suggestions (Heathfield, 2013):

1. Meet with employees following management staff meetings to update them about any company information that may impact their work. Changing due dates, customer feedback, product improvements, training opportunities, and updates on new departmental reporting or interaction structures are all important to employees. Communicate more than you think is necessary.
2. Stop by the work area of employees who are particularly affected by a change to communicate more. Make sure the employees are clear about what the change means for their job, goals, time allocation, and decisions.
3. Communicate daily with every employee who reports to you. Even a pleasant "good morning" enables the employee to engage with you.
4. Hold a weekly one-on-one meeting with each employee who reports to you. They like to know that they will have this time every week. Encourage employees to come prepared with questions, requests for support, troubleshooting ideas for their work, and information that will keep you from being blindsided or disappointed by a failure to produce on schedule or as committed.

GROWTH AND DEVELOPMENT

As previously identified, individuals spend approximately one-third of their life at work. Therefore, much of one's personal and professional growth and development potentially occurs at work. For organizations, this is an excellent opportunity to embrace and identify nurse leaders or potential leaders, nurture an environment that is supportive of its nurses, and recognize opportunities for mentorship, coaching, and succession planning. The support and nurturance of nurses' growth and development are a win–win situation for everybody involved.

Organizations that are chosen as career mainstays for many nurses have and should take every chance to nurture, support, and develop nurses' knowledge base, interpersonal and emotional skills, job competencies, and advanced educational interests and endeavors. The investment of the organization in its nurses reveals many benefits, not only for the organization as a whole but for its nurses as well.

An organization can receive many fringe benefits for supporting the growth and development of its nurses. A nurse's increased repertoire of skill sets, expertise, performance, and successive growth is what strengthens the integrity, capacity, and even the reputation of an organization. Furthermore, an organization's attention and interest in its nurses' growth and development positively reinforce recruitment and retention efforts, enhance cost-saving measures, increase the benchmark of quality care output, and build the organization as having a known reputable interest in its staff in general. Finally, they can increase goal commitment and attainment, in addition to job satisfaction (GM@W, 2012).

For individual nurses, the outcome can also be phenomenal. It not only promotes a sense of value, commitment, and dedication but also provides a challenge to nurses to remain interested, needed, and engaged. Finally, it encourages and promotes the development of self for nurses, and it also promotes skill acquisition, advances employment opportunities for nurses to progress in their careers, and promotes their sense of well-being (GM@W, 2012).

In the absence of opportunities for growth and development, nurses can often feel not valued, bored and disinterested, not appreciated, and not respected, and their performance, interest, and drive decrease. Hence, their sense of self-value and self-respect becomes compromised, and the testing of their own distressed mental health occurs (GM@W, 2012).

Organizationally, productivity decreases, conflict and poor morale flourish, and nurses become disengaged in the organization's efforts, mandate, and performance. As a result, organizational productivity suffers, and its bottom line as a reputable leader in health care services and delivery becomes tarnished.

LEGISLATION

Occupational Safety and Health Acts

Occupational health and safety acts are the cornerstone legislation for providing and ensuring healthy and safe workplaces. For most countries, occupational health and safety acts or some derivative thereof are perhaps the key legislation that organizations are required to follow. The main purpose of an occupational health and safety act is to protect workers from health and safety hazards on the job. It sets out duties for all workplace parties and rights for workers. It establishes procedures for dealing with workplace hazards and provides for enforcement of the law when compliance has not been achieved voluntarily (Ontario Ministry of Labour, 2009). Because they are government-legislated acts or statutes, they are mandatory for organizations to follow. It is from such legislation that organizations can then develop and implement accompanying policies and procedures that will help enforce such acts/statutes in business or health practice.

Workers have a general duty to take responsibility for personal health and safety, which means they should not behave or operate equipment in a way that would endanger themselves or others. More specifically, duties can include the following (Ontario Ministry of Labour, 2009):

- Work in compliance with the act and regulations
- Use any equipment, protective devices, or clothing required by the employer
- Tell the employer or supervisor about any known missing or defective equipment or protective device that may be dangerous
- Report any known workplace hazard or violation of the act to the employer or supervisor
- Not remove or make ineffective any protective device required by the employer or by the regulations

The profession of psychiatric/mental health nursing is no different from any other professional or workplace setting. Although psychiatric/mental health nursing can be perceived as dangerous and potentially volatile, it is probably just as safe as or even safer than other nursing settings because of the level of skill and expertise among nursing staff, which can work to defuse situations and deescalate client conflict. In any event, psychiatric/mental health nurses are legally obligated and expected to uphold the tenets of the Occupational Safety and Health Administration Act so that the setting remains safe and secure for clients, visitors, and colleagues.

Most organizations also have occupational safety and health departments or programs to assist employees and workplaces encountering occupational issues and concerns. They play an active role in health promotion and injury/disease prevention among employees (Sorensen & Barbeau, 2006; Zikovic, 2014). From a mental health care perspective, they can engage in the following activities to help promote mental health (MHCC, 2013):

1. Analyzing data related to mental health on absenteeism, disability, injuries, and use of services for employees at work or off work
2. Partnering with finance and human resources to contribute to the mental health data collection
3. Establishing supportive stay-at-work and return-to-work programs that assist employees
4. Advocating, where appropriate, for effective access to treatment and resources
5. Ensuring that healthy lifestyle programs are in place for healthy eating, sleep, exercise, and stress management, and linking these to good mental health
6. Including mental health and psychological safety in the work of joint health and safety committees

Under an occupational health and safety act or legislation, there are often many rights and responsibilities for people to be aware of and follow. They are categorized as:

1. Worker responsibilities
   a. Report all unsafe conditions and hazards.
   b. Follow safe work procedures.
   c. Use personal protective equipment when necessary.
   a. Cooperate with the health and safety committee or representative.

2. Worker rights
   a. The right to know about potential hazards.
   b. The right to participate in making the workplace safe and healthy. This participation can be in the form of being a safety representative or consulting with the employer, supervisor, or representative.
   c. The right to refuse unsafe work. There is also often a protocol that employees must follow if they are refusing unsafe work:
      i. Inform the supervisor.
      ii. If the supervisor is unable to resolve the problem, call in the safety committee for an opinion.
      iii. If the issue is still unresolved, the worker or the safety and health committee may call in the workers compensation board, as well as the occupational safety and health officer. The worker concerned must stay in the workplace while the officer is called in to make a determination. The employer has the right to assign the worker to alternate work. Another worker can be asked to do the work that was refused, provided that that worker is informed of the safety concerns and refusal.

3. Employer responsibilities
   a. The act requires employers to ensure health and safety of persons at the workplace. They are required to do the following (Workers Compensation Board of Prince Edward Island, 2009):
      i. Provide and maintain equipment, machines, and materials in a safe manner.
      ii. Provide the training and supervision necessary to ensure the health and safety of workers.
      iii. Ensure that workers, particularly supervisors, are familiar with workplace hazards and the procedures to minimize risks.
   b. Operate the business in such a way that workers are not exposed to health or safety hazards.

Employment Standards Acts

Some states, countries, and provinces also have what has been typically called an employment standards act. This, again, is legislation that is mandated by governments to help ensure that certain minimum standards are identified and met by both employees and employers. It seeks to provide fairness and justice equally to all employees and recognizes that fairness to all employees is a right.

Typically, the Ministry of Labor or some derivative thereof will oversee the fulfillment of the employment standards act (Government of Ontario, 2013). This is achieved through the completion of various roles of the ministry, such as:

1. Enforcing the employment standards act and its regulations
2. Providing information and education to employers and employees, making it easier for people to understand and comply voluntarily
3. Investigating possible violations
4. Resolving complaints

THE ROLE OF OCCUPATIONAL SAFETY AND HEALTH COMMITTEES

As a requirement of an occupational health and safety act, organizations are mandated to establish occupational health and safety committees. The requirement to have an occupational health and safety committee within your organization applies to every employer in a federal jurisdiction who is required to establish a workplace health and safety committee for each workplace controlled by the employer that has 20 or more employees.

The roles and duties of an occupational health and safety committee are many. They are:

1. Consider and expeditiously resolve health and safety complaints
2. Participate in all of the inquiries, investigations, studies, and inspections pertaining to employee health and safety
3. Participate in the implementation and monitoring of a program for the provision of personal protective equipment, clothing, devices, or materials, and if there is no policy committee, participate in the development of the program
4. Participate in the implementation of changes that may affect occupational health and safety, including work processes and procedures, and if there is no policy committee, participate in the planning of the implementation of those changes
5. Inspect all or part of the workplace each month, so that every part of the workplace is inspected at least once a year
6. Participate in the implementation and monitoring of programs for the prevention of workplace hazards
7. Participate in the development, implementation, and monitoring of programs to prevent workplace hazards if there is no policy committee in the organization
8. Participate in all of the inquiries, investigations, studies, and inspections pertaining to employee health and safety
9. Ensure that adequate records are kept on work accidents, injuries, and health hazards
10. Cooperate with health and safety officers
11. Participate in the implementation of changes that may affect occupational health and safety, including work processes and procedures, and if there is no policy committee, participate in the planning of the implementation of those changes
12. Assist the employer in investigating and assessing the exposure of employees to hazardous substances

13. Inspect each month all or part of the workplace, so that every part of the workplace is inspected at least once a year
14. Participate in the development of health and safety policies and programs if there is no policy committee

There are usually at least two members of an occupational safety and health committee. They are appointed by the employer, in accordance with the following conditions: At least half of the committee members are employees who do not exercise managerial functions. These members are selected by the trade union representing the employees in consultation with any employees who are not so represented. If they are not members of a union, then the employees at large will select their committee representatives. The occupational safety and health committee is led by two chairpersons, one of whom is chosen by the employer members and the other by the employee members. The terms of office are not to exceed 2 years (Government of Canada, 2013a).

The primary purpose of the committee is to facilitate communication on health and safety issues. An effective committee will help reduce losses associated with accidents and occupational illness. One of the main benefits of occupational health and safety committees is the role it plays in communication. Communication is the key to an effective health and safety system. The committee provides a link between the people doing the work and the people directing it. This brings a broad range of expertise and experience to assist with identifying hazards and finding solutions. Committees bring health and safety issues out into the open to have them resolved. The improved communication reduces accidents, benefits production, and contributes to the sense of teamwork in the workplace.

Furthermore, an optimally functioning occupational health and safety committee can help to ensure that accidents are reduced, awareness of health and safety is improved, a broad base of expertise and experience is available for solving problems, cooperation is encouraged through better communication, and all workers have a way to express concerns and have them addressed.

SUMMARY

As highlighted in this chapter, there is a significant amount of action that an organization can complete to help develop and foster a mentally healthy workplace for nurses. In addition to the legislation that an organization must follow, the internal workings and existing culture around staff engagement prove to be fundamentally important. Health promotion strategies for an organization are paramount to help build and sustain a mentally healthy workplace for nurses, all of which can achieve a less stressful environment. As figureheads of an organization, the leaders play a critical role in how an organization builds a positive, mental health–promoting environment.

DISCUSSION QUESTIONS

1. What are some of the different strategies that organizations can implement to help foster a mentally healthy workplace?

2. What value can a workplace mental health champion have, and what roles can this person play to help nurses at work?
3. What legislation in your state, province, or country can help steer organizations toward building and maintaining positive workplace mental health?
4. How can the internal workings of an organization, such as communication, morale, recruitment and retention, and recognition and reward, help to build positive workplace mental health?
5. What value do culture, psychological job fit, staff engagement, shared governance, and respect have in building a mentally healthy workplace?
6. How can organizations motivate and engage nurses to create higher retention and recruitment rates?
7. What are some of the health promotion strategies that an organization can offer to its nurses to help build and strengthen workplace mental health?
8. Of what value are leaders in helping to build an organization that has positive mental health?

REFERENCES

American Psychiatric Foundation. (2014). *Partnership for workplace mental health.* Retrieved from http://www.americanpsychiatricfoundation.org/what-we-do/public-education/partnership-for-workplace-mental-health

Athabasca University. (2012). *Protected disclosure (whistleblower) policy.* Retrieved from http://ous.athabascau.ca/policy/administration/whistleblower.htm

Bailey, J. E. (2011). Does health information technology dehumanize health care? *Medicine and Society, 13*(3), 181–185.

Bassett, S., & Westmore, K. (2012). How nurse leaders can foster a climate of good governance. *Nursing Management, 19*(5), 22–24.

Berry, L., & Curry, P. (2012). *Nursing workload and patient care.* Retrieved from http://nursesunions.ca/sites/default/files/cfnu_workload_paper_pdf.pdf

Callaghan, M. (2003). Nursing morale: What is it like and why? *Journal of Advanced Nursing, 42*(1), 82–89.

Canadian Mental Health Association. (2010). *Workplace mental health promotion.* Retrieved from http://wmhp.cmhaontario.ca/workplace-mental-health-core-concepts-issues/issues-inthe-workplace-that-affect-employee-mental-health/stress

Charthouse Learning. (2013). *Welcome to the official home of the FISH! philosophy.* Retrieved from http://www.charthouse.com/productdetail.aspx?nodeid=11986

Clavelle, J. T., O'Grady, T. P., & Drenkard, K. (2013). Structural empowerment and the nursing practice environment in Magnet® organizations. *Journal of Nursing Administration, 43*(11), 566–573. doi:10.1097/01.NNA.0000434512.81997.3f

Colosi, B. (2013). *2013 National Healthcare & RN Retention Report.* Retrieved from http://www.nsinursingsolutions.com/Files/assets/library/retention-institute/NationalHealthcareRNRetentionReport2013.pdf

Dale Carnegie. (2012). *What drives employee engagement and why it matters.* Retrieved from http://www.dalecarnegie.com/assets/1/7/driveengagement_101612_wp.pdf

Davies, N. (2012). Attention, courtesy and patience: How to talk to patients effectively. *Nursing Standard, 27*(4), 69.

Decision-Wise. (2013). *Decision-Wise uncovers strong correlation between employee engagement and customer satisfaction.* Retrieved from http://www.decision-wise.com/press-release/employee-engagement-and-customer-satisfaction.html

Dishman, L. (2013). *Secrets of America's happiest countries.* Retrieved from http://www.fastcompany.com/3004595/secrets-americas-happiest-companies

Elmqvist, C., Fridlund, B., & Ekebergh, M. (2012). Trapped between doing and being: First providers' experience of "front line" work. *International Emergency Nursing, 20*(3), 113–119. doi:10.1016/j.ienj.2011.07.007

Equality and Human Rights Commission of Britain. (2010). *An employer's guide to creating an inclusive workplace.* Retrieved from http://www.equalityhumanrights.com/uploaded_files/publications/an_employer_s_guide_to_creating_an_inclusive_workplace.pdf

Finkelman, A. (2006). *Leadership and management for nurses: Core competencies for quality care* (2nd ed.). Upper Saddle River, NJ: Pearson.

Funk, M., Gale, E., Grigg, M., Minoletti A., & Yasamy, M. (2005). Mental health promotion: An important component of national mental health policy. In H. Herrman, S. Saxena, & R. Moodie (Eds.), *Promoting mental health: Concepts, emerging evidence, practice* (pp. 216–225). Geneva, Switzerland: World Health Organization.

Goar, C. (2013). *Canada sets world's first standard for mentally healthy workplaces.* Retrieved from http://www.thestar.com/opinion/editorialopinion/article/1316732–goar-canada-sets-world-s-first-standard-for-mentally-healthy-workplaces

Gordon, A. (2013). *Canada launches workplace standards for mental health and safety.* Retrieved from http://www.thestar.com/news/world/2013/01/16/canada_launches_workplace_standards_for_mental_health_and_safety.html

Government of Canada. (2013a). *Health and safety.* Retrieved from http://www.hrsdc.gc.ca/eng/labour/health_safety/committees/workplace.shtml

Government of Canada. (2013b). *The Human Rights Act.* Retrieved from http://laws-lois.justice.gc.ca/eng/acts/H-6/page-1.html#h-2

Government of Ontario. (2013). *Employment standards.* Retrieved from http://www.labour.gov.on.ca/english/es

Guarding Minds @ Work. (2012). *A workplace guide to psychological health and safety.* Retrieved from http://www.guardingmindsatwork.ca/info/index

Harber, B., & Ball, T. (2003). *Redefining accountability in the healthcare sector.* Retrieved from http://www.ipac.ca/documents/Redefining%20Accountability%20in%20the%20Healthcare%20Sector.pdf

Haydon, R. (2013a). *Catch 22: When rapid growth leads to employee disengagement.* Retrieved from http://www.tlnt.com/2013/07/25/catch-22-when-rapid-growth-leads-to-employee-disengagement

Haydon, R. (2013b). *Show me the money: The bottom line impact of employee engagement.* Retrieved from http://www.tlnt.com/2013/06/11/show-me-the-money-the-bottom-line-impact-of-employee-engagement

Heathfield, S. M. (2013). *7 Ways to foster employee motivation—today.* Retrieved from http://humanresources.about.com/od/motivationrewardretention/a/employee_motivation.htm

Hudspeth, C. (2013). *Can we be polite without some people mistaking it for flirting?* Retrieved from http://thoughtcatalog.com/2013/can-we-be-polite-without-some-people-mistaking-it-for-flirting

Irvine, D. (2011). *Recognition & reward program best practices.* Retrieved from http://www.recognizethisblog.com/index.php/2011/04/recognition-reward-program-best-practices

Irvine, D. (2013a). *4 ways to a happier and more engaged workforce.* Retrieved from http://www.tlnt.com/2013/01/10/4-steps-to-a-happier-and-more-engaged-workforce

Irvine, D. (2013b). *What top companies know: The 5 basic rules of happy employees.* Retrieved from http://www.tlnt.com/2013/01/11/what-top-companies-know-the-5-basic-rules-of-happy-employees

Johnstone, M. J. (2009). *Bioethics: a nursing perspective* (5th ed.). Sydney, Australia: Churchill Livingstone.

Johnstone, M. J. (2012). Workplace ethics and respect for colleagues. *Australian Nursing Journal, 20*(2), 31.

Kanwit, S. W. (2008). *"Transparency" in principle and in practice: Health insurance plan perspectives.* Retrieved from http://www.ftc.gov/bc/healthcare/hcd/docs/Kanwit.pdf

Keleher, H., & Armstrong, R. (2005). *Evidence-based mental health promotion resource.* Report for the Department of Human Services and VicHealth, Melbourne. Retrieved from http://docs.health.vic.gov.au/docs/doc/9BBC986EBEEC1932CA257B2C0022ABE9/$FILE/mental_health_resource.pdf

Kramer, M., Schmalenberg, C., & Maguire, P. (2004). Essentials of a magnetic work environment: Culture, the unifying essential of magnetism, part 4. *Nursing, 34*(9), 44–48.

Lahtinen, E., Joubert, N., Raeburn, J., & Jenkins, R. (2005). Strategies for promoting the mental health of populations. In H. Herrman, S. Saxena, & R. Moodie (Eds.), *Promoting mental health: Concepts, emerging evidence, practice* (pp. 226–242). Geneva, Switzerland: World Health Organization.

Lee, D. (2012). *Improving engagement: Do workers know the game you want them to play?* Retrieved from http://www.tlnt.com/2012/02/03/improving-performance-do-your-workers-know-the-game-you-want-them-to-play

London, R. (2011). A new idea to combat workplace stress: Mental healthy days. *Psychology Today.* Retrieved from http://www.psychologytoday.com/blog/two-minute-shrink/201112/new-idea-combat-workplace-stress-mental-health-days

Maslow, A. H. (1962). *Towards a psychology of being.* Princeton, NJ: D. Van Nostrand Company.

Mental Health Commission of Canada. (2013). *The role of a champion.* Retrieved from http://www.mhccleadership.ca/identify-a-champion/the-role-of-a-champion

Merriam-Webster's Collegiate Dictionary. (2014). Retrieved from http://www.merriam-webster.com/dictionary

Montoro-Rodriguez, J., & Small, J. A. (2006). The role of conflict resolution styles on nursing staff morale, burnout, and job satisfaction in long-term care. *Journal of Aging and Health, 18*(3), 385–406.

Morneau Shepell. (2013). *What is Canada's National Standard for Psychological Health and Safety in the Workplace—and what does this mean for your business?* Retrieved from http://www.morneaushepell.com/sites/default/files/assets/pages/575-resources-workplace-mental-health/canadianpsychologicalhealthsafetystandardfaqs.pdf

New South Wales Government. (2009). *Protected disclosure policy.* Retrieved from http://www.records.nsw.gov.au/about-us/accessing-state-records-information/state-records-policy-documents-and-tabled-documents-1/protected-disclosures-policy

NIOSH. (2008). *Exposure to stress: Occupational hazards in hospitals.* Retrieved from http://www.cdc.gov/niosh/docs/2008-136/pdfs/2008-136.pdf

Ontario Ministry of Labour. (2009). *Laws of health and safety.* Retrieved from http://www.labour.gov.on.ca/english/hs/laws

Porter O'Grady, T. (2004). Shared governance: Is it a model for nurses to gain control over their practice? *OJIN: Online Journal of Issues in Nursing, 9*(1). Retrieved from http://www.nursingworld.org/MainMenuCategories/ANAMarketplace/ANAPeriodicals/OJIN/TableofContents/Volume92004/No1Jan04/Overview.html

Scott-Clarke, A. (2011). *Will mental health standards improve workplaces?* Retrieved from http://www.benefitscanada.com/benefits/health-wellness/will-mental-health-standards-improve-workplaces-18018

Sorensen, G., & Barbeau, E. M. (2006). Integrating occupational health, safety and worksite health promotion: Opportunities for research and practice. *La Medicina Del Lavoro, 97*(2), 240–257.

Spence-Laschinger, H. K., Wong, C. A., & Greco, P. (2006). The impact of staff nurse empowerment on person–job fit and work engagement/burnout. *Nursing Administration Quarterly,* 30(4), 358–367.

Sturgeon, S. (2012). Promoting mental health as an essential aspect of health promotion. *Health Promotion International,* 27(2), 220–229. Retrieved from http://heapro.oxfordjournals. org/content/21/suppl_1/36.full

Sullivan, E. J. (2012). *Effective leadership and management in nursing* (8th ed.). Boston, MA: Pearson.

The Health Communication Unit, University of Toronto. (2004). *The psychosocial work environment, the organization of work and the management culture of the workplace have the most dramatic impact on employee stress and health outcomes.* Retrieved from http://www.thcu.ca/ workplace/documents/intro_to_workplace_health_promotion_v1.1.final.pdf

Toth, M. (2012). *The facts on engagement.* Retrieved from http://manpowergroupblogs.us/ employment_blawg/2012/04/26/the-facts-on-engagement

Towers Watson. (2012). *Pathway to health and productivity.* Retrieved from http://www. towerswatson.com/DownloadMedia.aspx?media=%7B7BE638F3-9EA0-4BAE-A048- 7587BF501C1F%7D

Wilkerson, B. (2013). *Discussion paper: Mental health in the workplace.* Retrieved from http:// www.mentalhealthroundtable.ca/aug_13/San_Fran_Speech_June_26_2013.pdf

Williams, R. (2010). *Employee engagement: Define it, measure it and put it to work in your organization.* Retrieved from http://www.workforce.com/articles/employee-engagement- define-it-measure-it-and-put-it-to-work-in-your-organization

Williams, R. B. (2012). *The silent tsunami: Mental health in the workplace.* Retrieved from http://www.psychologytoday.com/blog/wired-success/201209/the-silent-tsunami- mental-health-in-the-workplace

Workers Compensation Board of Prince Edward Island. (2009). *Guide to workplace health and safety committees.* Retrieved from http://wcb.pe.ca/DocumentManagement/Document/ pub_guidetoworkplacehealthandsafetycommittees.pdf

Workplace Mental Health Promotion. (2013). *Work-life balance.* Retrieved from http://wmhp.cmhaontario.ca/workplace-mental-health-core-concepts-issues/ issues-in-the-workplace-that-affect-employee-mental-health/work-life-balance

World Health Organization. (2001). *Mental health: Strengthening mental health promotion (fact sheet no. 202).* Retrieved from http://www.who.int/mediacentre/factsheets/fs220/en

Yoder-Wise, P. S., & Kowalski, K. E. (2006). *Beyond leading and managing: Nursing administration for the future.* Philadelphia, PA: Mosby.

Zikovic, S. (2014). The role of occupational safety and health specialist in safety promotion and implementation: Case study. *International Journal of Injury Control and Safety Promotion* [Epub ahead of print]. No abstract available.

5

The Roles of Leadership and Management in Building a Mentally Healthy Workplace

Confucius recognized that "leading by example" was important to strong leadership, as well as honing virtues such as respect and humility.

LEARNING OBJECTIVES

By the end of this chapter, the learner will be able to:

1. Identify and discuss numerous strategies that a nursing leader can implement to help build a mentally healthy workplace.
2. Identify some of the key attributes that leaders possess to make them effective at building a mentally healthy workplace.
3. Discuss ways in which a nurse leader can influence, understand, and build a professional practice environment and foster engagement, commitment, and respect.
4. Discuss how change management can be orchestrated so as to avoid conflict.
5. Highlight some simple and miscellaneous strategies that nurse leaders can use to strengthen nurses' positive mental health in the workplace.

The panoramic landscape of health care corporations is forever changing, leading to the identification of more complex issues and concerns than ever before. Furthermore, as members of society become increasingly educated about their own rights and responsibilities and as the call for health care professionals and organizations to become more accountable and transparent continues, the adherence to an evidence-informed leadership theory is advisable, particularly as organizations become challenged daily to continue to promote optimal and quality patient and client care, services, programs, and resources to best meet the needs of the society and catchment population within which they serve.

The role of nurse leader is one of the most difficult in health care today. Nurse leaders juggle patient care issues, staff concerns, and medical staff relationships; address inadequacies and idiosyncrasies; and promote organizational initiatives. Then they balance all of this with a personal life (Wiley, 2001). The list of roles and

143

responsibilities of a nurse leader in trying to promote, create, and maintain a mentally healthy workplace is endless. In most cases, it is the nurse leader's core attributes, characteristics, and approach that make him or her effective and successful in sustaining a mentally healthy workplace. In addressing some of these core features, it should become more readily apparent how nurse leaders, by mere virtue of their existence, are able to build and foster a workplace where nurses' mental health is optimal. The nurse leader of any unit, setting, pod, or facility is in a pivotal position to help promote good mental health in the workplace. Nurses become leaders for numerous reasons, and it is these very attributes, styles, and roles that help foster a workplace environment for nurses that is respectful, collegial, and safe.

While it is respected that nurse leaders and managers can often fulfill very similar roles, they do so for very different reasons, as will be highlighted later. However, for the purposes of this book, the nurse leader and nurse manager will be considered one in the same, as someone who is positioned to guide, coordinate, and direct front-line nurses in their day-to-day workplace and who can help them achieve a respectful work environment. This chapter will address how a nurse leader can help build a workplace that is mentally healthy. It will provide some proactive strategies that can help nurse leaders prevent some of the most challenging situations they face that are counterproductive to the establishment of a mentally healthy workplace.

WHAT MAKES A LEADER AN EFFECTIVE LEADER?

We often ask ourselves what truly makes a leader a good leader. There are numerous attributes that help to define who will and who will not become effective leaders. The possession of these traits truly varies depending on the leaders' own lived experiences, work experiences, current personality traits, and even their upbringing and values that were inherited through their development, life experiences, and maturity. The effectiveness of a leader and the possession of these traits plays a significant role in how to build a respectful and mentally healthy workplace for nurses. The DNA of a leader is not something that is found in everyone, but instead consists of those characteristic attributes, whether learned or inherited, that make the leader who he or she is today as a successful or potentially successful one. The helical DNA strands symbolic of a leader are their genuine presence, concern, integrity, attitudes, character, determination, and energy, as well as their values, respect, and presence, all of which contribute significantly to the promotion, development, and growth of others, the organization, and self.

The nurse leader's *concern and respect for others* is one such admirable trait. Nurse leaders want to see nurses grow and succeed, and they recognize other nurses' strengths and weaknesses, but in doing so, they align nurses with rewarding tasks, fitting roles, and achievable goals that can foster a great autonomy and independence (Balovich, 2006). They focus on what is best, not worst, in people and believe in them (Covey, 1992). Their belief and faith are uplifting and motivational for others; openness, honesty, willingness, and commitment build one's level of trust and equally make oneself trustworthy that together promote progress, equality, and respect. Compassion is the most important quality in a leader (Nishar, 2013). This compassion generates loyalty, productivity, genuine interest, people involvement, and a just or blameless culture where encouragement comes from the heart. Leaders show a genuine concern for others and are caring and supportive of their efforts, values, and achievements while recognizing their struggles and challenges (Kouzes & Posner, 2007; Sullivan & Decker, 1997). If the nurse–nurse leader relationship is fractured in any way, then no amount of benefit, perks, or on-site health facilities will persuade the nurse to stay and perform. It is better to work for a great leader in an old-fashioned, resource-tight company than for a terrible leader in a company offering an enlightened, employee benefit-focused culture (Balovich, 2006). Providing a genuine warm welcome to all people who enter the workplace will entice them to stay and create an opportunity for further involvement (Wadud, 2013). For example, welcoming a float nurse to your unit for the first time may encourage the nurse to want to come back.

Nurse leaders are *visionaries*. They are concerned with the common good and how to bridge the human capital with the tasks and goals at hand to achieve the most successful outcomes for the organization and patients alike. They inspire a shared vision and promote people to be their creative selves and to embrace their dreams and share and believe in others to achieve goals and grow as persons and professionals (Kouzes & Posner, 2007). Leaders see beyond people's weaknesses and inefficiencies and embrace them as a nonpunitive opportunity to strengthen the nurse and/ or team, promote truth, and abolish naysayers, rumors, and gossip (Covey, 1992).

Nurse leaders typically have a *good work–life balance* (Yoder-Wise, 2011). By juggling and meeting the needs of the nurses, patients, organization, and society, they also engage in a self-renewal process to foster a sense of self. They are lifelong learners and see life as an adventure while constantly increasing their own knowledge base and skill set to enhance their natural abilities (Covey, 1992). They understand their own strengths, weaknesses, values, and attitudes (Daft, 2011; Sullivan & Decker, 1997) and believe in and take care of themselves, enjoy the role and its journey, and enthusiastically embrace the vision, the process, and the supportive followers.

Nurse leaders are *energetic and enthusiastic*. They radiate a positive energy and set the tone for a positive atmosphere that is abounding with enthusiasm, interest, and a drive and determination to get things done. Their view of life as an adventure is intriguing and motivating for others. Synergistically, they see things holistically, not as the sum of different parts (Covey, 1992). They are highly motivated with an intrinsic drive for success, task completion, and progress that effectively builds teams, achieves goals, and produces effective and appropriate and desired outcomes (Daft, 2011; Sullivan & Decker, 1997). As suggested by Sergeant and Laws-Chapman (2012), their emotional resilience helps to build a positive workplace culture, and their abilities to adapt to various adverse conditions while maintaining a sense of purpose, balance, and positive mental and physical well-being help to better achieve and understand self-awareness, the triggers that create negative emotional responses, default behaviors, linkage of negative triggers to the value or need, alternative choices, and changes in behavior.

Nurse leaders are *insightful, flexible, and adaptable*. They have a great deal of courage and audacity. They are tolerant of frustrations, disappointments, and naysayers yet are accepting of the consequences of their own actions (Daft, 2011). They exhibit a great deal of emotional stability, staying focused during change and adversity and insightfully seeing beyond the obstacles (Covey, 1992). Their personality is one that is adaptable, open to suggestions, and alert, and that has a strong sense of integrity or an ability to be candid and sincere with others (Daft, 2011). They use patience to foster a more productive and supportive environment for work to be completed and goals to be achieved, unlike impatience, which can be detrimental to the leader's success (Sullivan & Decker, 1997).

Nurse leaders are also *innovative and creative.* They are very charismatic in their actions and behaviors, yet find much strength in responding to stress. Their social initiative structures, teams, and motivates others as their confidence and self-assuredness help others understand and engage in creative problem-solving processes (Daft, 2011). They challenge the status quo, take risks in unprecedented territory, learn from their mistakes, and seek new learning opportunities (Kouzes & Posner, 2007). They drive the interpersonal aspects of morale and team spirit and help to guide, coach, and motivate people to do their best (Clark, 2011). Drawing from the philosophical paradigms of nursing as both an art and a science, nurse leaders are well-informed, well-grounded, pragmatic leaders who are flexible and adaptable to change, criticism, and group dynamics. Empirically, with science, they practice objectively to consider and process all information presented to make a well-informed, unbiased decision. Research and evidence-informed practices keep them abreast of the changes that occur in nursing. Artistically and interpretatively, nurse leaders genuinely understand why people act the way they do and actively engage their nurses and/or colleagues with empathy, sympathy, and compassion. Armed with the art and science of nursing leadership, nurse leaders are well on their way to implementing change and effective leadership skills. They understand what it takes to translate that research knowledge into holistic practice and in a manner that their followers understand.

Nurse leaders are highly *influential* people (Daft, 2011; Sullivan & Decker, 1997). They use persuasion rather than coercion and share ideas, reasons, and rationale that support their stance and position on a particular topic or issue that respect others' viewpoints (Sullivan & Decker, 1997). Integrity is valued over dishonesty so that honesty, fairness, and respect describe the integrity of the leader's efforts to garnish support from others. Integrity of character is the hallmark of leadership that seeks to make things better without caring who gets the credit (Sullivan & Decker, 1997), which levels the playing field between two parties and avoids control, manipulation, and coercion. Leaders enable others to act because of the clear directions, expectations, and trust they put into their nurses. Nurse leaders who trust and invest in their nurses will help compensate for any organizational inadequacies (Balovich, 2006). Their team building helps to promote this trust and collaboration through the use of influence and persuasion, so that followers feel empowered, strong, and committed to the cause (Kouzes & Posner, 2007). They maintain a sense of command that guides the organization with well-thought-out visions that make the organization effective and communicate the visions or goals to the people who can implement them, develop new knowledge, and refine the visions along the way (Clark, 2011).

Communication is key to being an effective nurse leader, as in, for example, developing a nursing governance structure to address all nursing practice issues; providing opportunities for nurses to enhance their individual leadership skills within a defined role; and creating mechanisms to help nurses manage professional role conflict effectively, as it arises, on a one-to-one and collective basis.

Closely related to communication is the need for nurse leaders to be very clear with their directions and the mission of their organization. Let people know what they are contributing to and the opportunities and benefits their contribution can bring to them. This commitment can help them fulfill their own goals, as well. Leaders can share with nurses how they got to where they are today as a result of commitment (Wadud, 2013). With clear vision and adaptive personalities, nurse leaders are able to demonstrate responsibility, accountability, and creativity (Daft, 2011). Their problem solving is innovative and open to suggestions; their understanding of colleagues, others, and events is candid, sincere, and responsive to the needs of the people and task at hand; and their array of confidence and initiative is met with much tolerance of disappointments, frustrations, and resistance. Finally, their admirable sense of charisma, positive attitude, cooperation, and collaboration serves well to influence others, build trust, and model respect, equality, and fairness.

Active listening is a powerful tool for good communication, so you need to listen, listen, listen and do so with respect, interest, sincerity, and good eye contact. Remember, everyone can use someone to listen to them. Listening shows you have faith and confidence in other people and what is important to them, and that you genuinely care about them (Wadud, 2013). As astute communicators who evince much honesty, sincerity, and integrity, nurse leaders welcome and are comfortable providing constructive criticism. However, they do so in a manner that keeps everyone informed and engages others in an open manner that is positive, inviting, and uplifting (Daft, 2011).

Not listening is costly to the individual and/or the organization. Employers should be able to cut their productivity and staff losses due to mental health issues by about a third by improving their management of mental health at work (ACAS, 2012).

The very nature of the many attributes of nurse leaders described above captures well how they can be influential in establishing and maintaining a positive workplace environment. The behaviors they model, the beliefs they share, the attitudes they demonstrate, and the sincerity, trust, and respect they have toward the cause and the people all promote positive mental health for nurses.

Finally, an effective nurse leader is *eager, positive, and uplifting.* According to LaBrosse, you need to leave the black hat (the negatives of what is going wrong, weaknesses, and what is not right) at home and wear the blue hat (the strengths, faster results, happiness, and opportunities of what is working) and build on it (LaBrosse, 2012). A positive relational leadership style further translates into higher levels of patient satisfaction and lower levels of patient mortality, medication errors, restraint use, and hospital-acquired infections (Wong, Cummings, & Ducharme, 2013).

Nurse leaders are a very *engaging* individuals. Their open, honest, positive, inviting, and uplifting manner (Daft, 2011; Sullivan & Decker, 1997) and their astute, multiple, and powerful communication skills keep everyone informed, welcome criticisms and feedback, and allow a two-way communication loop (Yoder-Wise, 2011). Hold staff meetings periodically, attend department meetings and/or patient or nursing rounds regularly, and communicate your presence and interest by visiting work areas to engage staff (Towers Perrin/Watson, 2012). Their openness fosters receptivity, collaboration, and cooperation with which work goals can be achieved, rationale can be discussed, and strategies and bridges can be built (Sullivan & Decker, 1997).

The *level of intelligence* of nurse leaders promotes the sound effectiveness and appropriateness of their judgment, decision making, knowledge, and fluency in all that they do. Their abilities promote cooperation, popularity in their position, and tactful approaches (Sullivan, 2012). They are well-trained critical thinkers who are able to assess a situation from all angles. Their knowledge, skills, confidence, and competence position them as an admirable role model from which everyone can learn and grow (Kouzes & Posner, 2007). They further identify opportunities to challenge their nurses, in turn boosting motivation so that the nurses feel included, valued, involved, and as if they have helped to contribute to the cause at hand (Wadud, 2013).

Finally, effective nurse leaders are typically *role models* for their followers. Nurse leaders who demonstrate a commitment to maintaining their own physical and psychological health can influence the health of employees as well as the health of the organization as a whole. Your own commitment as a leader will often show through in your attitude, behaviors, beliefs, and actions; others will contagiously follow your lead (Wadud, 2013).

Each of these attributes helps nurse leaders to continue to be effective by strengthening their integrity, energy, character, and outlook. Furthermore, such attributes can help strengthen their sense of achievement, prevent burnout, and promote and maintain self-development and success by enabling them to keep on track with a focus on their followers (Yoder-Wise, 2011). However, none of these works in isolation from the others. They actually work synergistically to help nurse leaders achieve success. When all are connected and fully functioning, they serve many purposes, but when one falls out of synchrony, deficiencies occur, superior leadership becomes compromised, and an imbalance dominates (Clark, 2011).

The introduction to this chapter indicated that the difference between leadership and management would be addressed. This is important to understand because not all managers are leaders and not all leaders are managers, so the impact they can have on developing and maintaining a mentally healthy workplace will vary. Some differences between nurse leaders and nurse managers are identified in Table 5.1.

However, there are also many similarities between managers and leaders. This common ground enables them to fulfill similar aspects of roles and structure such that patient care and organizational processes do not become jeopardized. Both have some degree of authority over others to ensure that the job gets done; are team heads; strive for effective communication; set objectives and goals to be achieved; require resources to achieve those goals; use strategies, action, and style to achieve results and operationalize goals; engage in some form of negotiation to fulfill their roles; and amicably resolve arising conflicts. Whereas management has been proved to use primarily the left brain of science and objectivity, the leader uses more of the right brain functions, which include sensitivity, intuition, and abstract thinking. The ability to use both sets of skills then requires the whole brain to be thinking.

As suggested by Balovich (2006), many managers are promoted from the rank and file with little, if any, preparation; therefore, they are less confident in their abilities, finding themselves in management and/or leadership positions for which they

TABLE 5.1 Differences Between Nurse Leaders and Nurse Managers

LEADERS	MANAGERS
Produce change and movement	Produce order and consistency
Establish direction	Plan and budget
Create vision	Establish agendas
Clarify the big picture	Set timetables
Set a strategy	Allocate resources
Align people	Organize and coordinate staff
Communicate goals	Provide structure
Seek commitment	Make job placements
Build teams and coalitions	Establish rules and procedures
Motivate and inspire	Control and solve problems
Inspire and energize	Develop incentives
Empower subordinates	Generate creative solutions
Satisfy unmet needs	Take corrective action
Are followed because people want to follow them	Are followed because people have to follow them
Are respected because of their knowledge and skills	Are respected because of their powers
Have a mission	Have a goal
Look for effectiveness	Look for efficiency

are not ready (Huston & Brox, 2004) and merely acting as "retire on active duty" or ROAD warriors, as named by Balovich (2006). As the insecurity, lack of confidence, and lack of competence of these leaders/managers rise and are fueled because they are now faced with a group of nurses who are quite confident and competent in their areas of expertise, they unfortunately feel threatened and abuse their power of position. This growth in jealousy, envy, and defensiveness very often leads to bullying, disrespectful antics, and therefore unethical, unprofessional, and poor leadership behaviors (Huston & Brox, 2004).

As more pressures are put on health care professionals, especially those in management roles, and as more opportunities are available for unchecked unethical practices, it is important for everyone to take stock and be vigilant. It is too easy to ruin careers and reputations, particularly in the "virtual" work settings that are becoming more and more common. Whether taking credit or assigning blame, nurse leaders must ensure that they are following their respective codes of practice. Everybody prefers to work for someone who acts ethically, not one who just "appears" to be ethical. It is not right just to look away in the hope that the unethical behavior may go away. Nurse leaders need to understand the value of whistle-blowing procedures and authentication without punishment, and the consequences of needlessly ruining careers. All nurse leaders must rise above the temptation to engage in such disrespectful behaviors and "step out of the line of mediocrity and away from what has become acceptable apathy" (Harmon, 2000). If the right thing is done, even at a professional price, personal integrity can remain intact. Nurse leaders need to take their positions of power, influence, and ethics seriously because the values and principles of "competence, integrity, honesty, trust, compassion, dedication to others, and courage are needed to set good examples" (Harman, 2000).

THE THEORETICAL AND PHILOSOPHICAL UNDERPINNINGS OF NURSING LEADERSHIP

Theory provides a guiding framework for and structured knowledge of how nurses can be effective leaders. It functions to help address important questions, adding to evidence-based care and management practices, and directing and sharpening the ability to predict or guide clinical and organizational problem solving and outcomes (Yoder-Wise, 2011, p. 7). For nurse leaders, the focus now is on how best to guide them toward using their personal attributes to constructively and productively influence the provision of optimal and quality nursing care, and to maintain the standards and integrity of the profession and the goals and strategic directions of the organization.

Nursing leadership theories are continually evolving in response to the changing climate of health care. As patient demographics change, technological advances increase, and the complexity of patient/client care and organizations grow, so too does the theory of what is needed in an exemplary leader because there is no "one size fits all" phenomenon. An individualized approach is needed that depends on the leader's own goals, values, aspirations, setting, context, subordinates' characteristics, performance, and values, as well as on the organizational expectations.

Many theoretical perspectives exist for how nursing leadership can be guided. While some have proposed that the use of one theory is best, others contend that components of several different theories (or a pragmatic approach, as eluded to above) work best in providing nursing leadership. While Transactional Leadership, Transformational Leadership, Emotional Intelligence, and Shared Leadership are the most newly created and recognized theories of nursing leadership, other, older theories, such as Trait Theory, Expectancy Theory, and Situational-Contingency Theory, were also common.

Transformational Leadership

Transformational leadership, one of newer leadership theories, emerged in the 1980s and 1990s in response to organizational needs for more emphasis on values, open communication, organizational commitment, and increased leadership, not management. The focus of this leadership theory is to change the actions and behaviors of followers and to better appreciate them as valued people, professionals, and employees by focusing primarily on open communication, staff engagement, empowerment, respect, and collaboration. Here, the leader is an inspirational and supportive role model who has the hearts, minds, and emotions of his or her followers at the forefront of priorities and progresses to build on their strengths to increase motivation, work satisfaction, morale, and engagement.

Shared Leadership Theory

Although Shared Leadership Theory is not yet well established, it is becoming common in Magnet hospitals. It was founded as a result of the numerous consolidations, reorganizations, decentralization, and increasingly complex problems that large conglomerate organizations experience. It is not so much about what leaders do, but more about what arises out of social relationships. It emphasizes both participative and transformational leadership theories and comprises relationships, open dialogue/discussion, communication, partnerships, and collaboration, in which leadership is a shared responsibility and accountability. These leaders have an admirable sense of confidence, independence, authenticity, optimism, courage, respect, responsibility, and professionalism, and their aim is to instill in their followers a sense of empowerment, work satisfaction, engagement, cooperation, and positive interpersonal relationships. Furthermore, they do so in a manner that is participative, such that they are equally involved in the interests of the organization, patients/clients, and profession.

The Paradigm of Emotional Intelligence

Emotional Intelligence as a leadership theory also has very recent roots (1990–1995). It relates to both personal and social competence and to how we manage ourselves as leaders with self-awareness, self-regulation, and motivation, and how we manage our relationships with others by using empathy and social skills. The ultimate goal is to create a harmonious work atmosphere and an increased sense of self that encourages praise, support, and intrinsic motivation. This leader has increased self-confidence and empathy, is a visionary and change catalyst, and is very "people-oriented," able to recognize and understand emotions and the awareness of self to skillfully manage his or her own emotions and relationships with others. The leader does so by using core skills of knowing self, maintaining control, reading others, perceiving accurately, communicating with flexibility, and being a visionary who aims to create harmony, democratic to build commitment, a coach who builds strengths and develops others, and a pacesetter who sets and meets high standards.

In addition to the most current theories presented here, numerous other theories have played a role and continue to influence nursing leadership and its philosophical foundations. Trait Theory, or Great Man Theory, for example, is perhaps one of the earliest leadership theories, rooted in history from 1900 to 1950. It originated from Aristotle's philosophy that certain people are born with leadership traits, and that these individuals are destined to succeed in whatever they choose as a result of these innate traits.

Situational-Contingency Theory, emerging from the early 1960s, is based on the premise that three key relationship factors influence the effectiveness of a leader: the task at hand, one's interpersonal skills, and the favorableness of the work situation. This theory is credited for including trust and respect, the task structure for clarity of goals and complexity of problems, and position power for influence (Yoder-Wise, 2011, p. 9).

Expectancy Theory, which began around 1994 (Vroom), suggests that one's behavior is a direct result of perceiving needs and becoming motivated to fulfill those needs. A positive relationship between hard work and good performance and outcomes/rewards increases this behavior (Yoder-Wise, 2011, p. 9).

Transactional Leadership arose out of the 1970s and the social exchange theory principles of the 1960s. It does not seem to depict what a leader needs to do to be effective, and here is why. The premise of this leadership theory reflects the historical image of "the boss"—one superior person, the leader, who has all the power and authority to make decisions and is in control over followers, who have no power or authority and who are not invited to give feedback. In a competitive, task-focused approach with an established hierarchy, the goals are determined by the leader and are designed to achieve a status quo or equilibrium through a "trade-off" with followers, with poor performance penalized and/or criticized. The dichotomy between the leader and subordinates is clear and does not necessitate much follower–leader interaction.

As you can see from these many different leadership theories, they all can play a role. However, the key philosophical underpinnings in nursing continue to be collaboration, participation, genuineness, engagement, authenticity, respect, open communication, and empowerment, as found in emotional intelligence, transformational leadership, and shared leadership.

OUT OF SIGHT, OUT OF MIND

All too often today, we hear and see for ourselves how nursing leaders are being placed farther and farther away from the very units they are expected to supervise. Looming workloads, a program management model of care delivery, and increased committee involvement are often the causes. The "presence" of the nursing leader or being in close proximity to the staff she or he oversees, and being genuinely present emotionally and spiritually for nurses are often met with challenges. Traditionally, the physical presence of the nursing leader was a normal expectation of the nurses whom she or he supervised and led. Today, however, conglomerates of health authorities and health care settings compromise the nurse leader's presence in every sense of the word.

Emotionally and spiritually, nurse leaders are able to show appreciation to their staff through a demonstration of their artistic endeavours. Nurse leaders are able to be focused yet sincere and empathetic. They are able to exude a presence of just "being there" for their staff/followers, a presence that suggests, "I am here to listen, help, support, and guide." They are typically acutely aware of the need for good mental health and so would be expected to behave accordingly for their staff. However, the workload, acuity of issues, and onerous responsibilities of nurse leaders, in addition to changing legislation, have absorbed much of their time, leaving little for anything else, such as staff recognition.

Physically, other challenges emerge. Many regional health authorities and hospitals now have opted to use the program management structure of care delivery. For example, one hospital may specialize in obstetrics, mental health, and gerontology, while another hospital may offer acute care medicine and surgery programs. This structure has often resulted in the nurse manager being physically moved away from the nursing units and staff he or she is expected to lead, and an opportunity for fostering good leadership is missed as the visibility, interactions, and presence of the manager decrease. Furthermore, the leader/manager of your nursing unit may no longer necessarily be a nurse, but rather a psychologist or social worker, creating an even bigger challenge in nursing clinical leadership, or should I say the potential for "lack thereof"?

CHANGE MANAGEMENT

Change is a naturally occurring process for everyone. By mere virtue of the role, scope, competencies, and position of nurse leaders, they are advocates for change for their nurses as well. As nurses are inundated with changing technology, client medications, staff, policies, and procedures, with complexities of care, and finally with changing client populations and demographics, change can enhance or disrupt workplace morale. In addition, other factors can threaten the workplace mental health of nurses, so that the nurse leader's approach is critical for making sure that nurses remain engaged and involved.

As instrumental agents of change, nurse leaders function and engage in activities that assist in the creation, coordination, and management of change to best address and reach the desired specific outcomes. The five key self-explanatory functions of a nurse leader are planning, organizing, implementing, evaluating, and seeking feedback (Yoder-Wise, 2011).

Nurse leaders need to build an environment that encourages innovation, creativity, independence, and autonomy so that everyone and the organization can grow. They also need to foster and sustain a positive environment of energy, connectedness, collaboration, and strength, where quality client care and staff satisfaction and pride flourishes. However, staff willingness, readiness, and involvement; existing culture; current attitudes, values, and beliefs; current group dynamics; source of change (internally or externally driven); level of group cohesiveness; and enforcement of change need to occur (Yoder-Wise, 2011, p. 332).

Out of Harvard University, John Kotter's model of change management is just one of many leadership frameworks that have proved helpful in effectively inducing change. The Kotter (2012) model suggests that you need first to establish a sense of urgency so that people see the need for change, and this should be followed by the creation of a guiding coalition whose members have the power to lead the change effort, encourage the group to work, and develop a vision to help direct the change effort and strategies for achieving that vision. The leader must then communicate the vision for buy-in so that nurses accept the vision and the strategy; empower actions by removing obstacles that undermine the vision; generate short-term wins that are visible, recognized, and rewarded with follow-through; never let up minimizing structures and policies that do not fit the vision; and finally incorporate change in a culture linking behaviors with organizational success.

While change may be perceived as good, productive, and needed, it can also be perceived as unwelcomed, frustrating, dissatisfying, and detrimental (Donahue as cited in Yoder-Wise, 2011, p. 325). Nurses' reactions to change or suggested change are in large part due to how the change is first introduced and the process it requires. Nurse leaders can become more skillful at introducing and implementing change by using change theory to plan for the implementation of organizational change. They can serve as agents of change by being open, honest, and supportive of staff and their inquiries; recognizing their own reactions to change and remaining open to others' ideas; and adapting their leadership style to meet the needs of the situation (Donahue as cited in Yoder-Wise, 2011, p. 325).

PERFORMANCE REVIEWS AND EVALUATION

The performance review and evaluation process is a critical piece that helps guide the relationship between the nurse leader and the nurses and enables him or her to use them to their fullest. It is an opportunity for the nurse and nurse leader to identify, discuss, and highlight an action plan to address any concerns the nurse or leader may have regarding the nurse's practice. Nurse leaders need to use this as a time to motivate nurses and to engage them in some open and honest dialogue with assured confidentiality. Although performance reviews can cause anxiety, they can also inspire, motivate, engage, and coach because they provide an opportunity for honest, open conversation about positive and negative results. Although motivation is not something that comes to mind for many when they think about a performance review, from a mental health perspective, a performance appraisal is motivating, productive, and beneficial for all involved.

INFLUENCING AND BUILDING HEALTH POLICY

Policies are crucial to the operation of an organization. They provide guidance and direction on practices, decision making, organizational goals, and desired outcomes, yet they allow reasonable flexibility, provide a means of control and consistency of approach, and help ensure fairness. Effective nurse leaders demonstrate commitment to following through on policy expectations as well as to being integral players for identifying and developing policy directions, bringing to the table their valuable expertise, knowledge, and perspective to meet organizational strategic directions and quality care services. As the value of a policy is often determined by the degree to which it was effectively communicated, the nurse leader's role here is again vital and represents yet another indicator of effective leadership.

UNDERSTANDING DIFFERENT GENERATIONAL COHORTS

Nurses come from very different walks of life and generational cohorts, each with its own values, work ethic, attitudes, beliefs, approaches, perceptions, and even skill sets. Different generational cohorts can represent another but different challenge in the workplace environment that nurse leaders need to understand. The leader needs to build and strengthen communication, understanding, and acceptance among generational cohorts so as to promote and establish a healthy workplace environment. Understanding these cohorts is an important first step. For example, baby boomers (1946–1965) expect their leader to be professional and supportive. They have a great work ethic, work very hard, and believe in the collective action of power, but they do not trust superiors. The members of Generation X (1965–1976) are hard workers but are not confident in leaders and organizations, so be ready to address their concerns and issues. They are not easily understood by baby boomers because they change jobs frequently to meet their personal aspirations and goals. Millennials (Generation Y) are technologically savvy, optimistic, and interactive, but they don't have much loyalty to their position, leader, or organization, or much professional stature (Evans as cited in Yoder-Wise, 2011, p. 43).

Trying to build acceptance, progress, and productivity in a workforce made up of different generations is challenging, so leaders need to identify with, understand, support, and accept the generational differences they face. Their five rules of maintaining balance, generating self-motivation, building self-confidence, listening to the members of the team, and maintaining a positive attitude are important to remember when leading nurses of different generations, dealing with them effectively, and sustaining them on a path to achievement. Just remember, you may have to tailor or modify your leadership style to best meet everyone's needs.

INSPIRING AND HELPING NURSES SUCCEED AND EXCEL

Too often, nurses feel as if they have reached a plateau with respect to sustaining an interest in what they do. Stressful work environments, difficult colleagues, and the complexities of client care can challenge their spirit, strength, and motivation to keep going. Inspiration is a rarity but a valuable asset if you have what it takes and the know-how to implement it. Simply understanding the importance of inspiration and making that conscious effort to do so can make all the difference. Inspirational figures such as Martin Luther King, Jr., Mother Teresa, Albert Einstein, Aristotle, and Nelson Mandela are proven testaments.

Trying to inspire, energize, and instill self-confidence in nurses and others can be a significant challenge for nurse leaders, particularly if they are not interested and not motivated, have a cumbersome task, and are met with much resistance. However, Olson (2012) identifies a four-step inspiration action plan to help people achieve success in inspiring others toward success. Briefly, these steps are as follows: First, define your audience; be clear about whom you want to inspire and you will succeed in doing so. Second, choose the right feeling; inspiration involves feelings, so determine what feelings your nurses want to experience, such as confidence, creativity, and respect. Third, inspire by example because cultivated and expressed inspiration can be contagious. Finally, be authentic, genuine, open, and sincere to make your message stick because honesty builds trust, gets others to believe, and inspires. LaBrosse (2012) adds that having fun and the sound of laughter are powerful and inspiring. Also, have a clear goal with a reasonable, enthusiastic approach while acknowledging people's contributions. Focus on their strengths and be sure to get the slackers off the team, roll up your sleeves and work "with" the team, address obstacles to show you've "got their back," and model accountability and show and communicate your progress.

Building Civility and Respect

Civility and respect in a workplace are the mainstay of a successful business (Williams, 2013). Unequivocally, a civil and respectful workplace for nurses is a necessity, perhaps even more so because the lives of others are at stake. Although we often hear about the prevalence of uncivil and disrespectful workplaces for nurses at work, a nurse leader can undertake many actions to help build and strengthen a workplace that breathes civility and respect. As "people don't leave companies, they leave managers" (Balovich, 2006), leaders are in an integral position to take ownership of this initiative and consistently ensure its maintenance and sustainability.

A workplace environment that boasts respect, courtesy, and appreciation also helps to build commitment, connectedness, engagement, interest, desire, motivation, and so a mentally healthy workplace and a positive culture. Although this seems simple and important, it is easily forgotten. Nurse leaders need to model respect and appreciation for their nurses. The Golden Rule of "treating others as you would like to be treated yourself," expressing appreciation for all that they do, and even a short "thank you" can go a long way toward making people feel respected and appreciated and that their efforts are being noticed. Focus on what is going well and have a "moment of recognition" at your staff meetings of the good that nurses do every day. Although some people may be surprised when you do it, everyone likes to be appreciated.

During tense moments and/or conflicts, respect has to be maintained. Conflicts, errors, and disagreements are experiences to grow from as lessons learned, so avoid blaming or finger pointing. Conflicts can be important growing periods.

Recognition and Reward

Nursing leaders are in a very strategic position to endorse actions of recognition and reward for their nurses. Nurse leaders, nurses, patients, and organizations all benefit from building and supporting a work morale that fosters nurses' intentions to stay in a professional work environment. During any day, month, or hour, there are many measures nurse leaders can use to achieve this with their nurses. These include providing nurses with regular feedback about clinical work (Sveinsdottir & Blondal, 2013) and showing recognition and reward through displays of appreciation as "small surprises and tokens of your appreciation spread throughout the year help the people in your work life feel valued all year long" (Heathfield, 2013).

Well-known human resources expert Susan Heathfield (2013) suggests that as leaders you need to praise your coworkers, use social niceties such as "please" and "thank you," and make general personal inquires such as about how their families are doing, what their hobbies are, or how their weekends are spent. Your genuine interest causes people to feel valued and cared about. You can also offer flexible scheduling, if feasible. If possible, give year-end bonuses, attendance bonuses, quarterly bonuses, and gift certificates to say "thank you"; go out to lunch with your staff; create a fun tradition for a seasonal holiday, such as a secret Santa gift exchange or a "gift grab"; bring in bagels, doughnuts, or another treat for staff and coworkers; and support training opportunities.

Nurse appreciation is never out of place. Any reason at all is a good reason to celebrate because it gives nurses the opportunity to share, interact socially and connect, relax, and enjoy one another as people. Any excuse will do; a victory, an organization's anniversary, a time to give out prizes or certificates to volunteers or workers, and a cultural sharing time are all good reasons for people to get together, relax, and enjoy one another's company. In fact, in many organizations, nurse appreciation is often a scarce commodity. Make your workplace the exception. Use every opportunity to demonstrate your gratitude to employees (Heathfield, 2013). As testament to its impact, giving rewards and recognition to nurses from their leader was negatively associated with mental health problems, such as anxiety and depression (Mark & Smith, 2012).

Understanding Teams and Group Dynamics

Group dynamics help to describe the communication processes and behaviors that occur during the life of a group. The purpose of a group or team is contingent on individual membership traits as well as group characteristics (Arnold & Boggs, 2011). Aspects of individuals, group characteristics, and group processes can all affect whether the group achieves its goals and mandates (Figure 5.1).

The process that takes place in groups, how they function effectively, and the dynamics that occur are integral for nurse leaders to recognize because they help to set the context for how a team or group of people can achieve their goals, make decisions, and build relationships. The group dynamics that occur can be productive or dysfunctional to any task or mandate a team is trying to achieve.

How a team functions, communicates, and sets and achieves objectives is critical and can easily influence the degree to which dynamics occur. Teams serve a vital function of any organization in how goals are achieved or strategic directions are met. In nursing especially, teamwork is a critical component of providing nursing

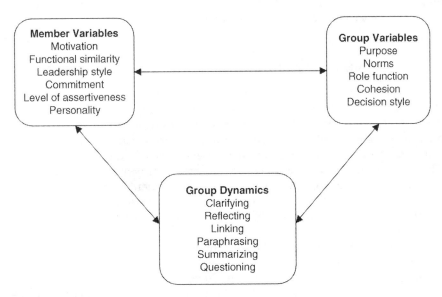

FIGURE 5.1   Understanding group processes.

Adapted from Arnold and Boggs (2011).

care to patients and collaborating with others. Teams in nursing settings may take the form of interdisciplinary rounds, multidisciplinary rounds, a code 9 team, or a code white team, just to name a few.

In regard to concepts of conflict resolution, singleness of mission, willingness to cooperate, and commitment (Yoder-Wise, 2011, p. 353), all have to be clear and in agreement about what they wish to achieve as a part of the team, interact and work with one another, and coordinate efforts to accomplish a shared goal or purpose (Daft, 2011, p. 294). The working environment is informal, relaxed, and comfortable; open discussion and communication occur, and people can speak their mind, express opinions, and even criticize and disagree so that objectives are ultimately understood and accepted, with a clear sense of direction and goals (Daft, 2011; Yoder-Wise, 2011). In addition, there is a focus on solutions and high-performance leaders. Members also act as leaders, protocols are abided by, and there is a supportive management system. Furthermore, there need to be efficient operating procedures, constructive interpersonal relationships, an active reinforcement system, and constructive external relationships; collaboration is used to develop, operationalize, and achieve goals; power is equally distributed and shared among members and is flexible and adaptable. Making processes among members where consultation is also invited, equal balance in what members set out to complete and the function of the group as a whole, mutual respect among members, and diversity and contributions of all members are also encouraged (Arnold & Boggs, 2011; Tomey, 2009, p. 376).

Although teams can encounter many obstacles (Daft, 2011, p. 297), the leader can engage many strategies to promote effective team functions and membership. They can do so by identifying common goals and making sure the goal is clear to everyone. There has to be commitment from each member to do what he or she does best (Fink, 2007). This is "not about YOU"; communication is vital, you need to work as a team and play as a team, and not everyone can lead.

BUILDING A PROFESSIONAL PRACTICE ENVIRONMENT

A professional practice environment for nurses is critical to how they perform their job and its associated roles and responsibilities. A highly engaged, well-educated, and committed nursing workforce, nurtured by a strong leadership team, is needed to create a positive professional practice work environment characterized by low turnover and high retention (Sanders, Krugman, & Schloffman, 2013). It can further enhance the degree of nurse engagement and empowerment (Wang & Liu, 2013).

A quality professional practice nursing environment is defined as one that has the organizational and human support allocations necessary for safe, competent, and ethical nursing care (Canadian Nurses Association, 2001). Research shows that the quality of the practice environment directly impacts the quality of care that registered nurses (RNs) and other health professionals can provide and so impacts patient safety (Aiken, Clarke, Sloane, Sochalski, & Silber, 2002; Aiken, Clarke, Sloane, Lake, & Cheney, 2008; International Council of Nurses, 2001). Indicators such as job satisfaction, productivity, recruitment, and retention impact significantly the quality of registered nurses' practice environments (Brooks & Anderson, 2005; Canadian Council on Health Services Accreditation,

2007; Canadian Nurses Association, 2001, 2010; Nurses Association of New Brunswick, 2011).

A quality professional practice setting supports nursing practice, fosters professional development, and promotes the delivery of quality care. As partners to achieve quality care, nurses and organizations have a shared responsibility to create practice environments that support competent nurses in providing quality outcomes for clients. You need to *support nurses' leadership* (Wadud, 2013), and all nurses are leaders to some extent, regardless of their experience, seniority, and the setting in which they work. They all have patient assignments or nursing roles, responsibilities, and accountabilities they are expected to fulfill that have to be achieved in a manner that is accountable, responsible, and competent. Tap into nurses' strengths, interests, and capabilities and invite them to chair a meeting or working group so that they can feel a sense of ownership and success. Always remember that nurses all have their own talents, strengths, interests, skills, and values that they would like to use to help contribute, so tap into and offer them increased roles, such as chairing a meeting, so they can improve if so desired.

The American Association of Colleges of Nursing (2013) has identified many hallmarks of a professional practice nursing environment. It is these hallmarks that can best support nursing professional practice and enable all nurses, regardless of setting, age, expertise, and education level, to reach their fullest potential. First, there is an organizational philosophy of clinical care that emphasizes quality, safety, interdisciplinary collaboration, continuity of care, and professional accountability, and nurses are given the opportunity to provide feedback and to play a role in policy development and in operational issues related to clinical quality, safety, and clinical outcomes evaluation. Second, there is recognition of nurses' contributions of knowledge and expertise to clinical care quality and patient outcomes. These contributions often manifest themselves through such things as educational preparation, certification, and recognizing, compensating, and rewarding role distinctions among staff and specialty nurses are supported, utilized, and respected by an organization to enhance nursing care. Third, executive-level nursing leadership is promoted as nurses participate in governing bodies and committees, report to the chief executive officer or president, and have authority and accountability. Fourth, empowering nurses' participation in clinical decision making and care systems through their involvement in committees, communication structures, performance improvement, utilization reviews, and patient safety concerns, and the authority to develop, execute, and control their practice are also reflective of an organization's effort to involve and engage nurses to build professional integrity and practice. Fifth, maintaining advanced clinical practice programs pertaining to education, certification, and advanced preparation is a professional practice must. Incentives, opportunities for promotion and longevity, and peer, patient, and manager performance evaluations are greatly needed. Sixth, providing professional development support for nurses through continuing education opportunities, resource support, preceptorships, orientation programs, refresher programs, residency programs, internships or other educational programs, and specialty certification and advanced credentials is also encouraging to entice the development of a professional practice environment. Creating collaborative relationships, participating in standing organizational committees, and using peer reviews from a qualitative perspective of patient errors are essential. Finally, the use of technology to its utmost where and when possible is the final hallmark of professional nursing practice, such as through electronic documentation and the use of appropriate equipment, supplies, and technology to optimize the efficient delivery of quality nursing care.

A quality professional practice nursing setting also supports the effective utilization of nurses and organizational resources and considers other critical elements as well: effective and timely communication systems; evidence-informed care delivery processes; leadership; organizational supports that have collaboration, accountability, transparency, and quality assurance and review processes in place; professional development systems around orientation, preceptorship, and mentorship; response system to external demands such as changes in legislation, consumer demands, health care trends, accreditation, and health and safety requirements; and finally facilities and equipment and the physical environment needed to support and increase the efficiency and effectiveness of client care, services, and programs (Canadian Nurses Organization [CNO], 2011). Finally, as found by Sanders, Krugman, and Schloffman (2013), a standardizing culture change of uninterrupted meal breaks needs to occur, as well as strategies to better manage increased patient volumes, provide best practices for facility design, enhance physician–nurse relations, and offer a hospital wellness program.

THE VALUE OF NURSING STANDARDS OF PRACTICE

Knowledge and practice of nursing standards also help nurses become more effective leaders. As a self-regulated profession, the development of standards of practice occurs at a higher political level of one's province, state, county, and country and should apply to all nurses of that jurisdiction, regardless of their practice setting. Nurse leaders must know the accurate standards of clinical competency for the safe care of their unit's patients, understand key quality and safety improvement measures, lead staff training to ensure the safest care for patients, and ensure staff access to necessary equipment (U.S. Department of Health and Human Services, 2012).

There are many different versions of standards of nursing practice as well as expected competency listings, with each state, province, etc. having their own. The standards provide a guide to the knowledge, skills, values, judgment, and attitudes that are needed to practice safely. They reflect a desired and achievable level of performance with which actual performance can be compared. Their main purpose is to promote, guide, and direct professional nursing practice. The competency listings provide a brief overview and list of the various skills and competencies that nurses are expected to uphold in their practice.

Standards of practice in nursing typically revolve around key expectations and themes that include accountability, continuing competence, ethical work behaviors, the development of knowledge, the application of knowledge and leadership, and professional relationships and demeanors. Their evidence-informed basis helps to ensure that the best current treatment and care are provided.

The primary purpose of standards is to identify for nurses, the public, the government, and other stakeholders the desired and achievable level of performance benchmarks expected of nurses in their practice from which actual performance can be measured. They serve to protect the public and to regulate nursing practice, practice consultations, nursing education, and administration guidelines. They also serve as a legal reference for public information and research and policy.

The American Nurses Association (ANA) standards of nursing practice cover every aspect of nursing practice as played out in nurses' roles and responsibilities as well as the nursing process. These standards include assessment, diagnosis, outcomes identification, planning, implementation, coordination of care, health teaching and health promotion, consultation, prescriptive authority, and treatment and evaluation. Also regarding professional nursing, performance standards of ethics, education, evidence-based practice and research, quality of practice, communication, leadership, collaboration, professional practice evaluation, resource utilization, and environmental health are included (ANA, 2010).

ENGAGEMENT

Engagement is a must for nurse leaders. It is defined as "the level of commitment, trust, and motivation that staff within a business have" (Culture Consultancy, 2013). Most nurse leaders struggle with the topic of engagement. While 70% of people in the U.S. workforce do not feel fully engaged in the workplace, almost 55% feel they are doing what they have been asked to do and are expected to do because they feel undervalued and so are hesitant to exert any further effort than is necessary. Poor engagement breeds hostility, disrespect, and bullying, and such negative behaviors undermine the confidence, competence, and accomplishments of coworkers. Similar to bullying, disengagement creates losses in productivity, increased accident rates, increased absenteeism, and increased staff turnover, not to mention a damaged organizational reputation that jeopardizes future patient relations, services, and revenue (Dale Carnegie, 2013). To the contrary, engaged nurses drive business, relations, and productivity as they go above and beyond their call of duty. Furthermore, they increase patient satisfaction (Davidson & Brown, 2014; Freeney & Fellenz, 2013), patient safety (Davidson & Brown, 2014; Spence Laschinger & Leiter, 2006), and increase profit margins (McCormack, 1994). Employee engagement is a win–win situation for everyone, yet 75% of organizations have no engagement plan or strategy in place (Enterprise Coaching Solutions, 2014).

There are numerous ways that nurse leaders can engage their nurses. Nursing leaders are the visible faces and heard voices of an organization. About 60% of employees who state they have every confidence in the skills, style, and abilities of their leader to lead an organization in the right direction are fully engaged (Dale Carnegie, 2013). Nurse leaders need to let their nurses know they are valued and supported. Get to know your nurses on a personal level so that you can tap into and complement their strengths and accomplishments and overcome their weaknesses to develop and support their professional growth. Remember, as a leader you are their coach and mentor. According to human resource expert Derek Irvine (2013), you need to build a strong fabric and relationships with others to accomplish work "together." Second, engage in activities that fit their strengths, values, and lifestyle to increase efficiency, effectiveness, and mood. Third, you need to practice gratitude so that your nurses know they are valued. Finally, you need direction of the greater mission and how to achieve it.

Irvine (2013) adds that a culture of recognition supported by strategic social employee recognition encourages everyone to notice, appreciate, and recognize others for living the organizational values and strategic directions. Detailed messages of praise from peers and managers alike give us the perspective we need on the importance, value, and meaningfulness of what we do every day.

Emerging trends of higher levels of absenteeism, more complaints between members of staff, frequently missed deadlines, and lower levels of accountability from staff are often visible, so ask around your management team to see what other people's perceptions are and look out for certain behaviors. If you think you are spotting signs of a low level of employee engagement, you need to take steps to repair this and get your company's staff attitudes and relations back on track. This impacts organizational productivity levels and quality patient care (Culture Consultancy, 2013).

INVOLVEMENT AND INFLUENCE

Nurse leaders must remain focused on ensuring that patients receive the best care possible and that they remain motivated and enriched by their work. Take the time to understand what motivates individual nurses because recognizing and celebrating their achievements can energize them. Inexpensive and simple measures to do so include employee-of-the-month awards, luncheons, and staff recognition days. Furthermore, leaders who serve their staff by "pitching in" and helping out energize nurses and improve morale because they set a personal example of good work ethic and motivation. They allow their staff "to see how their efforts have paid off when it comes to the patients they serve" (Dye & Garman, 2006).

PREVENTING WORKPLACE CONFLICT

Any organization in which people work together is bound to have conflict, and the profession of nursing is no exception. Conflict occurs when two or more people view a situation, event, or issue from very different perspectives that may not be similar or consistent. At its worse, conflict can represent a power struggle, with one person trying to harass, demean, injure, or neutralize another. The profession of nursing, which bases much of its work on teamwork, collaboration, and interprofessional relationships, and that regularly interacts with patients, families, and visitors, brews much potential for conflict. Although conflict is often associated with negative outcomes, it does serve positively to influence personal, organizational, and professional growth (College of Nurses of Ontario [CNO], 2009).

All nurses have the potential to demonstrate leadership in their professional roles. However, nurses in formal leadership positions making decisions have particularly important roles to play and are key to the prevention and resolution of conflict. Nurses in formal leadership positions are responsible for supporting nurses in effective conflict management. For example, nurse administrators should establish systems that facilitate the development of conflict resolution skills for all members of the health care team (CNO, 2009). Preventing conflict amongst nurses is a key task for any nurse leader. Give your nurses an opportunity to air their grievances with each other in a controlled environment. Help them to resolve the ongoing conflict and to create a partnership (McKinney, 2011; Thomas & Hynes, 2007). There are many strategies that a nurse leader can engage in to help prevent the development of conflict before it escalates out of control.

According to the CNO (2009), the aim of establishing a quality work environment is to develop a culture in which nurses prevent conflict from escalating or address it in a meaningful way. Nurses must be able to work in cooperation with colleagues to deliver safe, competent, effective, and ethical client care. All nurses lead by example. When nurses in formal leadership positions actively promote behaviors that prevent the escalation of conflict, nurses see the value of conflict management firsthand. Unresolved conflict hinders communication, collaboration, and teamwork, all of which negatively affect patient care. In a quality work environment, employers provide mechanisms that nurses can readily use to intervene in conflict before it escalates.

Conflict resolution needs to be a priority among nurse leaders. They need to empower nurses to resolve problems among colleagues; provide them with greater autonomy by participating in decision making and opportunities for professional development; foster positive relationships, trust, and respect among staff members; promote a work environment in which conflict-creating forms of behavior (for example, exclusion or dysfunctional cliques) are not tolerated; recognize precipitating factors and promptly intervene; help staff members to develop conflict management interventions; encourage positive attitudes; and seek learning opportunities to increase comfort levels of staff (CNO, 2009).

Nurse leaders can develop and implement policies that do not tolerate abuse of any kind; ensure that policies against workplace conflict are directed at combating any form of discrimination; ensure that professionalism is modeled; establish and uphold organizational values, vision, and mission that acknowledge the health, safety, and well-being of staff; educate managers and staff in communication, as well as in conflict prevention and management; support effective collaboration and communication among health care team members, especially between nurses and physicians (for example, interprofessional rounds); implement strategies to ease the impact of change and decrease stress among staff; identify and address staffing needs as soon as possible, especially at peak times; and ensure a comfortable and safe physical environment (for example, use safety mirrors, security guards, protective barriers, surveillance cameras, or an alert system when urgent help is needed). Furthermore, they can promote a respectful work environment by modeling professional behaviors, attitudes, and beliefs; mentor, support, and integrate new staff members into the practice setting; reflect on personal attitudes, motivators, values, and beliefs that affect relationships with colleagues; identify personal areas in need of improvement and strive to alter their own behavior in situations that have previously ended in conflict; and recognize that personal stress may affect professional relationships and take steps to manage that stress (CNO, 2009).

Conflict among colleagues escalates for various reasons. This can be reflected in a misuse of power, bullying, or horizontal violence; barriers to collaboration; different perspectives accentuated by factors such as age, gender, length of service, generational differences, culture, and education level; nonsupportive team members; poor psychological job fit; unsupported novice nurses; orientation practices; fear of reprisal; and lack of awareness about the need to anticipate and manage conflict. By recognizing these contributing factors, nurses can seek constructive and collaborative approaches to resolving differences and preventing the development and escalation of conflict (CNO, 2009). For leadership strategies that can best deal with and manage conflict once it occurs and escalates out of control, please see Chapter 13.

PREVENTING CONFLICT WITH PATIENTS

Conflict can also arise with patients, families, and visitors. With a focus of providing client-centered care, it is important that this circle of care include the patient and families in an open, honest, seamless, and collaborative way. Recognize extraneous variables; the patient may be intoxicated, restrained, fatigued, overstimulated, confused, anxious, worried, or fearful, or may have a history of noncompliance or aggression, ineffective coping techniques, or difficulties in communication (CNO, 2009). Similarly, a nurse who is disrespectful, inattentive, judgmental, or loud and threatening to a patient, or who is not culturally competent and fails to provide an adequate standard of practice to the patient, can also precipitate conflict.

Although measures of preventing conflict vary depending on the individual patient and/or family member encountered and the demeanor and presentation of the nurse, there are some common threads that can be applied. Following the client's lead about information giving and decision making and understanding the meaning behind the client's behavior, use proactive communication strategies that focus fully on the client; employ client-centered care strategies to prevent behaviors that contribute to the escalation of conflict; seek to understand the client's health care needs and perspectives; and ask open-ended questions to establish the client's concerns (CNO, 2009). Furthermore, use active listening and open body language to display a calm, respectful, and attentive attitude; respect and address the client's wishes, concerns, values, priorities, and point of view; anticipate conflict in situations where it previously existed and create a plan of care to prevent its escalation; and reflect to understand how one's own behavior and values may negatively affect the patient, family member, or visitor.

BUILDING COMMITMENT

Commitment is the backbone of an organization because it provides strength, attracts peoples' attention, and helps to increase confidence, cooperation, trust, camaraderie, and motivation (Wadud, 2013). It reflects the degree of dedication an individual has to whatever it is he or she is doing, working on, or invested in. Committed nurses typically have an intrinsic drive and determination to succeed at whatever cause, belief, or organization they are interested, invested, or employed in. These nurses are typically ready, willing, and able to initiate progress and complete the task or cause at hand.

Commitment is one indicator that nurse leaders can build upon, model, and demonstrate to promote a mentally healthy workplace. Nurses who are committed tend to go that extra mile to do things not quite included in their position description, in the hope of boosting morale, generating momentum, increasing the quality of patient care, or benefiting the organization as a whole. They believe in the goals and values of the organization and are willing and want to get involved; they show up, they follow through, and they stick to the cause, no matter what challenges they face along the way.

Commitment is important to foster and encourage (Wadud, 2013) because the more committed people are, the more effective they are in influencing others; they are less easily deterred by discouragement, they cooperate at a higher level, showing camaraderie, trust, and caring, and they learn how to be effective. Nurses need to try things out, make mistakes, and then figure out a strategy that works.

The absence of commitment breeds tension, conflict, and discontent, so that a "no one seems to care" and a "so what?" attitude develops. Efforts, staff, and required tasks seem to dwindle. As a result, the absence of commitment creates a low level of work satisfaction, decreased cooperation, and increased tension, cumulatively adding to the many stressors nurses already experience. Finally, it infectiously lowers existing morale and challenges the existing culture. Leaders focused on producing outcomes, and not psychosocial dynamics within the organization, are more likely to hear about staff health complaints and set a negative example that can undermine the legitimacy of any organizational program, policy, or service intended to support employees. Middle managers are at greater risk for lacking commitment because "they must be leaders and be led simultaneously; a role conflict that can lead to feelings of powerlessness and stress" (Guarding Minds @ Work, 2012).

Complacency, or "self-satisfaction accompanied by unawareness of actual dangers or deficiencies," can also set in because of a failure to complete performance reviews, poor oversight, better-than-expected performance, overconfidence, stagnant responsibilities, monotonous work or tasks, group think, and tunnel vision, and it can exert a detrimental impact on everything from employee turnover to the bottom line. To avoid complacency, a nurse leader needs to enhance a sense of urgency through creativity, involve nurses in decision-making processes (Kotter, 2013), treat individual employees as "leaders," and encourage them to educate, mentor, and coach others and share your big company vision (Kotter, 2013).

Nurses need to know that their work is vital to the success of the organization because this will increase their sense of accomplishment, value, and trust. These all equate to employees who are hard-working and passionate about their work and their employer, lower turnover, fewer employee problems or issues, a higher degree of teamwork and cooperation, lower operating and labor costs, a higher level of customer satisfaction, and the ability to attract and retain nurses.

Commitment should always be built and sustained as it evolves and grows. Working, making decisions, facing challenges, and enjoying successes together, as well as learning from each other and mistakes made, all build a strong sense of commitment (Wadud, 2013). Although you need to have fun and play together and overcome obstacles and support each other's leadership, you also need to hold each other to high standards, appreciate and respect one another, challenge each other, build relationships, and experience a victory together. If you view your nurses as leaders, they will view the group as theirs and have a pride of ownership. Even the person who gets everyone in the room laughing when the energy bogs everyone down is performing an important leadership function. Help nurses recognize their leadership talents because everyone has talents to share (Wadud, 2013).

You need to always invite and encourage people to do more, so they know that their contribution matters and you are interested. When you ask people to commit to an effort, cause, or organization, you are offering them something of great value (Wadud, 2013). The invitation to others to become involved translates into offering them an opportunity to work on an issue that is important to them, benefits the community, expands their skills, makes them part of a team, teaches them to lead, raises them to meet a challenge and high standards, and gives them something significant to achieve. Numerous strategies can help build different degrees of commitment if you provide a genuine, warm welcome to all nurses, are open and clear about the mission, model commitment, give people work to do, match the level of the challenge with the person, communicate and listen attentively, build a respectful workplace culture, celebrate their successes, and support "their" leadership (Wadud, 2013).

PROMOTING POSITIVE MENTAL HEALTH AT WORK

Promoting positive mental health is not as hard as it first seems. While almost 50% of managers have no training in managing workers with mental health issues (Williams, 2012), there are numerous ways that this can be achieved by the nurse leader (Mental Health Commission of Canada [MHCC], 2013), such as the following: increase your ability to recognize mental distress and spot its signs; ensure your own competency in the skills necessary to support employees with mental health concerns; effectively communicate with employees about accommodation needs; engage the problem and help nurses understand their role in the duty to accommodate and develop the skills/approaches to manage the performance of mentally distressed nurses; discuss stay-at-work and return-to-work plans; ensure direct reports; understand mental health policy; provide educational opportunities about mental health in the workplace; ensure employees receive encouragement and support to develop interpersonal, emotional, and job skills; tackle the stigma around mental health (Advisory, Conciliation, and Arbitration Service [ACAS], 2012; MHCC, 2013); and develop solutions by listening because sometimes all people need is someone to listen to them, so be empathetic (ACAS, 2012).

BE AWARE OF BOUNDARIES

Nurse leaders need to remain cognizant of professional boundaries and recognize when they begin to move into a personal realm. They can become friends with their nurses and socialize with them; however, actions that cross the barrier of professionalism need to be attended to immediately. An isolated episode of such behaviors is not as concerning as a pattern of those behaviors, at which point reporting is necessary, disciplinary action may result, and the nurse leader will have to withdraw from the relationship (College of Nurses of Ontario, 2006).

Don't be your own worst enemy; discuss your behaviors and emotions with a close colleague. As a leader, you can easily become to close, too caring, and biased. You have to keep your distance from your front-line nurses so that objectivity is maintained, responses are nonbiased, and boundaries are respected. Respect for professional boundaries is needed to avoid a perception of favoritism and leniency. Furthermore, emotions often get in the way and consciously or unconsciously influence decisions concerning raises, layoffs, assignments, and promotions, as well as unrealistic or inappropriate expectations your "friend" nurse has of you, the leader, or that you as the leader have of your "friend nurse." Also, it makes it harder for you as a leader to judge, discipline, and/or give constructive feedback to the "friend nurse," and you may expose yourself to the risk for discrimination lawsuits (McCarthy, 2011).

As a nurse leader, you are not immune to complaints from your staff nurses, so don't take them personally. Finally, in social settings, friends often do silly things because they are in a safe place, but when managers model such silly and unprofessional actions outside work, it is not regarded as "setting an example," and, yes, do not upload those pictures of your staff party onto your Facebook page, as I so embarrassingly once did (McCarthy, 2011). You need to tread very carefully when socializing with your "friend" nurse. From the opposite perspective, it should also be remembered that some employees may find your attempts to be a friend as personally intrusive, inappropriate, or even hostile, possibly prompting legal action. They might even find your "advances" to be creating a hostile work environment, and again, you would be exposing yourself and your company to that old lawsuit thing (McCarthy, 2011).

According to Harvard professor Dr. Linda Hill and known business executive Mr. Kent Lineback (Hill & Lineback, 2011), leaders need to harness the collective power of the group to improve individual performance and commitment, and having close personal ties with your staff nurses will cause you to struggle as a leader. Making necessary people decisions or evaluating others will be tough. You cannot be on good terms with some and not others. "If you're reluctant to discipline or terminate someone because of the harm it might do to your relationship, then your ties to that person will prevent you from doing your job as the boss" (Hill & Lineback, 2011). Therefore, it is important to remember that "friendship exists for itself"; as social beings, we need close, supportive connections with others, and the nurse–boss relationship exists to accomplish work. "If something prevents a direct report from doing his or her job, then the relationship must end." Second, friends are typically equals, but nurse leaders and staff nurses cannot be equals because they fulfill completely different roles and so have status inequality. Third, friends accept each other as they are and don't actively evaluate and try to change each other, whereas a nurse leader must constantly assess nurses' performances and abilities and encourage change if needed. Fourth, friends don't check up on each other all the time as a nurse leader needs to do to obtain progress reports, evaluations, and commitment. "Friends do have expectations of each other," but they are instead mutual and less demanding. Fifth, you cannot be friends with all nurses equally or with some and not others, as it would make for bad relations and create a divide. Sixth, you need to be caring but focused on the work as your relationship with your nurses should not be driven by control, friendship, affection, or authority, but yet as an effective leader you need to use genuineness, compassion, and caring (Hill & Lineback, 2011).

According to McClain and Romaine (2007), the need to belong is basic to human beings so they can survive and thrive. Friendships at work can produce many benefits for each of the nurses, the unit/department, and the organization a whole because they can make work more fun, increase satisfaction and productivity, and even help employees weather the inevitable downs and hard times of work life and boost retention rates.

McClain and Romaine (2013) add that a break in friendships at work between the nurse leader and the nurse can "divide and disrupt a department or work group." As a result, "cliques" can form to exclude some and not others, depending on your interests and relationship, that threaten possible harm, undermine nurses' efforts, and turn vicious office politics, rumors, and gossip into workplace destruction and sabotage.

The electronic and tech-savvy world we live in today has brought with it much invasion into our privacy if you are so inclined. Making friendships with the nurses who report to you as the nurse leader, or with your own superiors and/or physicians, is something that technology has made easier and tempting. As found by Peluchette, Karl, Coustasse, and Emmett (2012), nurses do not seem to mind that their superiors have seen their Facebook page and would accept a friend request from their superiors, and 40% of them had even already invited their superior to be their "friend"; however, they did not want patients to see such information or to become friends. In addition, nurse "leaders should encourage staff to take their eyes off the latest technology long enough to make sure their contacts with colleagues and patients are positive ones" (Bowman, 2012).

OTHER MISCELLANEOUS MEASURES NURSE LEADERS CAN USE

As we highlighted in Chapter 1, stress is a direct source that impacts our mental health and well-being. If we can learn to prevent stress or keep it under control, then this is surely a step in the right direction and one that a nursing leader can help support, coordinate, and facilitate to curb the impact of nurses' stress in the workplace; included are such issues as "workload modification, non–ward-based initiatives, changing shift hours, forwarding suggestions for change, music, special events, organizational development, ensuring nurses get breaks, massage therapists, and acknowledgement from management and leadership within wards" (Happell, Martin, & Pinikahana, 2003). Moreover, nurse leaders need to involve nurses in identifying initiatives to reduce occupational stress and develop stress-reduction initiatives.

Nurse leaders need to recognize existing working relationships among nurses and how they are key to optimizing patient care, service delivery, and the recruitment and retention of competent and skilful nurses (Laschinger, Leiter, Day, Gilin-Oore, & MacKinnon, 2012). Furthermore, they need to make it a priority to prevent discontent, ambiguity, and distrust among nurses and also to promote respect, civility, and collegiality and in so doing realize the value of humanness in the running of their organization/unit.

The workplace of nurses should be structurally empowering (Laschinger et al., 2012), one where "employee access to social structure in the workplace enables employees to accomplish their work in a meaningful way" and that fosters trusting and civil working relationships, enhances work effectiveness, and boosts access to support, guidance and/or mentoring from peers or supervisors, resources, information, and opportunity (Kanter, 1993). It provides benefits of engagement (Laschinger et al., 2012), commitment (Laschinger et al., 2011), nurse retention (Laschinger & Finnegan, 2005), nurse job satisfaction (Laschinger, Finnegan, & Wilk, 2011), decreased burnout (Cho, Laschinger, & Wong, 2006), increased feelings of respect and fairness (Laschinger & Finnegan, 2005), increased trust in management (Laschinger & Finnegan, 2005), increased mental and physical health (Laschinger, Finnegan, & Shamian, 2001), increased turnover intentions (Nedd, 2006), and decreased levels of nursing supervision and coworker incivility (Smith, Andrusyszyn, & Laschinger, 2010).

As administrators in acute care facilities consider strategies for organizational and staff interventions to reduce medication errors, it is important to consider physical environmental factors to have a comprehensive understanding of the issue (Mahmood, Chaudhury, & Valente, 2011).

Implement an open-door policy for staff members to talk, share ideas, and discuss concerns. Make sure managers understand that the problems they can and should solve will be directed back to them, but it is the executives' job to listen (Towers Perrin/Watson, 2012)

Again, each of these leadership strategies can successfully create a workplace atmosphere that is characterized by collaboration, openness, cooperation, collegiality, respect, and most importantly, the heart. With this nurse leader at the helm, nurses should feel a strong sense of respect, autonomy, teamwork, and involvement.

According to Weston (2010), nurse leaders are also in an integral position to help enhance their level of autonomy and control over their own nursing practice. These can occur through such actions as clarifying expectations and expected behaviors; embedding nursing knowledge into clinical practice processes; recognizing and rewarding autonomous practice; role modeling expected behaviors; coaching nurses not demonstrating expected behaviors; enhancing competence in nursing practice; and creating a learning environment that supports and enables formal and informal educational opportunities.

Enhancing nurses' control and autonomy over their practice is also a significant strategy to engage. For example, nurse leaders need to establish participative decision making to involve nurses and minimize bureaucracies; enhance competence in decision making by teaching nurses about the decision; create and ensure strong and visible nurse leaders who have much autonomy and professional control; work upstream to influence social, political, and economic factors; and publicly describe nursing's unique expertise and contribution. As found by Mark and Smith (2012), the expectation by nurse leaders of their nurses to use their own skill discretion was also negatively associated with mental health problems, such as anxiety and depression.

Using a relational style of leadership, nurse leaders can orchestrate the logistics and seamless functioning of the nursing practice setting. Ensure that appropriate staffing and other resources are in place (Wong, Cummings, & Ducharme, 2013) and that senior nurse executives contribute to strategic directions in senior-level decision making (Huston, 2008; Wong, Laschinger, Cummings, Vincent, & O'Connor, 2010); at the department and unit levels, engage front-line nurses in decision making about patient flow and staffing, quality improvement activities, and continuous learning opportunities to improve overall care delivery (Thompson et al., 2011; Tregunno et al., 2009).

THE NO-NO'S

Up to now, we have focused on what nursing leaders should do to try to promote positive workplace mental health for nurses and how best to foster a workplace environment that prides itself on respect, collegiality, and collaboration. Having uncovered and discussed in depth some of the must-haves for nursing leaders, some of the pitfalls of nursing leadership should also be addressed and highlighted. According to Balovich (2006), leaders need to be attentive to actions that may be disrespectful to coworkers and customers and take timely steps to either correct the offensive behavior or terminate the offender. Some of these offenses are listed below.

- Loud telephone conversations
- Showing up late for work or meetings
- Scheduling excessive personal appointments (medical, etc.) during work hours
- Wearing too much perfume or cologne
- Blaming someone else rather than acknowledge being at fault
- Taking credit for someone else's work
- Sending unwanted e-mail
- Searching for non–work-related information on the Internet
- Having a condescending or rude attitude toward others
- Talking behind someone's back
- Not communicating important information to coworkers
- Telling offensive jokes and stories
- Gossiping
- Not pulling one's own weight
- Providing false or incorrect information to customers or coworkers
- Playing personal radios, recorders, or telephone messages loudly

Dave Kerpen (2013), chief executive officer of Likeable Local and *The New York Times* best-selling author and keynote speaker, suggests that "Leaders must be sensitive to the fact that the whole team is looking up to them. Everything the boss says is magnified because it's the boss saying it." For example, when a leader uses such phrases as "that client drives me nuts" (or in our case that patient or that colleague), "I'm the boss," "I'm too busy," "What's the latest gossip?" "What's wrong with you?" "You're the one with the problem," "I don't care about that," and "Don't argue with me," it ultimately sends the wrong message to the nurses. As a result, the nurses feel less motivated, lose sight of what's important, and lose respect. Trust and commitment are lost, empathy is lacking, the nurses feel undervalued, and a negative and even toxic atmospheric tone is set, leaving leaders frustrated and nurses isolated, less empowered, and discouraged, with poor communication. While all of these are very damaging phrases, the tone used, the circumstances under which the boss is speaking, the semantics behind the spoken words, the speed of talking, and the dynamics between the two parties are also significantly important to consider for interpretation (Kerpen, 2013).

SUMMARY

The nursing leader plays a critical role in the development of a workplace that fosters respect, collegiality, and a kindred spirit, all of which help to build a workplace that promotes mental health among nurses. Leaders are not leaders if they are not effective at what they do and what they are expected to do. While many theories about superior leadership abound in nursing, only a selected few, it seems, really focus on the goal of engaging nurses and building respect among nurses. Nurse leaders are instrumental in leading initiatives such as change, reviews, health policy, commitment, and the prevention of conflict, and they must do so in a manner that uses rewards, involvement, engagement, and an appropriate level of power and politics. In essence, there are numerous interventions a nurse leader can implement so that civility, respect, boundaries, and a mentally healthy workplace are built and maintained, one where nurses do not feel stressed.

SAMPLE QUESTIONS

1. What are some strategies that a nursing leader can complete to help build a mentally healthy workplace?
2. What are some key attributes that leaders possess to make them effective at building a mentally healthy workplace?
3. What are some ways in which a nurse leader can influence, understand, and build a professional practice environment where engagement, commitment, and respect are fostered?
4. How can change management can be used to avoid conflict?
5. What are some simple and miscellaneous strategies that nurse leaders can use to strengthen nurses' positive mental health in the workplace?

REFERENCES

Advisory, Conciliation, and Arbitration Service (ACAS). (2012). *Promoting positive mental health at work.* Retrieved from http://www.acas.org.uk/media/pdf/j/2/Promoting-positive-mental-health-at-work-accessible-version.pdf

Aiken, L. H., Clarke, S. P., Sloane, D. M., Lake, E. T., & Cheney, T. (2008). Effects of hospital care environment on patient mortality and nurse outcomes. *Journal of Nursing Administration, 38*(5), 223–229.

Aiken, L. H., Clarke, S. P., Sloane, D. M., Sochalski, J., & Silber, J. H. (2002). Hospital nurse staffing and patient mortality, nurse burnout and job dissatisfaction. *Journal of the American Medical Association, 288*(16), 1987–1993.

American Association of Colleges of Nursing. (2013). *Hallmarks of the professional nursing practice environment.* Retrieved from http://www.aacn.nche.edu/publications/white-papers/hallmarks-practice-environment

American Nurses Association. (2010). *Nursing: Scope and standards of practice.* Silver Spring, MD: Author.

Arnold, E., & Boggs, K. U. (2011). *Interpersonal relationships: Professional communication skills for nurses* (6th ed.). St. Louis, MO: Saunders.

Balovich, D. (2006). *Respect in the workplace.* Retrieved from http://www.creditworthy.com/3jm/articles/cw81706.html

Bowman, D. (2012). *Your career is a business, so run it like one.* Retrieved from http://www.ttgconsultants.com/articles/careerbusiness.html

Business Wire. (2013). *Dale Carnegie Training uncovers major drivers of employee engagement in US workforce.* Retrieved from http://www.businesswire.com/news/home/20130211005999/en/Dale-Carnegie-Training-Uncovers-Major-Drivers-Employee#.UvVLyGJdX4s

Canadian Nurses Association. (2001). *Quality professional practice environments for registered nurses: Position statement.* Ottawa, Ontario, Canada: Author.

Canadian Nurses Organization. (2011). *RN and RPN practice: The client, the nurse and the environment.* Retrieved from http://www.cno.org/Global/docs/prac/41062.pdf

Cho, J., Laschinger, H. K., & Wong, C. (2006). Workplace empowerment, work engagement and organizational commitment of new graduate nurses. *Nursing Leadership, 19*(3), 43–60.

Clark, D. (2011). *The four pillars of superior leadership.* Retrieved from http://www.nwlink.com/~donclark/leader/LMCC.html

College of Nurses of Ontario. (2006). *Practice standard: Therapeutic nurse–client relationship, revised 2006.* Retrieved from http://www.cno.org/Global/docs/prac/41033_Therapeutic.pdf

College of Nurses of Ontario. (2009). *Conflict prevention and management.* Retrieved from http://www.cno.org/Global/docs/prac/47004_conflict_prev.pdf

Covey, S. R. (1992). *Principle-centered leadership.* New York, NY: Simon & Schuster.

Culture Consultancy. (2013). *Should I worry about employee engagement?* Retrieved from http://www.cultureconsultancy.com/links/should-i-worry-about-employee-engagement/#sthash.YfLKHkRb.dpuf

Daft, R. L. (2011). *The leadership experience* (5th ed.). Mason, OH: South-Western Cengage Learning.

Davidson, J. E., & Brown, C. (2014). Evaluation of nurse engagement in evidence-based practice. *AACN Advanced Critical Care, 25*(1), 43–55. doi:10.1097/NCI.0000000000000006

Dye, C., & Garman, A. (2006). *Exceptional leadership.* Chicago, IL: Health Administration Press.

Enterprise Coaching Solutions. (2014). *Engagement and retention.* Retrieved from http://www.positivecoach.com/pdf/employee-engagement-and-retention.pdf

Fink, N. (2007). *The high cost of low morale: How to address low morale in the workplace through servant leadership.* Retrieved from http://www.roberts.edu/Academics/AcademicDivisions/BusinessManagement/msl/Community/Journal/TheHighCostofLowMorale.htm

Freeney, Y., & Fellenz, M. R. (2013). Work engagement as a key driver of quality of care: A study with midwives. *Journal of Health Organizational Management, 27*(3), 330–349.

Gallagher, A. (2007). The respectful nurse. *Nursing Ethics, 14*(3), 360–371.

Guarding Minds @ Work. (2012). *A workplace guide to psychological health and safety.* Retrieved from http://www.guardingmindsatwork.ca/info/index

Happell, B., Martin, T., & Pinikahana, J. (2003). Burnout and job satisfaction: A comparative study of psychiatric nurses from forensic and a mainstream mental health service. *International Journal of Mental Health Nursing, 12*(1), 39–47.

Harman, L. B. (2000). Confronting ethical dilemmas on the job: An HIM professional's guide. *Journal of the American Health Information Management Association, 71*(5), 53–54.

Heathfield, S. M. (2013). *Top 10 ways to show appreciation to employees from food to favors for employee and coworker appreciation.* Retrieved from http://humanresources.about.com/cs/rewardrecognition/a/appreciation.htm

Hill, L. A., & Lineback, K. (2011). *Be the boss, not a friend.* Retrieved from http://management.fortune.cnn.com/2011/01/18/be-the-boss-not-a-friend

Huston, C. (2008). Preparing nurse leaders for 2010. *Journal of Nursing Management, 16,* 905–911.

Huston, J. L., & Brox, G. A. (2004). Professional ethics at the bottom line. *The Health Care Manager, 23*(3), 267–272.

International Council of Nurses. (2002). *ICN Position Statement on Patient Safety.* Retrieved from http://www.icn.ch/pspatientsafe.htm

Irvine, D. (2013). *4 steps to a happier and more engaged workplace.* Retrieved from http://www.tlnt.com/2013/01/10/4-steps-to-a-happier-and-more-engaged-workforce

Kanter, R. M. (1993). *Men and women of the organization.* New York, NY: Basic Books.

Kerpen, D. (2013). *17 things the boss should never say.* Retrieved from http://www.linkedin.com/today/post/article/20131007134515-15077789-17-things-the-boss-should-never-say?trk=mp-details-rc

Kotter, J. (2012). *The 8-step process for leading change.* Retrieved from http://www.kotterinternational.com/our-principles/changesteps/changesteps

Kotter, J. (2013). *5 tips for getting complacent employees urgent.* Retrieved from http://www.forbes.com/sites/johnkotter/2013/01/29/5-tips-to-get-complacent-or-frantic-employees-truly-urgent

Kouzes, J. M., & Posner, B. Z. (2007). *The leadership challenge* (4th ed.). San Francisco, CA: Jossey-Bass.

LaBrosse, M. (2012). *10 ways to inspire your team.* Retrieved from http://www.cheetahlearning.com/PMMC/download/Nov2007KnowHow.pdf

Laschinger, H. K. S. (2010). Staff nurse work engagement in Canadian hospital settings: The influence of workplace empowerment and six areas of work life. In S. Albrecht (Ed.), *The handbook of employee engagement: Perspectives, issues, research and practice* (pp. 309–322). Cheltenham, UK: Edward Elgar.

Laschinger, H. K. S., & Finnegan, J. (2005). Using empowerment to build trust and respect in the workplace: A strategy for addressing the nursing shortage. *Nursing Economics, 23,* 6–13.

Laschinger, H. K. S., Finnegan, J., & Shamian, J. (2001). Promoting nurses' health: Effect of empowerment on job strain and work satisfaction. *Nursing Economics, 19,* 42–52.

Laschinger, H. K. S., Finnegan, J. E., & Wilk, P. (2011). Situational and dispositional influences on nurses' workplace well-being: The role of empowering unit leadership. *Nursing Research, 60*(2), 124–131.

Laschinger, H. K. S., Leiter, M. P., Day, A., Gilin-Oore, D., & MacKinnon, S. P. (2012). Building empowering work environments that foster civility and organizational trust. *Nursing Research, 61*(5), 316–325.

Mahmood, A., Chaudhury, H., & Valente, M. (2011). Nurses' perceptions of how physical environment affects medication errors in acute care settings. *Applied Nursing Research, 24*(4), 229–237. doi:10.1016/j.apnr.2009.08.005

Mark, G., & Smith, A. P. (2012). Occupational stress, job characteristics, coping, and the mental health of nurses. *British Journal of Health Psychology, 17*(3), 505–521. doi:10.1111/j.2044-8287.2011.02051.x

McCarthy, D. (2011). *I'm your boss, not your friend: 10 reasons why your boss shouldn't be your friend.* Retrieved from http://www.greatleadershipbydan.com/2011/03/im-your-boss-not-your-friend-10-reasons.html

McClain, G., & Romaine, D. S. (2007). *The everything managing people book.* Avon, MA: F & W Publications.

McClain, G., & Romaine, D. S. (2013). *Working relationships.* Retrieved from http://www.netplaces.com/managing-people/socializing-at-work/workplace-relationships.htm

McCormack, D. (1994). Marketing strategies nurses can employ to promote health. *Canadian Journal of Nursing Administration, 7*(4), 21–34.

McKinney, B. K. (2011). Withstanding the pressure of the profession. *Journal of Nurses Staff Development, 27*(2), 69–73. doi:10.1097/NND.0b013e31820eee6a

Mental Health Commission of Canada. (2013). *A leadership framework for advancing workplace mental health.* Retrieved from http://www.mhccleadership.ca/identify-a-champion/actions-by-department/actions-related-to-managers-and-supervisors.html

Nedd, N. (2006). Perceptions of empowerment and intent to stay. *Nursing Economics, 24,* 13–19.

Nishar, D. (2013). *Want to be a compassionate leader? Call your mom!* Retrieved from http://www.linkedin.com/today/post/article/20131007054942-554288-want-to-be-a-compassionate-leader-call-your-mom?trk=mp-details-rc

Nurses Association of New Brunswick. (2011). *Quality practice environment for registered nurses.* Retrieved from http://www.nanb.nb.ca/downloads/Quality%20Practice%20Environment%20for%20Registered%20Nurses_E%20(1).pdf

Olson, A. (2012).*Why inspiring others is the secret to success.* Retrieved from http://blog.brazen-careerist.com/2012/03/27/why-inspiring-others-is-the-secret-to-success

Peluchette, J., Karl, K., Coustasse, A., & Emmett, D. (2012). Professionalism and social networking: Can patients, physicians, nurses, and supervisors all be "friends"? *The Health Care Manager, 31*(4), 285–294. doi:10.1097/HCM.0b013e31826fe252

Sanders, C. L., Krugman, M., & Schloffman, D. H. (2013). Leading change to create a healthy and satisfying work environment. *Nursing Administration Quarterly, 37*(4), 346–355. doi:10.1097/NAQ.0b013e3182a2fa2d

Sergeant, J., & Laws-Chapman, C. (2012). Creating a positive workplace culture. *Nursing Management, 18*(9), 14–19.

Smith, L., Andrusyszyn, M. A., & Laschinger, H. K. S. (2010). Effects of work incivility and empowerment on newly-graduated nurses' organizational commitment. *Journal of Nursing Management, 18,* 1004–1015.

Spence Laschinger, H. K., & Leiter, M. P. (2006). The impact of nursing working environments on patient safety outcomes: The mediating role of burnout/engagement. *Journal of Nursing Administration, 36*(5), 259–267.

Sullivan, E., & Decker, P. J. (1997). *Effective management in nursing.* Boston, MA: Addison-Wesley.

Sullivan, E. J. (2012). *Effective leadership and management in nursing* (8th ed.). Boston, MA: Pearson.

Sveinsdottir, H., & Blondal, K. (2013). Surgical nurses' intention to leave a workplace in Iceland: A questionnaire study. *Journal of Nursing Management.* doi:10.1111/jonm.12013. [Epub ahead of print].

Thomas, M., & Hynes, C. (2007). The darker side of groups. *Journal of Nursing Management, 15*(4), 375–385.

Thompson, D. N., Hoffman, L. A., Sereika, S. M., et al. (2011). A relational leadership perspective on unit-level safety climate. *Journal of Nursing Administration, 41*(11), 479–487.

Tomey, A. M. (2009). *Guide to nursing management and leadership* (8th ed., Chapter 5). St. Louis, MO: Elsevier-Mosby.

Towers Perrin/Watson. (2012). *Global workforce study.* Retrieved from http://towerswatson.com/assets/pdf/2012-Towers-Watson-Global-Workforce-Study.pdf

Tregunno, D., Jeffs, L., McGillis Hall, L., Baker, R., Doran, D., & Bassett, S. (2009). On the ball—Leadership for patient safety and learning in critical care. *Journal of Nursing Administration, 39*(7/8), 334–339.

U.S. Department of Health and Human Services. (2012). *The role of the nurse manager.* Retrieved from http://www.ahrq.gov/legacy/cusptoolkit/nursing/slnursing.htm

Wadud, E. (2013). *Building and sustaining commitment.* Retrieved from http://ctb.ku.edu/en/tablecontents/sub_section_main_1136.aspx

Wang, S., & Liu, Y. (2013). Impact of professional nursing practice environnent and psychological empowerment on nurses' work engagement: Test of structural equation modelling. *Journal of Nursing Management.* doi:10.1111/jonm.12124. [Epub ahead of print].

Weston, M. J. (2010). Strategies for enhancing autonomy and control over nursing practice. *Online Journal of Issues in Nursing, 15*(1). Retrieved from http://www.nursingworld.org/MainMenuCategories/ANAMarketplace/ANAPeriodicals/OJIN/TableofContents/Vol152010/No1Jan2010/Enhancing-Autonomy-and-Control-and-Practice.html#Autonomy

Wiley, K. (2001). The nurse manager's role in creating a healthy work environment. *AACN Clinical Issues, 12*(3), 356–365.

Williams, D. K. (2013). *Great leaders know respect is the keystone of a successful business.* Retrieved from http://www.forbes.com/sites/davidkwilliams/2013/05/29/great-leaders-know-respect-is-the-keystone-of-a-successful-business

Williams, R. B. (2012). *The silent tsunami: Mental health in the workplace.* Retrieved from http://www.psychologytoday.com/blog/wired-success/201209/the-silent-tsunami-mental-health-in-the-workplace

Wong, C. A., Cummings, G. G., & Ducharme, L. (2013). The relationship between nursing leadership and patient outcomes: A systematic review update. *Journal of Nursing Management, 21*(5), 709–724. doi:10.1111/jonm.12116

Wong, C. A., Laschinger, H. K., Cummings, G. G., Vincent, L., & O'Connor, P. (2010). Decisional involvement of senior nurse leaders in Canadian acute care hospitals. *Journal of Nursing Management, 18*(2), 122–133.

Yoder-Wise, P. S. (2011). *Leading and managing nursing* (5th ed.). St. Louis, MO: Elsevier-Mosby.

6

The Role of the Nurse as a Person and a Professional

> *Be the change you want to see in the world.*
> —*Mahatma Gandhi*

LEARNING OBJECTIVES

By the end of this chapter, the learner will be able to:

1. Discuss the importance of the role of the nurse as a person and a professional in maintaining a mentally healthy workplace.
2. Highlight and discuss various coping strategies and principles that can help an individual face and deal with stress.
3. Discuss why it is important to understand concepts such as the power of knowledge, the rumor mill, perception, empowerment, attitude, and selectively picking your own battles.
4. Identify and discuss why it is important to maintain a work–life balance.
5. Better understand how your nursing professional standards of practice and your governing legislation can guide your practice.
6. Discuss how you as an individual and the various lessons, values, beliefs, and morals that you bring with you can help you be resilient against the impact of stress.

Good mental health means one is able to live and to address, perform, and complete tasks that are appropriate, accurate, safe, and timely without any impairment of judgment, concentration, thought processes, and behaviors. This of course applies to both our personal and professional lives and how we ready ourselves to deal with stress and stressors; the impact is certainly individualized, and no one size fits all. Being aware of and promoting our own mental health better prepares us to deal with occupational stressors and to foster good mental health in the workplace. In Chapter 1, we identified stress and the many different sources of stress. Now we will examine stress from the perspective of how we, as nurses, can better prepare ourselves and our minds to deal with whatever life, work, and society throw our way. These practices, behaviors, and commitments are many and varied because

177

what a nurse can do personally should support what she can do as a professional as well, so it is through the lens of both that we will investigate how individuals can help promote their own mental health and prevent mental health challenges.

Nurses focus not only on themselves and what they can do to foster a mental healthy workplace but also on how they can protect themselves. Maintaining good mental health and engaging in activities to help foster and strengthen personal mental health is crucial to our overall well-being. In the absence of good mental health, we find it difficult to deal with life's challenges, cope with changes, interact, think clearly and coherently, and even perform some everyday routines. All of these processes help in our functioning and survival in life and work. We may be nurses, but we are also humans. As humans, nurses are not immune to the effects of stress and deteriorating mental health.

As human beings, there is much nurses can do to promote their optimal mental health and much in which they can engage to avoid mental health challenges. I am not going to lecture you on the rights and wrongs of living, but I am going to point out to you some things, simple things, that we as human beings can do to foster and strengthen our own mental health. Having a solid foundation of good mental health helps us to deal better with stressors at home and work. Making direct, evidence-informed research links to the physiological processes of the brain that impact mental health, I will walk you through practices pertaining to diet, exercise, rest, social interaction, work–life balance, and other personal and professional behaviors and practices that help to solidify and strengthen your good mental health.

To protect themselves from the clutches of work evil, dishonesty, and political propaganda, nurses can participate in a number of strategies. Quite simply, they all revolve around certain key themes of being smart, thinking before you speak and do, and being savvy. Just because your body is fit, that doesn't necessarily mean that your mind is fit. Sometimes we let our mental hygiene slip and then problems can begin, we forget about caring for ourselves, and feel as if we need to get our head back on "straight." However, for you and most others, that journey has begun. You know something has not been quite right recently, and here are some things that are going to help you get over this mountain in life.

In the position of nurse, as one who provides care, support, and life-altering and even life-saving measures and interventions, good mental health is integral. When dealing with the lives and health of other people, it is important for nurses to be clear, precise, and alert to ensure good clinical judgment, best practices, and competence.

Nurses who work in any particular setting, be it a hospital, private clinic, or community setting, have the power and capability within themselves to help build a mentally healthy workplace. As both a person and professional, the nurse brings strengths, characteristics, fortitude, and integrity to help build this environment. This chapter will help identify some measures that a nurse can take proactively at a personal and professional level to sustain a workplace environment that promotes good mental health for all.

Good personal mental health arms you to promote good mental health in the workplace. You are in no position to support a mentally healthy workplace if your own mental health is not on solid footing. First, your own personal mental health strengthens your mind for how you interact and handle difficult situations involving others; second, it models for many others an admirable sense of self and how confidence, competence, and esteem are promoted in the workplace. Professionally, fostering good mental health in the workplace is also very important to achieve if you wish to maintain and sustain your own good mental health.

When the mental health of a nurse becomes jeopardized, the potential for negative results increases. The nurse works with blurred vision and impaired judgment, so that the safety and health risk of patients can be compromised. Hence, all the more reason for why building a mentally healthy workplace is unequivocally critical.

THE ESSENCE OF COMMUNICATION

Communication is a vital tool for everyone to build, foster, and sustain relationships. It makes up a significant portion of who we are as human beings and professionals. Communication is defined as a complex array and exchange of information in which verbal and nonverbal behaviors are used for the purposes of sharing information (Buck & Van Lear, 2002). Within this exchange of information, nonverbal communication consists of a series of gestures, tone of voice, body movements, and facial expressions that help to give context and understanding to the spoken words. As stated by Sonnenberg (2013), actions often speak much louder than words.

Communication among nurses is a crucial aspect of their being able to perform their job completely, safely, and with a high degree of quality. Nurses often rely upon different forms of communication to complete such actions as patient assessment, advocacy, therapeutic interventions, and patient education. It is also important as nurses interact with colleagues on such matters as clarifying a patient's status, hand-off reporting, asking for help with a heavy or uncertain task or skill, and even passing surgical instruments during an operating room procedure. The point is that communication is integral to nursing in every manner possible. Without communication, nurses can easily find themselves uncertain of actions being taken, unsupported by colleagues, and even at risk for making errors and hence jeopardizing patient care. The very foundations of communication—respect, trust, status equity, and time availability—are needed as a first step toward improving communication (Tschannen & Lee, 2011).

Communication is vital for teamwork to occur, and teamwork is often cited as a critical component of health care delivery (Happell, Platania-Phung, Scott, & Nankivell, 2014). Nonetheless, many errors in health care are born as a result of a lack of communication (Dunn et al., 2007; Sutcliffe, Lewton, & Rosenthal, 2004), such as was found in the Joint Commission report of 2010, in which 82% of sentinel events originated from poor or lack of communication. Similarly, Rucker, O'Connor, and Buxbaum (2006) found that up to 75% of patient care decisions were often made in the absence of all needed data and information.

Any struggles, difficulties, or barriers encountered in the communication process can potentially impact a nurse's mental health. In the absence of effective communication, a nurse's mental health can become strained. Unequivocally, the presence of a toxic workplace environment can drive a nurse into seclusion, withdrawal, and even depression, in which communication becomes compromised or further limited. In any event, communication remains an important component of nursing practice and the functionality and effectiveness of nursing as a competent, safe, and knowledgeable profession. Only through effective communication can a nurse's confidence, integrity, and respect be maintained to help ensure competent, safe, and quality professional practice. As nurses play a valuable role in health care teams, effective communication also helps to ensure collegial collaboration, timely evaluations of interventions, accurate coordination, and effective delegation when needed.

So important is communication among health care professionals that in studies the lack of it significantly correlated with poor patient outcomes, medical/clinical errors, and even sentinel events (Chant, Jenkinson, Randle, & Russell, 2002). Similarly, research focused on improving communication has resulted in improved quality of patient care (Hamric & Blackhall, 2007; Kramer & Schmalenberg, 2003), increased patient and professional satisfaction (Boyle & Kochinda, 2004; Hamric & Blackhall, 2007), and greater retention rates (Boyle & Kochinda, 2004; Krairiksh & Anthony, 2001).

For you, the nurse as a person and a professional, your communication should be clear, honest, open, concise, focused, and respectful. These are the key elements that individuals need to remember when interacting and working with others. You have to be aware of both your verbal and nonverbal communication in how you interact with others. What you say, where you say it, how you say it, and to whom you say it determine everything in how those messages are perceived, interpreted, and responded to. Of course in nursing, we also have to be astutely aware of the circumstances in which we work. For example, after a 999, a 666, a code white, or any other emergency distress code that a facility utilizes is called, you may very well observe people yelling, ordering, and demanding, but these are of course for obvious emergency situations. However, when we refer to patients as the "hip fracture" in room 250 or the "drug addict" in room 102, these are neither professional nor appropriate phrases of communication, nor do they say a lot about the nurse speaking them.

MAKING ASSUMPTIONS

At both a personal and a professional level, assumptions are just downright dangerous. If you are making assumptions, you are playing with fire. Assumptions serve two main purposes: they make you look as if you don't know what is happening at the moment, compromising and wreaking havoc with your own mental health, and they can serve to damage the mental health and character of someone else. Technically, assumptions are a breakdown in communication and one of the biggest pitfalls in communication that can occur. An assumption is generally defined as something taken for granted or accepted as true without proof.

For you as a person, assumptions achieve nothing positive. They are embarrassing (Crouteau, 2014), and they destroy relationships, violate the trust people develop, signify disrespect, create an alarming sense of discomfort, and are often inaccurate representations of information (Lue, 2010). As a person, you can literally destroy yourself over assumptions. You can run yourself down and even become depressed over it (Lue, 2010). You try to convince yourself that you know what others are thinking about you, which in turn colors what you actually "think" they feel about you. You try to make real in your own mind thoughts and feelings that actually have no substantive truth for being real. So what happens is that you continuously torment yourself and even ruminate over what "might" be. This is truly a case in which mind has to be over matter, so what you think exists and what actually exists do not match, and you have to draw on the strength of your mind to correct such false assumptions because the matter just don't exist.

Reality check: You do not, nor will you ever, have the ability to read people's minds, and no, you can't think for someone else either.

For the individual nurse, the practice of making assumptions is even more dangerous as the lives of people may be at stake and the support you receive from colleagues to maintain and sustain that life can become jeopardized. Literally, assumptions can create a highly stressful work atmosphere that truly tests one's mental health and integrity. For you as a professional, the negativity of making assumptions continues. They are often not accurate, and they stifle your growth and development because they are missed opportunities to optimize yourself as a better person and a better nurse. Furthermore, they hinder your creativity by dampening your spirits, innovativeness, and imagination; you are so preoccupied with trying to analyze the assumption that you lose a great deal of time ruminating over its false existence, and these opportunities pass you by. Ultimately, they can cause errors in our clinical judgment and detract from our focus of quality patient care delivery and competent performance of skills and procedures. In addition, they create misunderstandings and can even heighten one's sensitiveness or create a sense of paranoia or increase self-consciousness because people think they are being talked about.

Although assumptions function to give us some sense of certainty in a generally uncertain world and save us the energy of trying to find out the truth of the matter, they ultimately work with imprecise data or findings and create an unsettled, uncomfortable sense at work. For nurses, it is necessary to find out the facts first and avoid judging a book by its cover based on what you "think" to be true. When you are working with the lives of others, the trust of the public, and the constraints of a busy, fast-paced, and often critical care environment, you can't make assumptions. Assumptions only serve to misrepresent the truth, increase your risk for error, and damage the collegial relationships you rely on to perform at your best. Let it be another golden rule for you never to assume anything.

THE POWER OF KNOWLEDGE

In the words of the 16th-century philosopher Sir Francis Bacon, "knowledge is power." The phrase implies that knowledge or education increases one's potential or abilities in life. It is the basis for improving one's reputation and influence, and thus acquiring power. Paraphrasing Proverbs 24:5, "A wise man has great power, and a man of knowledge increases strength." If you are a nurse or studying to become a nurse, you have already taken on one of life's greatest yet rewarding challenges. Regardless of the nursing college or university program, you may at first feel overwhelmed and even threatened by the amount of content that has to be learned, the long hours of clinical rotations, the long hours of study, and the depth of under-standing that is expected. For many, I am sure, the anatomy, physiology, and pathol-ogy courses were/are perhaps the greatest sources of stress for you. However, by the time you finish your nursing program, you feel empowered by what you have learned.

Seeking out new and different knowledge is stimulating, rewarding, fun, and empowering. You already have a great knowledge base, but we can never learn too much. The building of new knowledge keeps the mind in check and active. Neu-rons are forced to keep mobile, seeking and building new connections of internal information highways. Knowledge is power, and you, my friend, are a knowledge broker with a great deal of power, so use it wisely.

Nursing knowledge helps define nursing as a profession and is central to the issue of professional accountability. It is vital to attempt to answer questions, inform nursing practice, acknowledge the importance of all knowledge not just anecdotal accounts or scientifically informed practice, personal understanding, and interpre-tation of moral and ethical reasoning (Hall, 2005).

Feeding your mind with knowledge is like spreading fertilizer on your grass; it promotes growth and strengthens and builds resiliency. It further improves social relations, fosters close, trusting relationships with others, and builds on warmth and love with others. Feeding your mind with the mental foods of knowledge enhances your purpose and confidence, decreases boredom, and can even prevent both inter-nal and external conflict (Boyd et al., 2013).

On the other hand, knowledge can also be the enemy of nurses. The mere nature of the knowledge that nurses have acquired through their education and experi-ence around signs and symptoms, behaviors, treatment, and general health and well-being can work to their disadvantage. To their potential detriment, it is often identified as a reason why nurses feel they are invincible. They know all too well how to stay healthy and what it takes to keep well, but they don't always practice what they preach. They are always there to advocate for and to educate a patient on health promotion and disease prevention, but the very confidence and competence that affirm their nursing practice do not translate so well in identifying and taking care of their own needs. All nurses have this power of knowledge; however, it is up to the individual nurse how to use it to his or her advantage. Let it be known, then, that just as someone can try to abuse you with power, you too have the exact same weapon of knowledge to deploy and resist those using knowledge power to intimi-date, bully, and humiliate you.

AVOID THE RUMOR MILL AND GRAPEVINE

No matter where you work, you will always run into rumors. Although rumors may be the mainstay of workplaces, they can infiltrate and poison morale and tax your own mental health. Best practice would be to "take everything you hear with a grain of salt." In other words, do not pay too much attention when you hear information being said about someone else, because where there is smoke there is not always fire. When you see and hear someone talking about a person who is not present (behind the other person's back, so to speak), it says a lot about that someone. What you need to be asking yourself is, "If this person is talking about Sally when she is not present, then what could he or she possibly be saying about me when I am not around?"

Rumors actually represent a form of great stress for individuals at work, particularly nurses. Although the grapevine can be the main conduit for the benefit of sharing information (Rosenberg McKay, 2013), it generally consists of unwelcoming responses to and comments about somebody else, or something someone did or is suspected of doing. It is taking a small amount of information and translating it destructively into false or inaccurate assumptions that catch peoples' attention, make you the center of attention with increased power for being privy to this information, and then go on to destroy someone's reputation.

To *avoid* getting entangled in the grapevine, there are a few suggestions that Rosenberg McKay (2013) says are good practice. Briefly, they are as follows: Take everything you hear with a grain of salt and find out the facts and truth first, because everything you hear is not always true. Carefully choose what it is you share with others and do not share with anyone any information you would not want anyone else to know about; you may be great at keeping a secret, but not everyone is. Finally, use the grapevine to your advantage to make known any information that is positive and uplifting, such as a success, scholarship, or other positive event.

YOU: YOUR HISTORY, LIFE EXPERIENCES, PHILOSOPHY, VALUES, MORALS, BELIEFS, ETHICS, SUPPORTS, HABITS, SENSITIVITIES, ATTITUDE, AND LIFESTYLE BEHAVIORS

Our personal life is a well-founded source of stress for all of us who work. We engage in many activities outside work with friends, families, and the community; this helps many of us to fulfill a positive sense of self and value and is an interest/ activity in which we seek comfort and relaxation. Although many of these events may have positive value and can actually help to buffer unwanted stress, they still exist as a form of stress for the nurse. Regardless of the personal roles nurses play outside work, it is important to recognize that these can possibly be adding to their already mounting work stress.

As individuals and functioning human beings, it is important for us to know ourselves first and to be aware of our limitations; strengths; sensitivities; our own values, beliefs, and philosophy; and how our past experiences have contributed to these domains. All of these foci enable us to guide and monitor our expectations, our aspirations and goals in life and work, and what coping skills do and do not work for us.

Donahue (1996) suggests that the development of one's values, self-knowledge, self-control, and a good quantity of common sense helps one decide about the conditions of one's mental health. Enjoying life helps to promote positive mental health, and drawing from your common sense, past experiences, daily interactions, and what you observe in others and their environment helps to achieve this. This will help you plan for the future in how you react and respond and control unnecessary worries about the future, and so achieve a work–life balance.

Your Supports

Social support among nurses is a necessity; we are, after all, social beings. The old adage "no man is an island" is so true in every respect. As Daiski (2004) found, social support is often lacking among nurses, but it must come from each of them to the others, not from the hospital. While nurses are taught to be support persons and advocates of their patients and patients' families, they fail in fulfilling these roles for one another. Vonfrolio (2005) adds that perhaps nurses are so exhausted and drained physically, emotionally, and spiritually that they have very little, if anything, left to give each other. As added by Woelfle and McCaffrey (2007), if nurses make every effort to honestly care about one another, professional relationships can improve. For example, social support from colleagues and superiors, in particular, has a protective effect against the development of posttraumatic stress disorder (Adriaenssens, de Gucht, & Maes, 2012).

Your Attitude

Attitude means everything when you are working with and for others and taking care of external parties like patients, families, and key stakeholders. Having a positive attitude in the workplace can help with potential promotions, build collegial relationships, and boost your confidence. Employers promote employees who can not only produce but also motivate others in the workplace. A positive attitude is an "I can" attitude.

We can change our attitudes indirectly by spending more time in more positive thoughts and actions (Williams, 2007). Replace every negative, fearful, angry thought with positive, uplifting, and productive ones and with hobbies, volunteer work, church and club activities, and so forth. Other actions that can improve our attitudes are exercise programs, donating money to worthy causes, letting others go first, holding the door open for someone coming behind you, helping neighbors and strangers, and tipping excessively. You will be pleasantly surprised by the outcome as it improves our experience of life and replaces stress and anger with joy and satisfaction. In the words of the Christian apostle Paul, "Be gentle and not anxious about anything. Think about things that are true, praiseworthy, noble, right, pure, lovely and admirable ... and you will have peace" (Philippians 4:1–9).

According to Shiota (2013), a positive attitude improves work performance, work ethic, and confidence; impresses leaders; increases productivity and outputs; and makes work enjoyable. Its infectious nature enhances communication, is esthetically uplifting for coworkers, increases friendliness, and makes work more enjoyable. A positive attitude will help to motivate other employees, boost worker productivity, help to lower absentee rates, and cause the workplace to be less stressful, hence reducing the risk for stress-related diseases such as heart disease, digestive problems, depression, obesity, pain, and autoimmune diseases (Johnson, 2013).

Be Optimistic

Optimism goes a long way toward making us feel good about ourselves, our roles, and our achievements. Research from the Harvard School of Public Health recently found that "the most optimistic people had 50 percent less risk of a first heart attack when compared with the least optimistic" (Levit, 2013). Further, as reported by Levit (2013), "Other studies show optimists experience significantly less stress, less depression, and heal faster than pessimists," notes Dr. Nelson. "Not only that, but optimists outperform their own abilities. You may be good at something, but if you're an optimist, you'll be better at it. No matter what you undertake, you'll experience more success and joy by the simple decision to become an optimist."

Becoming an optimist is not difficult, it just takes much focus and concentration. The following are some suggestions by Dr. Nelson and others:

1. *Focus on what is working.* "If you are not getting along with your boss, instead of focusing on the negatives, look at the situation with a new lens. Is your boss getting the job done? If the boss is new, does it look like he is trying to manage well? If so, cut your boss some slack. Meanwhile, look for ways to maximize your skills and your contributions to the company" (Levit, 2013).
2. *Play the "what if?" game with a positive spin.* We all play the "what if?" game, but for the most part, we play it negatively—for example, "If I get fired, I'll go broke and my girlfriend will break up with me." Instead, ask yourself "what if?" in a hopeful direction. For example,"If I get fired, I have a good skill set. I've learned a lot at this job and I've made new connections. I'm sure I can parlay some of that into a new situation. Meanwhile, I'll put some extra effort into my current position so I'm not so dispensable" (Levit, 2013).
3. *Don't be so hard on people.* Everyone makes mistakes and fails at something from time to time. When coworkers do something wrong on the job, don't blame or complain. Figure out what you can do to help them succeed. This will enable you to value their efforts to do better, and they in turn will most likely value your help. And oftentimes, your boss will take notice (Levit, 2013).
4. *Lift your employees' spirits.* If you're the boss, do you tend only to point out things an employee does wrong? Start acknowledging your employees for doing things right. They will be more likely to repeat the good behavior they have been praised for, and their sense of competence and happiness on the job will increase. And in the end, so will your bottom line (Levit, 2013).
5. *Surround yourself with beauty.* Redecorate your house or garden. Do some spring cleaning. Put on some happy music. Do whatever helps you feel relaxed and at peace. Practice whatever form of spiritualism that appeals to you. This is a life coping skill and will help you recognize beauty and remain optimistic.
6. *Focus on the positive, not the negative.* You need to focus on what it is you have and you would like to have, things that are positive or have positively influenced your life somehow. As Koffman (2006) suggests, "Forget what you don't want and focus on what you want." Sometimes, what "you try to avoid you unconsciously create." We exert so much of our time and energy on it that it begins to engulf us completely.

A negative attitude has far-reaching effects as well. Negative energy can virtually exhaust you and drain every ounce of existence from you, so you have little or no energy left to achieve those positive things you would like to achieve. A bad or negative attitude can be hazardous to your career, decrease motivation, create a wandering mind, and in some cases cause people to lose their job. It induces stress with complaints and is hurtful to others. Behavioral issues in the workplace such as rudeness, yelling, shunning, mobbing, gossiping, refusing to talk to or acknowledge others, harassing, challenging conflict, incessant complaining to supervisors, ignoring directives, and working slowly are toxic to all who bear witness to it (Cross, 2013). Attitude problems manifest themselves differently in each individual. It is important, therefore, to address the problem head-on before resentment builds. Johnson (2013) adds that a negative attitude not only interferes with potential promotions but can also cost employees their jobs because their lack of interest, negativity, and lack of team spirit are dangerously toxic.

YOU ARE ONLY HUMAN

Humans spend approximately one third of their life working; therefore, the activity of work can be jeopardized when either physical or mental health is compromised. Living and working within your recognized limitations is something we all do; however, when mental health is compromised, because of its insidiousness, it can occur without our realization that it is happening. A string of busy days with heavy workloads, staff shortages, and you just finishing a couple of overtime shifts can quickly engulf you and become a new normal.

As practicing nurses, the lives and care of others are often placed in our hands, so that our good mental health and its accompanying cognitive processes, thinking ability, and astute concentration and judgment are critically needed. Good mental health for nurses helps to ensure they are able to engage productively in activities, fulfill collegial and caring relationships with others, have an affirmed comprehension of knowledge, and demonstrate skills and competency such that their responses to patient care are accurate, timely, knowledgeable, and evidence-informed. However, as a nurse and human being, one can perform only as well as one's mental health permits. Finally, good mental health provides flexibility to adapt to change and to cope with adversity, to an actualization of optimal self-esteem, confidence, courage, resilience, and growth.

The daily encounters of a nurse at work, such as maneuvering through vital signs, delegating tasks, facing angry family members, changing dressings, and dealing with increased patient acuity, whether they are related to workload, collegial relationships, or patient demands, all contribute to the buildup of stress. The mental health associated with a productive and adaptive response to stress does not always occur in a clear manner. You can and will make mistakes, but you will also learn from these mistakes because, again, you are only human.

Although it is important to recognize stress, many often do not. However, once you admit to yourself that you are dealing with high levels of stress, you can start doing something about it. If your organization has a stress management program, find out more about it, and communicate with your family and friends what you are experiencing, so they can understand (McNutt, 2008).

You need to quit being so hard on yourself; sometimes we can be our own worst enemy. We set our standards so high, so that sometimes they are almost unachievable, that we nearly kill ourselves trying to reach them. Not many stop to ask themselves why. And why am I trying to get there, when this will quite simply achieve the same goal?

This is just one example, and of course depending on our upbringing, values, and personality type, we don't like to take no for an answer too often, or at least we would prefer not to. But striving to be a perfect person is not going to make it happen. There is no perfect person in this world, except perhaps your religion authority figure, such as God in the case of Christianity. The Zen of letting go is not easy (Stack, 2013), and striving for perfection is actually counterproductive to what you set out to achieve. Letting go of perfection will free more time for yourself, make you feel better and happier, decrease your worry, promote self-growth, and help you to readily accept change and realize you cannot control others. This is then why it is important to not sweat the small stuff and love one day at a time, live each day to its fullest, follow your intuition, and do one thing at a time (Carlson & Carlson, 2013). As a recent survivor of cancer and brain surgery myself, having feared I was fatally ill, I have lived this experience and through this very philosophy learned how to let the stress go and live more happily and freely.

EMPOWER YOURSELF

Empowering yourself needs to happen to give you strength, confidence, and competence (Marston, 2013). Marston adds there are several ways you can empower yourself and beat any personal and professional challenges thrown your way. These include learning from every experience, never giving up in spite of letdowns, being respectful and thankful always, and taking responsibility and being accountable in all that you do. Today, we typically refer to this as protective empowering, which has an important role to play for nurses and how they practice through an ethical lens. Nurses may often encounter struggles in balancing their own power with those of the client's choices. To help address these challenges, protective empowering is something that nurses do in an effort to maintain their standards of practice and promote a balance between the safety of their clients and clients' choices and their own professional responsibility. Ethically, it means nurses seek to act and make decisions in the most responsible and professional manner possible, while at the same time promoting beneficence (doing good) and nonmaleficence (doing no harm) for clients' safety with clients' autonomy or the choices they should be allowed to make. Some of the theoretical underpinnings of the theory of protective empowering include that safety and choices are addressed simultaneously, that the possibility of health is sought within illness, and that clients' views and participation are invited (Chiovitto, 2009).

The theory of protective empowering further helps nurses to reflect on their own practices and the extent to which they provide standardized care for their clients, as it helps them to describe what it is nurses do on a day-to-day basis as they care for their clients and the actual experiences nurses have had in their day-to-day work with patients that represent how nurses accomplish caring with their patients and the outcomes or consequences of caring.

THE VALUE OF PERCEPTION

The behavioral patterns that accompany major depressive disorder stem partly from how a person perceives his or her life circumstances. How people perceive a situation affects their emotional responses, as well as their ability to process incoming information. The study by Milutinovic, Golubovic, Brkic, and Prokes (2012) focused on the different perceptions of stress among critical care nurses, and these perceptions varied depending on age, marital status, and education level. They state, "Most situations are subjective. Life events, examinations, or types of work can be very stressful to one person yet easier to cope with and 'water off a duck's back' to others. As with many forms of perception, scientists don't know the actual neural mechanisms that allow you to combine your prior experience with information coming in through your senses, and produce your brain's judgment that a situation is dangerous." However, from experience and practice, we know they exist.

Much of our stress comes from within us. How we interpret others' actions, conversation, nonverbal gestures, and behaviors all determine if something becomes a stressor for us. Even a negative self-talk or rumination of events and exchanges causes us to focus on self-criticism and pessimistic overanalysis, and to turn an innocent remark into a major source of stress. As expressed by the Canadian Mental Health Association (CMHA, 2014), "Understanding where your stress originates can help you decide on a course of action." While external stressors, like bereavement or career changes, can be managed over time and with the support of family and friends, internal stressors, caused by our own negative interpretation, require changes in attitude and behavior. Remember, a problem is a problem only if you perceive it to be (Koffman, 2006).

Our perception of stress is what can create its negative impact. As found by Nabi et al. (2013) in the Whitehall II study, people who believe stress is affecting their health "a lot or extremely" had double the risk for a heart attack compared with people who didn't believe stress was having a significant effect on their health. Further, psychological stress results from a subjective "cognitive appraisal" that an external demand made on the individual is excessive, conflicting, or unacceptably prolonged (McIntosh & Sheppy, 2013).

WORK–LIFE BALANCE

Achieving work–life balance is crucial to achieving good mental health. Because you spend a third of your life at work, you want to make sure your work and your personal life are balanced. The maintenance of a healthy work–life balance is something vitally important if you wish to continue to do the things you enjoy. Work–life balance is the "state of well-being that a person can reach or set as a goal in order to allow [him or her] to manage effectively multiple responsibilities at work, at home and in [the] community. Work–life balance is different for everyone, and it supports physical, emotional, family and community health and does so without grief, stress or negative impact" (Canadian Mental Health Association [CMHA] Ontario, 2010). Work–life balance touches every aspect of your life and helps you achieve equilibrium in all that you do.

Balancing personal and professional demands takes integrity, virtue, strength, and awareness of self. Although the key is not to become overwhelmed, sometimes nurses lose sight of this, avoiding the sources and impact of stress, and therefore not dealing with the stress and stressors they face every day. Further, nurses are one group of health care providers who believe they are immune to stress-related disease because they've studied it, nurtured clients dealing with it, and therefore feel they "know all about it." Deferred attention to one's own experience of stress and needs regarding stress and stressors can exert negative outcomes on nurses. Greater workplace flexibility enables employees to minimize work–life conflict by allowing them to accomplish the tasks necessary in their daily lives.

Work–life balance is so important to our everyday lives, particularly for nurses who work lengthy shifts. Whether you realize it or not, if you are trying to work harder to get everything done as soon as possible, reducing the quality time you spend with family and friends or sleeping less to do more, you probably don't have much balance. What ultimately happens is that many of those symptoms that we identified in Chapter 1 develop and mental health becomes impacted. Poor work–life balance can negatively impact an individual's mental health, and it can also hinder the prevention and management of mental illness. For example, if you are feeling overwhelmed and losing control of your life and are experiencing feelings of guilt, inability to focus and concentrate, chronic exhaustion, increased irritability, and bad temper, you are probably lacking a needed balance between your personal and professional life. These multiple roles can be enriching and allow for fulfillment of individual strengths and responsibilities, but conflicting responsibilities can lead to role conflict or overload.

The effects of workplace stress go far beyond the workplace and spill over into one's personal life. Heavy workloads, unsupportive managers, and work cultures can disrupt work–life balance (Todd, 2004). The technology of cell phones and e-mail keeps nurses connected to their work outside the office at all times, blurring the boundary between work and life. Some examples of effective workplace interventions to restore work–life balance include flexible working hours, time banking, providing child care services at work, study leave, employee assistance programs, leave without pay, career breaks, and supporting voluntary work as part of paid work time (Pollett, 2007; Todd, 2004).

Nurses must learn to take care of themselves, as well as their patients. By doing so, they will feel more valued and happier both at work and at home; have reduced stress; have better confidence, concentration, responsibility, and sense of control; have a greater sense of well-being, commitment, and job satisfaction; and have better organizational citizenship behaviors (behaviors of personal choice that benefit the organization) and job performance (Canadian Centre for Occupational Health and Safety, 2012).

Mentally, you build many self-accomplishments and have an increased sense of self, value, and concept as well as greater self-esteem, confidence, sense of success and achievement, and finally, sense of belongingness and importance.

Finding that balance between work and pleasure is often a challenge for many people. It means taking time out for "you." Typically, most nurses are working consistently on their feet, rushing around under pressure so much that their shift is often finished before they realize it. As a nurse, you need to proactively plan time for yourself as well. Whether this is time designated for your family, yourself, friends, or community, you need to embrace it and go with it; you may be surprised with how it makes you feel afterward. That book, puzzle, or Sudoku you never had time to do, the walk in the park with your dog, or the scrapbook you don't seem to have time for—take the challenge, it may be life-changing. Similarly, the movie, volunteer work, book club, and time with your children or dog that you keep putting off are all activities that can get you out of the house and workplace into an arena of fun and pleasure that refuels and refreshes your mind and lets you *have fun*. As a recent cancer survivor myself, my own philosophy is that life is too short. If you would like to do something that you feel would be fun and engaging and put a smile on your face, then go do it. As long as, of course, it is legally and morally conducive to your own values and beliefs. And always, think before you speak.

You have to remember, no one is going to take care of you and your needs the way you will. You know your strengths and limitations; sometimes you just need to remind yourself of them. Write them down and set little goals for you to help overcome some of these limitations, then do it. Nobody is perfect, so you aren't expected to be either. Sometimes as nurses we set our standards too high because society expects us to know a lot about everything. We know a lot, but we don't know everything and what is best for everybody. This is probably why we use collaboration in both our personal and professional lives.

Being a nurse who typically works long hours and night shifts in busy settings is hard work. There is no doubt about it. We are often so caught up with caring for others that we forget to take care of ourselves. Nurses, for example, are perhaps one of the worse populations at keeping doctors' appointments and at getting diagnostic tests done in a timely manner.

There are many different strategies you can employ to try to achieve a healthy work–life balance, many of which are quite similar to addressing and dealing with stress. For many, this is not an easy feat; however, you have to be in total control of your own endeavors, abilities, and obligations, so balance them wisely. A nurse can help achieve this balance by acting on basic advice and being proactive by living in a healthy manner, eating well, exercising, and getting lots of sleep. Further, you need to take breaks, take a vacation, and get away from work; don't overstretch yourself by setting unrealistic goals, say no every now and then, set your boundaries, and turn off that pager, BlackBerry, or iPod and explore your options as it will help you feel more energized, recharged, and productive (Tomey, 2009; Yoder-Wise, 2011). As found by Ruggiero (2005), nurses said factors that would help increase their job satisfaction were more weekends off, less depression and emotional stress, and better or more creative scheduling.

PROFESSIONAL STANDARDS OF PRACTICE

Knowledge and practice of nursing standards are other key indicators that help nurses become more effective, have better balance, and build a more respectful workplace that supports the mental health of nurses. One of the key characteristics of a self-regulating profession is the development of standards of practice, and they are the guiding force for many nurses. A standard is an authoritative statement that sets out the legal and professional basis for nursing practice (American Nurses Association [ANA], 2010).

Standards of practice in any profession are often developed at a higher political level of one's province, state, county, or country and should apply to all nurses of that jurisdiction regardless of the practice setting in which they are employed. They typically revolve around key expectations and themes that include accountability, continuing competence, ethical work behaviors, the development and application of knowledge, and leadership and professional relationships and demeanors. The standards of practice act as guidelines for nurses to follow when providing care to patients. As they are evidence-informed, they help to ensure that the best or most up-to-date treatment and care are being provided. Their primary purpose is to identify for nurses, the public, government, and other stakeholders the desired and achievable level of performance expected of nurses in their practice, against which actual performance can be measured. In addition, they help to protect the public by providing safe, competent, and ethical care; they help to regulate nursing practice and to regulate and approve nursing education; they provide guidelines for nursing leadership and quality control, a legal baseline, and public information; and they are involved in research and policy development. They are the expected benchmark to articulate the committed responsibility and accountability of nurses' professional practice.

PROFESSIONAL ETHICS

In nursing, ethical knowing concerns itself not just with moral questions of right and wrong but also with situational moral obligations. The foundation of the nurse's ethical knowledge is embodied in the college's or association's professional code of ethics, which includes nursing values and ethical responsibilities. However, considering "the complexity of the ethical issues in modern health care practice" (White, 2012, p. 209), ethical decision making is not often clear-cut, despite the importance of moral standards and codes of ethics. Doing what is "just" in theory does not always coincide with a practical orientation of doing what is "good" for the patient (White, 2012). Ethical knowing aids nurses in navigating situational and relational decision making and in morally conducting their practice—not only to provide the best care to patients but also to contribute to the good of society. Johnson (2013) adds that the moral aspect of nursing cannot be separated from the notion of competency and excellence in nursing.

The ethical practice of nurses often goes hand in hand with their legal practice. Ethical practice in nursing is forever at the forefront of nurses' decisions, practices, and policy implementation. It represents a science in which moral actions interface with moral values and beliefs. Ethics represents the systematic study of what a person's actions and conduct ought to be with respect to self, other human beings, and the environment (Guido, 2006) and the principles of morality of what we consider right or wrong (Yoder-Wise, 2011). Furthermore, as ethics applies more specifically to nursing, it is "concerned with motives and attitudes and the relationship of these attitudes to the overall care" of the client. It helps nurses to justify what is right or wrong and what one's life and relationships ought to be, not what they actually are (Marquis & Huston, 2012). The ultimate goal of ethics in nursing is to "provide a reasoned and best solution to situations that arise in everyday clinical practice" (Guido, 2006, p. 67). For example, while the law states you must do one thing, as outlined in legislation, your morals, values, and own personal and professional ethics may be pulling you in another direction or toward another option or decision. Quite often, you may feel drawn by this opposing force of morals, values, and ethics because you feel it is in the best interests of the vulnerable client at that time, or because it may be something you are not certain of or comfortable with, at a personal level.

The list is endless when it comes to the kinds of ethical situations that nurses may find themselves in when caring for individuals with mental illness. No matter what the setting, ethical issues span the continuum from geriatric psychiatry to acute adult care, to forensics, and yes, to pediatric psychiatry as well. However, there are many common principles of ethics in the nursing profession. Although there are many identified principles of ethics in nursing, the main ones include autonomy (to promote the good of all), beneficence, nonmaleficence (doing no harm), veracity (always telling the truth), fidelity (standing by your promise or commitment), respect, and justice (fair and equal treatment of all; Yoder-Wise, 2011, p. 89).

To help put nurses' own beliefs, values, and perceptions into perspective in a way that doesn't jeopardize the quality of care required for the client, an ethical decision-making framework can and should be utilized. The completion of a nurse's assessment (what is legally and morally right), exploration of alternatives (what the choices are and the pros and cons of each), analysis (what could result from my decision), application (does my choice do the greatest good, do no harm, and apply the Golden Rule), and action (you need to be ready to accept responsibility and act on it) can all guide the nurse to arrive at the best possible ethical solution or decision (Project Management Institute, 2012).

Geographical jurisdictions and countries have their own codes of ethics for practicing nurses. As taken directly from the ANA (2001), primary nursing values include providing safe, compassionate, competent, and ethical care; promoting health and well-being; promoting and respecting informed decision making; preserving dignity; maintaining privacy and confidentiality; promoting justice; and being accountable.

LEGISLATIVE REQUIREMENTS FOR LICENSED PROFESSIONALS

The law serves a number of functions in nursing. Like all other law-abiding citizens and members of a caring/giving profession, nurses are in positions of trust and are therefore expected to uphold all forms of the law, perhaps even more so because they are responsible for the care of vulnerable patients. These legally obligated functions relate to issues regulating the practice of nursing and the relationship between the nurse and the patient, especially in relation to the dignity of the human person, regulation of the nursing profession, the confidentiality of information between nurse and patient, and the important issue of consent. It is your standards of practice and code of ethics that guide your professional conduct in your professional nursing practice. Finally, they help to establish the boundaries of independent nursing action and assist in maintaining a standard of nursing practice by making nurses accountable under the law (Nmonu, 2008) because it is important to remember that your license to practice as a nurse is a privilege, not a luxury.

PSYCHOSOCIAL BEHAVIORS AND PRACTICES

In addition to your eating habits, there are some psychosocial behavior and practices you can use to promote mental health. Some of these, although the list is not exhaustive, include such things as social support, work–life balance, dealing with stress, sleep, taking on challenges, taking care of yourself, and exercise. Again, physiologically, we will also better understand their connection to building good mental health.

Social support. Social support and networking are perhaps among the most valuable measures to help foster and strengthen your good mental health. Having people around us that we engage, trust, and interact with lets us know and feel that we are not alone. Having good social supports with whom we frequently interact helps to boost our own mental health. Building strong relationships and avenues of social support greatly helps to enrich our life; it also gives us a greater sense of value, concept, and overall well-being, as well as an opportunity and safe place to talk, vent, and share with a trusted confidant.

Contribute to your community. Volunteering your time for a cause or issue that you care about, such as helping a neighbor, working in a community garden, or do something nice for a friend, not only improves the lives of others but also is sure to improve your life. Meaningful involvement helps to increase self-esteem, confidence, and your value as a member of society, and such preoccupation of your mind prevents you from dwelling and ruminating on the things that cause you stress.

Challenge yourself. To avoid getting too comfortable in a mundane job and creating plateaus of untapped energy, motivation, and interest, you need to reach out and grasp new and different challenges and opportunities. Learn a new skill or take on a challenge to meet a goal as learning improves your mental fitness, builds skills and confidence, and gives you a sense of progress and achievement (Koffman, 2006). You have to remember that there is always a challenge out there if you're willing to accept it (Mental Health Foundation, 2013). A new job, position, and slate of coworkers can give you an increased sense of meaning, new learning, and a feeling of belonging and being valued, not to mention self-worth and confidence. A career that motivates you emotionally to get excited in the morning is a coping skill. However, if your job is something you don't like, you can still deal with it. Although a problem is an external entity outside yourself and is creating an issue of discomfort for you in some respect, then you need to view it as a challenge, take hold of it, and go with it to address it. In this way, you can show your true colors, your skills, your knowledge base, and your leadership abilities (Koffman, 2006).

OTHER BEHAVIORS AND PRACTICES FOR YOURSELF

In addition to the many everyday practices and routines of daily life that apply to all humans, identified above, there are several other behaviors, tips, and practices that can help us as humans maintain and sustain good mental health. These include such things as resilience, being socially savvy, and integrity.

According to the American Psychological Association (2014), resilience is not a trait that people either have or don't have; it involves actions, thoughts, and behaviors that can be learned and developed in anyone. Building resilience can involve many simple things, such as accepting that change is part of living, making connections, accepting help if you need it, not being afraid to ask for it, avoiding seeing crises as insurmountable problems, taking decisive actions, creating realistic goals and moving toward them, grasping opportunities for self-discovery, nurturing a positive view of yourself and the future, being attuned to your body's needs, and keeping things in perspective.

Resiliency is closely related to coping. Everyone goes through hard times and suffers pain, it's all a part of life that causes us much stress, sadness, and anxiety. Resiliency becomes evident when individuals who have good mental health are able to bounce back from the adversity of a lost job, lost relationship, illness, sadness, or other setback (Elements Behavioral Health, 2013). They see the circumstance or situation for what it is and try to reestablish their emotional balance, and by doing so they ensure that they don't become trapped in negative mood states or in depression or anxiety.

Being Socially and Technologically Savvy

Social media have tremendously changed the way people interact and carry on with their everyday lives and work (Briscoe, 2013). However, they can also create much havoc in your life. Social media sites such as Twitter, Facebook, LinkedIn, and even dating network sites all possess some very valuable information about who you are as a person and as a nurse. As the market for BlackBerries, smartphones, iPods, and iPads takes off, the opportunity for interaction has increased substantially. However, there are two main concerns about how technology can impact your mental health: the risk of sharing unintended information about yourself and the risk of losing that face-to-face interaction and the role interaction plays in sustaining mental health.

Social media communication tools have profoundly changed our lives and how we interact and are influenced by one another and the world around us (Briscoe, 2013; Gordhamer, 2009). These tools increase one's reach and power when it comes to influencing others (Briscoe, 2013).

Social networking does offer many benefits, such as increased social networking and building alliances and friends. It not only helps people stay in touch with existing contacts but also aids in the formation of new alliances and sharing of common interests. It opens up the possibilities of discovering and learning new information, sharing ideas and interests, and interacting with others. LinkedIn, for example, allows people to create professional networks that help them search for jobs or get tips on how to enhance their careers, which frees up time spent looking for jobs (Briscoe, 2013). These sites and those of Twitter and Facebook are fun and make it possible to stay connected with colleagues, friends, and family, but caution should always be exercised. You have to be very careful about what information you are sharing with others and posting publicly for the whole world to see. The sites are an effective means to find and maintain both old and potentially new friendships and meet future loved ones, and they have led to telephone calls, meetings, and even marriages that have been very successful (Gordhamer, 2009).

The previous goal was to make sure that you appeared confident, knowledgeable, and in control. However, social media have shifted this paradigm so that you no longer try to appear perfect, but to be more transparent with your thoughts and feelings, to reveal your humanness. As the networks for sharing and amplifying information strengthen, the ability of each person to influence public opinion and policies increases. As a result, we feel much like active participants who have a voice in the events of our world (Gordhamer, 2009).

The advent of technology comes with a price. It decreases opportunity to talk to and interact with people face to face (Skype is just not the same, is it?). The removal of the face-to-face opportunity for interaction can decrease the amount of cognitive stimulation and socialization factors that we, as humans, strive to obtain, and it also infringes on the potential for exercise and leisure activity (Briscoe, 2013). Furthermore, what you post publicly has the potential to be seen by much of the world and used against you. Placing private pictures and personal information out into cyberspace can come with hefty costs, such as mental illness and addictions (Esposito, 2010) and even suicide (Agomuoh, 2012). Nurses need to be especially cognizant of what they post on social media sites for fear that patients' confidentiality and privacy of care may become breached. Whom they make friends or connections with, the comments they post, and the groups they join can all create personal and professional mentally challenging issues for nurses. Many nursing associations and colleges now have released position or policy statements about what is and is not acceptable for their members to be sharing on social media websites.

Respect 101

Our very existence does not hold any value if people do not respect us. Respect can and has been defined differently by various individuals and groups. It basically means consideration of self and of others and paying attention and valuing others' privacy, their physical space and belongings, and their different viewpoints, philosophies, physical abilities, beliefs, and personalities. Respect in the workplace is perhaps the most desired workplace attribute that people want. You know when you do and don't have respect from the people with whom you work, as it becomes clearly visible through their verbal messages and nonverbal behaviors and gestures. Although respect is often perceived as a difficult concept to address (Garrison, 2012), it is not hard to enforce, as some of the simplest and smallest of gestures and words can help.

Respect among nurses and the nursing profession in general is a significant item of discussion.

In order to gain respect and have respect for others, you must first have respect for yourself and realize that you are worthy of it. This can be achieved in many ways, such as refraining from "making jokes or negative remarks that demean their abilities, skills or other aspects of them." One can earn respect only by giving respect to oneself and to others (Balovich, 2006). Some simple suggestions on how respect can be demonstrated at work include the following: Treat everyone with courtesy, politeness, and kindness; encourage colleagues to express opinions and ideas; listen to others before expressing your viewpoint; use people's ideas to change or improve work and let them know you used their ideas; never insult people, name call, disparage, or put down people or their ideas; avoid nit-picking, constantly criticizing even over little things, belittling, judging, demeaning, or patronizing; and treat everyone the same regardless of race, religion, gender, size, age, and country of origin. Furthermore, include all of your coworkers in meetings, discussions, training, and events and do not marginalize; praise more, criticize less, rely on facts, not hearsay or chatter, treat others as you would like to be treated (the Golden Rule), take responsibility for your actions, own up and say you were wrong, and be empathetic (Heathfield, 2013; Richman, 2007).

Respect is not difficult to achieve, and it brings many great benefits to those who bear witness to it and become involved. Besides the familiar karma of "what goes around, comes around," it really is how you deal with, talk to, behave, and interact with others or in the presence of others. However, many workplaces are still struggling to achieve it among their employees. In one U.S. study cited by Richman (2007), "Americans view incivility as a serious problem that is getting worse. One study found that 60% of employees believe that coworkers' annoying behaviors negatively impact the workplace, and as a result, 40% reported that they are looking for new employment. These and other findings illustrate that disrespectful and uncivil behaviors drain productivity and negatively influence both an organization's bottom line and the overall economy" (Richman, 2007).

Things to do to show respect are many and varied. If every nurse develops an awareness of showing and speaking respect for others, then "employees will serve as role models and these behaviors will spread in the workplace and beyond." One of the golden rules in any relationship is to listen to people. Listen to their opinions, ideas, or qualms before giving your viewpoint. Do not butt in or cut them off while they are speaking. It is important for the other person to feel that his or her opinion is of value, and by interrupting the person, you will be showing disrespect. Do not have preconceived notions about what that person might be saying.

Respect produces many benefits. It breeds collegiality, collaboration, good morale, knowledge transfer (Hodge, 2010), cooperation, and even profitability for the organization. Most importantly, respect in the workplace can ward off mental health challenges and disorders and can promote customer/patient safety and satisfaction. Furthermore, it can decrease the incidence of workplace conflict (Hodge, 2010); produce an open and inviting atmosphere where people feel free to speak their mind; promote engagement and make people valued and involved (Hodge, 2010); and promote work security (Collins, 2010), loyalty (Collins, 2010), and greater retention of workers (Collins, 2010). In the absence of respect, we often feel that we are not appreciated or respected for our sincerity and talent, but instead demeaned and taken for granted.

THE VALUE OF COLLEGIALITY AND COLLABORATION

Interprofessional collaboration among health care workers is a critical element in today's health care systems. Collaboration among disciplines is just as important as collaboration among your nursing colleagues. Interprofessional collaboration can be defined as health care clinicians working together, bringing their own unique knowledge, skill set, and practices to the table with the common goal of providing optimal care, treatment, and recovery for the patient. It is underpinned by the values of honesty, directness, respect, and listening to others' viewpoints.

Interprofessional collaboration is a skill or competency, in itself, that is important for all to develop and respect. It truly represents the most complete approach needed to ensure holistic patient/client care and an amenable delivery of services to best meet the needs of patients/clients and their families. The six key principles that should be included in interprofessional collaboration include focusing on and involving the patient, taking a population health approach, ensuring quality of care and services, supporting access of the patient to the right professional, trust and respect, and regular, clear communication.

Finally, you need to be aware of workplace politics. Within the workplace as well, nurses are often confronted with the negativities that politics in the workplace often bestow upon them and that further threaten nurses' moral fiber. Politics of this nature still represents behaviors of individuals as they attempt to acquire, develop, and use power and other resources to obtain their preferred outcomes in a situation in which there is uncertainty about choices. It is frequently characterized by relationships within an organization that determine how a person will act in a given situation. It is closely associated with power; however, this type of politics can work to the detriment of the individual nurse, the leader, or the workplace morale in general.

As a practicing nurse, you too can exercise some legitimate power that will help you move your life and career forward. For example, learn to speak your organization's language and don't expect it to learn yours, learn the organization's priorities and how you can help meet these needs, learn the power lines and who has the power, become acquainted with those who are powerful, develop your professional knowledge and power skills, be proactive rather than passive or reactive, assume authority in your dealings, take risks, be verbal about your achievements to increase your visibility, meet your supervisor's needs, and take care of your emotional, physical, and spiritual self.

Knowing Your Boundaries

As a nurse, you also have to remain cognizant of your professional limitations. Ethically, boundaries, self-disclosure, and the use of touch are important to know and understand. The therapeutic relationship between a nurse and the client serves a significant role (College of Registered Nurses of British Columbia [CRNBC], 2006). It should be professional and serve a therapeutic purpose, in which the client's needs are first and foremost in the grand scheme of things. As patients seeking health care are considered vulnerable, it is the nurse's responsibility to maintain that focus on professionalism and therapeutic care, regardless of how the client responds or behaves.

Nurses need to remain aware of what differentiates a professional from a personal relationship. The College of Nurses of Ontario (CNO; 2006) suggests that there are five components of the nurse-client relationship: trust, respect, professional intimacy (such as when a nurse assumes closeness to complete nursing tasks such as bathing and dressing), empathy, and recognition of nurse–patient power imbalances. However, nurses also need to recognize when the therapeutic

TABLE 6.1   Differences Between Professional and Personal Relationships

CHARACTERISTIC	PROFESSIONAL RELATIONSHIP (NURSE–CLIENT)	PERSONAL RELATIONSHIP
Behavior	Regulated by a code of ethics and professional standards	Guided by personal values and beliefs
Remuneration	Nurse paid to provide care to client	No payment for being in the relationship
Length of relationship	Limited by duration of the client's need for nursing care	May last a lifetime
Location of relationship	Place defined and limited to where nursing care is provided	Place unlimited, often undefined
Purpose of relationship	Goal-directed to provide care to client	Pleasure-, interest-directed
Structure of relationship	Nurse providing care to client	Spontaneous, unstructured
Power of balance	Unequal, with nurse having more power due to authority, knowledge, influence, and access to privileged information about client	Relatively equal
Responsibility for relationship	Nurse (not client) responsible for establishing and maintaining professional relationship	Equal responsibility to establish and maintain
Preparation for relationship	Formal knowledge, preparation, orientation, and training of nurse required	Formal knowledge, preparation, orientation, and training not required
Time spent in relationship	Nurse employed under contractual agreement that outlines hours of work for contact between nurse and client	Personal choice for how much time is spent in relationship

Adapted from British Columbia Rehabilitation Society (1992).

relationship moves beyond the professional level. For example, nurses should avoid becoming "friends" with their clients, socializing with patients, and engaging in a romantic or sexual venture with their clients. An isolated episode of such behaviors is not as concerning as a pattern of those behaviors, at which point reporting is necessary, disciplinary action may result, and the nurse will have to withdraw from the relationship (CNO, 2006). A nurse's actions and behaviors that cross the barrier from professionalism should be addressed as soon as possible. A nurse may find it best to help discuss his or her behaviors and emotions with a close colleague. By doing so, the nurse may better understand the issue of professional boundaries with clients and the importance of maintaining those boundaries.

There are also areas of boundary concern that do not involve a romantic engagement. Such areas of caution include abuse of a verbal, financial, physical, sexual, and emotional nature, giving and receiving gifts from patients, and completing tasks for monetary gain. Table 6.1 outlines some differences between professional and personal relationships.

Self-Disclosure

Both verbal and nonverbal communication is the main vehicle through which care is provided to patients. How and what a nurse communicates to a patient serves many therapeutic purposes, such as achieving productive thinking for the patient, providing emotional support and endurance, and enhancing positive behavioral outcomes (Keltner, Schwecker, & Bostrom, 2007, p. 91).

With all good intentions in mind, when nurses engage in discussion and communication with clients who have mental illnesses, their well-meaning altruistic and empathetic drives to help their patient can place them in a compromising position. In efforts to relay support to clients, nurses want to let the clients know that they truly understand them because they, their friends, or their family may also have been there or encountered life-challenging obstacles such as the clients are experiencing now. As a result, it is at times like this that nurses are enticed to disclose their own personal information and experiences. According to the CRNBC (2006), it occurs when a nurse shares personal information with a client. Self-disclosure may be used in moderation as long as it is focused on the needs of the client. In these situations, disclosing personal information may have the therapeutic intent of reassuring, counseling, or building rapport with clients. Some self-disclosure can often be a therapeutic tool for the nurse–client relationship as it helps to foster and strengthen rapport, trust, and respect between the nurse and the client (CNO, 2006). Self-disclosure must be done for the client's benefit, not as a self-fulfilling venture for the nurse, who may seek to obtain personal gratification or fulfill desires and needs from the disclosure (Zur, 2011). In essence, excessive self-disclosure is important for a nurse to avoid, as others can perceive this information as one of your vulnerabilities and at times draw upon tactics of intimidation and humiliation to bolster their own self-esteem and confidence and therefore use the nurse's personal information against him or her.

In a very similar light, empathy is often a recognized common goal of self-disclosure. Communicating empathy is an essential skill of any nurse. Empathy can be defined as "the ability to recognize and understand a client's feeling and point of view objectively" (Keltner et al., 2007, p. 91). However, it must never imply or suggest that the nurse can fully "experience" the feelings of the client.

However, there are many concerns that arise when a nurse decides to self-disclose. The nurse must remain cognizant of the limits of that self-disclosure so that the client does not in turn use that information against the nurse and hence place the nurse in a highly vulnerable position. However, "disclosing personal information that is lengthy, self-serving or intimate is never acceptable" (Keltner et al., 2007, p.13).

The Use of Touch

The use of touch in nursing is an important issue to discuss ethically and legally. Although a nurse may feel a touch on the client's hand or a hug is appropriate and supportive for the client, it may not be without ethical or legal ramifications. Therefore, caution should always be exercised.

The use of touch is recognized as use of one's therapeutic self that conveys messages of caring, concern, support, empathy, and acceptance (Arnold & Boggs, 2011; Keltner et al., 2007). The caring nature of nursing will always involve some form of touch, whether it is to complete a task such as a dressing change or taking vital signs or just a touch that is a showing of support and is used therapeutically to provide comfort, calmness, or encouragement to the client (CRNBC, 2012).

There are many reasons why the use of touch with patients should be carefully considered. The use of touch by a nurse toward a client can be often misinterpreted, particularly by psychiatric or confused patients, who may experience touch as physical or sexual abuse and who may have symptoms of paranoia, ruminating thoughts, or sexual thoughts and obsessions. Hence, in these situations, touching can often be misunderstood and perceived as a violation of one's personal space or privacy, a sexual advance or gesture, or an aggressive move (Keltner et al., 2007), so it is best to avoid it or practice much caution.

SUMMARY

The role of the nurse as a person and a professional requires much integrity, adaptability, and commitment. Only you can have control over what you think, what you say, and how you respond and behave. While there are many strategies and principles of coping, it still requires an individualized approach so as to maintain a work–life balance. Above all, as a person and a professional, it is also your responsibility to help build and maintain a mentally healthy workplace, and you do so as long as you have morals, values, beliefs, and a good attitude and you remain cognizant of your governing standards of practice and the legislative framework that guides such practice.

DISCUSSION QUESTIONS

1. What is the role of a nurse as a person and a professional in maintaining a mentally healthy workplace?
2. What are some coping strategies and principles that can help an individual face and deal with stress?
3. Why it is important to understand concepts such as the power of knowledge, the rumor mill, perception, empowerment, attitude, and selectively picking your own battles?
4. Why it is important to maintain a work–life balance?
5. How do your nursing professional standards of practice and your governing legislation guide your practice?
6. How are you as an individual and unique human being, with your lessons learned, values, beliefs, and morals, able to be resilient against the impact of stress?

REFERENCES

Adriaenssens, J., de Gucht, V., & Maes, S. (2012). The impact of traumatic events on emergency room nurses: Findings from a questionnaire survey. *International Journal of Nursing Studies, 49*(11), 1411–1422. doi:10.1016/j.ijnurstu.2012.07.003

Agomuoh, F. (2012). Amanda Todd suicide doesn't end cyber torment for ridiculed teen. *International Business Times.* Retrieved from http://www.ibtimes.com/amanda-todd-suicide-doesnt-end-cyber-torment-ridiculed-teen-846827

American Nurses Association. (2010). *Nursing: Scope and standards of practice* (2nd ed.). Retrieved from http://nursingworld.org/Nursing-Scope-Standards

American Psychological Association. (2014). *The road to resilience.* Retrieved from http://www.apa.org/helpcenter/road-resilience.aspx

Arnold, E., & Boggs, K. U. (2011). *Interpersonal relationships: Professional communication skills for nurses* (6th ed.). St. Louis, MO: Saunders.

Balovich, D. (2006). *Respect in the workplace.* Retrieved from http://www.creditworthy.com/3jm/articles/cw81706.html

Boyd, R., et al. (2013). *How to have good mental health.* Retrieved from http://www.wikihow.com/Have-Good-Mental-Health

Boyle, D. K., & Kochinda, C. (2004). Enhancing collaborative communication of nurse and physician leadership in two intensive care units. *Journal of Nursing Administration, 34*(2), 60–70.

Briscoe, C. J. (2013). *How social media is playing a great role in our daily life.* Retrieved from http://www.webmasterview.com/2011/12/social-media-role-in-daily-life

British Columbia Rehabilitation Society. (1992). *Nurse–client relationships.* Retrieved from https://www.crnbc.ca/Standards/Lists/StandardResources/406NurseClientRelationships.pdf

Buck, R., & Van Lear, C. A. (2002). Verbal and nonverbal communication: Distinguishing symbolic, spontaneous, and pseudo-spontaneous nonverbal behavior. *Journal of Communication, 52*(3), 522–541.

Canadian Centre for Occupational Health and Safety. (2012). *Mental health—psychosocial risk factors in the workplace.* Retrieved from http://www.ccohs.ca/oshanswers/psychosocial/mentalhealth_risk.html

Canadian Mental Health Association. (2014). *Take control of stress.* Retrieved from http://www.cmha.ca/mental_health/take-control-of-stress/#.UvWXp2JdX4s

Canadian Mental Health Association Ontario. (2010). *Job burnout.* Retrieved from http://wmhp.cmhaontario.ca/workplace-mental-health-core-concepts-issues/issues-in-the-workplace-that-affect-employee-mental-health/job-burnout

Carlson, R., & Carlson, C. (2013). *Don't sweat the small stuff, and it's all small stuff.* New York, NY: Hyperion.

Chant, S., Jenkinson, T., Randle, J., & Russell, G. (2002). Communication skills: Some problems in nursing education and practice. *Journal of Clinical Nursing, 11*(1), 12–21.

Chiovitto, R. F. (2009). *The theory of protective empowering as a lens for health, healing and hope with individuals in acute psychiatric-mental health settings.* Retrieved from http://cfmhn.ca/sites/cfmhn.ca/files/media/2009Conf/2C2_-_Chiovitti.pdf

College of Nurses of Ontario. (2006). *The therapeutic nurse-client relationship: Revised 2006 practice standard: An overview.* Retrieved from http://www.cno.org/Global/4-LearnAboutStandardsAndGuidelines/prac/learn/modules/tncr/pdf/TNCR-Chapter2.pdf

College of Registered Nurses of British Columbia. (2006). *Boundaries in the nurse-client relationship.* Retrieved from https://www.crnbc.ca/Standards/Lists/StandardResources/406NurseClientRelationships.pdf

Collins, M. C. (2010). *Why respect matters in the workplace.* Retrieved from http://www.helium.com/items/2031114-why-respect-matters-in-the-workplace

Cross, S. (2013). *Attitude problems in the workplace.* Retrieved from http://www.ehow.com/about_7640641_attitude-problems-workplace.html

Crouteau, P. (2014). *The danger of making assumptions.* Retrieved from http://www.legacy-bowes.com/latest-blog-posts/entry/the-danger-of-making-assumptions.html

Daiski, I. (2004). Changing nurses' disempowering relationship patterns. *Journal of Advanced Nursing, 48*(1), 43–50.

Donahue, P. (1996). *Origin of nursing.* Retrieved from http://www.nursingpower.net/nursing/origen.html

Dunn, E. J., Mills, P. D., Neily, J., Crittenden, M. D., Carmack, A. L., & Bagian, J. P. (2007). Medical team training: Applying crew resource management in the Veterans Health Administration. *Joint Commission Journal on Quality and Patient Safety, 33*(6), 317–325.

Elements Behavioral Health (2013). *Resiliency and good mental health.* Retrieved from http://www.elementsbehavioralhealth.com/mental-health/how-to-promote-good-mental-health

Esposito, L. (2010). *In cyber bullying, depression hits victims hardest.* Retrieved from http://www.cfah.org/hbns/2010/in-cyber-bullying-depression-hits-victims-hardest

Garrison, M. (2012). *5 smart routes to gain respect in the workplace.* Retrieved from http://workawesome.com/office-life/5-smart-routes-gain-workplace-respect

Gordhamer, S. (2009). *5 ways social media is changing our daily lives.* Retrieved from http://mashable.com/2009/10/16/social-media-changing-lives

Guido, G. W. (2006). Fostering legal and ethical practices. In P. Yoder-Wise & K. Kowalski (Eds.), *Beyond leading and management* (pp. 77–98). St. Louis, MO: Mosby.

Hall, A. (2005). Defining nursing knowledge. *Nursing Times, 101*(48), 34.

Hamric, A. B., & Blackhall, L. J. (2007). Nurse-physician perspectives on the care of dying patients in intensive care units: Collaboration, moral distress, and ethical climate. *Critical Care Medicine, 35*(2), 422–429.

Happell, B., Platania-Phung, C., Scott, D., & Nankivell, J. (2014). Communication with colleagues: Frequency of collaboration regarding physical health of consumers with mental illness. *Perspectives in Psychiatric Care, 50*(1), 33–43. doi:10.1111/ppc.12021

Heathfield, S. M. (2013). *How to demonstrate respect at work: Ten tips.* Retrieved from http://humanresources.about.com/od/workrelationships/a/demo_respect.htm

Hodge, C. (2010). *Why respect matters in the workplace.* Retrieved from http://www.helium.com/items/1967537-why-respect-matters-at-work

Johnson, M. (2013). *Workplace effect on attitude.* Retrieved from http://www.ehow.com/facts_5921443_workplace-effect-attitude.html#ixzz27TzxKpeK

Keltner, N. L., Schwecker, L. H., & Bostrom, C. E. (2007). *Psychiatric nursing* (5th ed.). St. Louis, MO: Mosby.

Koffman, F. (2006). *Conscious business: How to build values through values.* Boulder, CO: Sounds True.

Krairiksh, M., & Anthony, M. K. (2001). Benefits and outcomes of staff nurses' participation in decision making. *Journal of Nursing Administration, 31*(1), 16–23.

Kramer, M., & Schmalenberg, C. (2003). Securing "good" nurse/physician relationships. *Nursing Management, 34*(7), 34–38.

Levit, A. (2013). *How to be more optimistic at work.* Retrieved from http://www.businessinsider.com/4-ways-to-be-more-optimistic-at-work-2013-3

Lue, N. (2010). *Life lessons: The danger of making assumptions about people and relationships.* Retrieved from http://www.baggagereclaim.co.uk/life-lessons-the-danger-of-making-assumptions-about-people-and-relationships

Marquis, B. L., & Huston, C. J. (2012). *Leadership roles and management functions in nursing: Theory and application* (7th ed.). Philadelphia, PA: Lippincott Williams & Wilkins.

Marston, R. (2013). *Five ways you can empower yourself to achieve.* Retrieved from http://greatday.com/nmot/features/five-ways-you-can-empower-yourself-to-achieve.html

McIntosh, B., & Sheppy, B. (2013). Effects of stress on nursing integrity. *Nursing Standard, 27*(25), 35–39.

McNutt, B. (2008). *How does stress associated with being a nurse affect your relationship with your family?* Retrieved from http://ezinearticles.com/?How-Does-Stress-

Associated-With-Being-a-Nurse-Affect-Your-Relationship-With-Your-Family?&id= 1416670

Mental Health Foundation. (2013). *How we can help ourselves.* Retrieved from http:// www.mentalhealth.org.uk/help-information/an-introduction-to-mental-health/ how-can-we-help-ourselves

Milutinovic, D., Golubovic, B., Brkic, N., & Prokes, B. (2012). Professional stress and health among critical care nurses in Serbia. *Arhiv za Higijenu Rada i Toksikologiju, 63*(2), 171–180.

Nabi, H., Kivimaki, M., Batty, G. D., Shipley, M. J., Britton, A., Brunner, E. J., et al. (2013). Increased risk of coronary heart disease among individuals reporting adverse impact of stress on their health: The Whitehall II Prospective Cohort Study. *European Heart Journal.* doi:10.1093/eurheartj/eht216

Nmonu, E. I. (2008). *Nursing ethics and jurisprudence.* Retrieved from http://www.nou.edu. ng/noun/NOUN_OCL/pdf/pdf2/NSS%20320%202.pdf

Pollett, H. (2007). *Mental health promotion: A literature review.* Retrieved from http://www. cmhanl.ca/pdf/Mental%20Health%20Promotion%20Lit.%20Review%20June% 2018.pdf

Project Management Institute. (2012). *PMI ethical decision-making framework.* Retrieved from http://www.pmi.org/~/media/PDF/Ethics/Ethical%20Decision%20Making%20 Framework%20-%20FINAL.ashx

Richman, B. (2007). *Ten tips for creating respect and civility in your workplace.* Retrieved from http://www.lorman.com/newsletter/article.php?article_id=694&newsletter_id=150

Rosenberg McKay, D. (2013). *Gossip: Does it have a place at* work? Retrieved from http://career-planning.about.com/od/bosscoworkers/a/gossip.htm

Rucker, D., O'Connor, B., & Buxbaum, J. (2006). *Reducing errors/improving care.* HIMSS Symposium and Exhibition, San Diego, CA.

Ruggiero, J. S. (2005). Health, work variables, and job satisfaction among nurses. *Journal of Nursing Administration, 35*(5), 254–263.

Shiota, L. (2013). *Why does your attitude affect your workplace?* Retrieved from http://www. ehow.com/facts_5882073_attitude-affect-workplace_.html#ixzz2hQgEKRC5

Sonnenberg, F. (2013). *ACTIONS speak louder than words.* Retrieved from http://www.frank-sonnenbergonline.com/blog/actions-speak-louder-than-words

Stack, L. (2013). *10 reasons why you need to quit trying to be perfect.* Retrieved from http://www. tlnt.com/2013/07/26/10-reasons-why-you-need-to-quit-trying-to-be-perfect

Sutcliffe, K. M., Lewton, E., & Rosenthal, M. M. (2004). Communication failures: An insidious contributor to medical mishaps. *Academic Medicine, 79*(2), 186–194.

Todd, S. (2004). *Improving work-life balance—What are other countries doing?* Ottawa, ON: Labour Program, Human Resources and Skills Development Canada.

Tomey, A. M. (2009). *Guide to nursing management and leadership* (8th ed., Chapter 5). St. Louis, MO: Elsevier-Mosby.

Tschannen, D., & Lee, E. (2012). The impact of nursing characteristics and the work environment on perceptions of communication. *Nursing Research and Practice.* doi:10.1155/2012/401905 http://www.hindawi.com/journals/nrp/2012/401905/

Vonfrolio, L. G. (2005). Get real: End horizontal violence. *Registered Nurse, 68*(2), 60.

White, J. (2012). Patterns of knowing: Review, critique, and update. In P. Reed & N. Shearer (Eds.), *Perspectives on nursing theory* (6th ed., pp. 207–216). Philadelphia, PA: Wolters Kluwer Lippincott Williams and Wilkins.

Williams, G. D. (2007). *Attitude and stress, effects on the body.* Retrieved from http:// EzineArticles.com/702403

Woefle, C. Y., & McCaffrey, R. (2007). Nurse on nurse. *Nursing Forum, 42*(3), 123–131.

Yoder-Wise, P. S. (2011). *Leading and managing nursing* (5th ed.). St. Louis, MO: Elsevier-Mosby.

Zur, O. (2011). *I love these e-mails, or do I? The use of e-mails in psychotherapy and counseling.* Retrieved from http://www.zurinstitute.com/email_in_therapy.html

7

Workplace Bullying

> *All that is required for evil to prevail is for good men to do nothing.*
> —Edmund Burke

LEARNING OBJECTIVES

By the end of this chapter, the learner will be able to:

1. Define workplace bullying and the various categories of bullying that can occur.
2. Have a better understanding of why workplace bullying occurs.
3. Discuss the irony of bullying in a caring profession.
4. Identify and discuss the individual, professional, and organizational impact of workplace bullying.
5. Identify and discuss some key strategies that can be used to address workplace bullying.
6. Discuss how existing legislation in your jurisdiction can help to address workplace bullying.

The occurrence of workplace bullying and other disruptive and toxic workplace behaviors is truly not a recent phenomenon. The very premise of such behaviors actually predates the Common Era (CE). Even before the time of Christ, it was acknowledged that "all cruelty springs from weakness" (Seneca, 4 BCE–CE 65). In essence, that is exactly what bullying portrays, as it represents cruel, malicious, and vindictive actions, words, and behaviors directed toward others in an attempt to make them feel belittled, humiliated, demeaned, incompetent, and useless, just to name a few. As organizations in this fiscal and economic climate struggle to maintain and sustain optimal service delivery, the occurrence of workplace bullying by the very professionals responsible for providing "care" deepens these struggles even more so. The study of bullying, oppression, and its effects has been ongoing for more than 20 years (Woelfle & McCaffrey, 2007).

In the context of this chapter, bullying will not be equated fully with violence. Although it is often referred to as horizontal or lateral violence and can be correlated with increased violence (Woelfle & McCaffrey, 2007), bullying does not always mean violence was involved. Based on the premise that workplace violence is an exercise of physical force or the attempt to exercise physical force by a person against a worker in a workplace that causes or could cause physical injury to the worker (Workplace Mental Health Promotion, 2013), bullying in the context as described in this chapter will not be referred to as violence, but as a separate entity with its own horrific existence.

By the time you finish this chapter, you will see how bullying can create effects that are worse than the impact of violence. When violence occurs, it is something we physically see and witness, is short-lived, and because of its obviousness can be adequately documented, addressed, and dealt with, regardless of who the perpetrator is—a nursing colleague, a doctor, a patient, or a visitor. However, bullying takes a more insidious, underhanded approach. As a result, it can often go unnoticed and not addressed—therefore promoting its propagation and impact over a prolonged period of time and a metamorphosis into what we come to accept as normal, yet destructive. The actual act of violence for nurses at work will be discussed further in Chapter 10.

This may be a difficult chapter to read for some, but all nurses and nursing students need to be aware of the potential of bullying so that they do not blame themselves for such bullying tactics directed toward them. Nurses need to remember that each and every day they work, they are doing amazing work, performing heroic miracles, and contributing significantly to the lives of the patients and families they touch every time they come to work. It is this message that nurses need to collectively believe, for it is with compassion, kindness, and collegiality that the evils of workplace bullying can be abolished. No matter if you are student nurse, a novice nurse, or a veteran nurse, you have all experienced or witnessed workplace bullying (Daiski, 2004).

WORKPLACE BULLYING 101

Bullying is called many things by many different people. Most often in legislative acts and statutes, it is referred to as psychological harassment. In research and the literature, it is often phrased as horizontal violence or hostility, lateral violence, workplace incivility, or mobbing. Most recently, it has been disturbingly referred to as "professional cannibalism," perhaps to capture the meaning of the phrase nurses so often hear, "nurses eating their young." Regardless of what you call it, the meaning and the effects are still the same. Bullying in nursing has emerged as a growing concern, touching every corner of nursing practice and care that nurses face and struggle with daily.

There are several defining criteria for workplace bullying. These are as follows (Quine, 2001):

1. *Impact on the individual.* Individuals are subjected to gestures, slurs, behaviors, or verbalizations that make them feel humiliated, intimidated, and harassed.
2. *There must be a negative effect on the individual.* As a result of the impact of bullying, people typically feel that their self-esteem, self-confidence, self-value, and self-concept have been undermined and are plummeting downward.
3. *Persistence.* The bullying is persistent and repetitive, so much so that it increases in frequency. This persistence of demeaning and downgrading of human beings

through vicious words and cruelty gradually undermines confidence and self-esteem (Adams, 1997). The repeatedly offensive, vindictive, cruel, or malicious behavior is used as an attempt to humiliate or undermine an individual or employee.

4. *Consistency.* There is a consistent pattern of behavior designed to control, diminish, or devalue a peer (or group) that creates a risk to the health and safety of that person or others. These remarks, behaviors, and gestures are marked by harmony, regularity, or steady continuity as the perpetrator has the same remarks, behaviors, and gestures and intention each time the bullying act occurs.

Defined, workplace bullying is the ongoing health- or career-endangering mistreatment of an employee by one or more peer or higher-up (Canada Safety Council, 2010). It can be the misuse of power or position that undermines a person's ability or leaves the person feeling hurt, frightened, angry, or powerless. Further, it is the engaging in a course of vexatious comments or conduct against a worker in a workplace that is known or ought reasonably to be known to be unwelcome, and repeated, unreasonable, or inappropriate behavior directed toward a worker or group of workers that creates a risk to health and safety (Workplace Mental Health Promotion, 2013).

As added by Dunn (2003), workplace bullying occurs when sabotage is directed toward coworkers or colleagues who are at the same level or a lower level within an organization's hierarchy. It is behavior that humiliates, degrades, or indicates a lack of respect for the dignity and worth of an individual (Rowell, 2008). Reinforced by the motto of the U.K. National Workplace Bullying Agency (2009), "Those who can, do; those who can't, bully."

THE PROFILE OF THE BULLY

In the past, bullying typically characterized the actions of children as they set out to hurt the feelings of other children in the confines of a playground or school. It was in the 1970s that Norwegian psychologist Dan Olweus began his study of what was happening among Norwegian school children. René Veenstra, a sociologist at the University of Groningen in the Netherlands, suggested that a train of reported suicides prompted the study (Pappas, 2010). Since that time, years of research have continued to illustrate the power imbalances between bullies and their victims as a crucial element. Veenstra adds that bullies strive for admiration, control, status, and dominance, so they strategically pick their victims wisely and focus on those whom they know few other people will defend. In spite of these desires for control and aggression, bullies also want affection because they are seeking the approval and admiration of the larger group or population at hand.

What occurs in adults who are nurses is not much different from what occurs on the playground or schoolyard among children. If anything, it is perhaps more intense and psychologically concerning because we are now referring to mature, fully developed adults, not children who are seeking approval from their peers to "fit in."

Bullies know what to say, what to do, whom to do it to, and when to do it. They can play mind games and reverse psychology with others and are often takers who are mean-spirited, insecure people with poor or nonexistent social skills and little empathy. They turn this insecurity outward, finding satisfaction in their ability to attack and diminish the capable people around them (Canada Safety Council, 2010). This person can be charming, shallow, and superficial yet deceptive, devious, and manipulative, and can be a pathological liar with sociopathic and/or psychopathic tendencies (U.K. National Workplace Bullying Agency, 2009). Bullies are typically individuals who feel they are owed an exaggerated degree of apparent respect from others (Harvey, 2002). It is as if the world owes them something and they intend to collect it, and the only way to do that is by putting people down, belittling them, and robbing them of every ounce of self-esteem and concept they could possibly have.

Bullies know when to act. They are shrewd enough to realize that bullying needs to be invisible and done behind closed doors without witnesses if at all possible. Unless, of course, bullying is part of the culture in the unit or setting and a gang mentality is prevalent and accepted. In the presence of a gang mentality, other nurses have adopted such practices, and out of feeling intimidated themselves and a fear of negative ramifications for themselves, they simply join in with the bully. Bullies typically know whom they can safely target, and while the bully seems to be primarily female, the victim is also typically female. Bullies are in supervisory roles or outrank their targets (Namie, 2009).

Many people often ask if bullies know or even realize what they are doing and saying to others. This is an interesting debate because some suggest that because they can have a mental illness, they do not realize what they are doing. However, others have asked that if the act is premeditated enough, then how can bullies not know what they are doing? If bullies have the cognitive capacity to plan ahead, identify potential targets, and understand the best time to perform the act, then that is accepting that they know exactly what they are doing. As found by Woelfle and McCaffrey (2007), there is actually a positive correlation; as the prevalence of bullying in nurses increased, so too did the bullies' own acknowledgement that they were being bullies.

CATEGORIES OF WORKPLACE BULLYING

According to Rayner and Hoel (1997), workplace bullying can be categorized into five different classes:

1. *Threat to professional status.* This includes professional humiliation in public, belittling, sarcasm, called someone lazy, etc.
2. *Threat to personal standing.* This includes such actions as gossiping about you, what you did, and what you said. It is also manifested through name calling, insults, teasing, mocking, and putdowns.
3. *Isolation.* Purposely depriving someone of activities or opportunities; failing to invite the person to staff parties; denying the person leave, vacation time, and training/learning opportunities; withholding of information.
4. *Overwork.* This results from undue pressure to work harder, work more, and get more done. It can also arise when a supervisor or colleague sets unrealistic job

demands and guidelines and repeatedly or unnecessarily interrupts someone to delay the person's work progress or schedule.
5. *Destabilization.* In essence, this is setting someone up for failure. One nurse exerts effort so that another nurse's goals at work are sabotaged. It can also mean assigning a nurse meaningless tasks or removing from a nurse some responsibility that previously gave him or her a sense of belongingness, value, and independence, or repeatedly reminding a nurse of past mistakes or near misses in a taunting sort of fashion to undermine the nurse's true capabilities.

Holloway and Kusy (2010) propose another unique approach to categorizing toxic behaviors in the workplace. These three quoted categories are as follows:

1. *Shaming.* Humiliates others, makes sarcastic remarks, takes potshots at others, and points out the mistakes of others.
2. *Passive hostility.* Distrusts the opinions of others, displays passive–aggressive behavior, protects own territory, has difficulty accepting feedback, and is clueless that such behaviors are toxic.
3. *Team sabotage.* Monitors team members' behaviors, meddles in teamwork, and uses authority to punish others.

PREVALENCE OF BULLYING

Bullying has now moved beyond the playground and schoolyard. Currently, it has no boundaries or affinity for any particular workplace setting. A quick search will reveal to you that bullying occurs not only among other health professionals but in nearly every imaginable workplace environment. Bullying and the effects of bullying make the headlines on a weekly if not daily basis somewhere in the world. Approximately 21% of all workers have been targeted by bullies (Brunner & Costello, 2003; Namie, 2009).

Many organizations and businesses feel that workplace bullying does not affect their workplace; however, the prevalence is staggering. When the Workplace Bullying Institute conducted a survey in 2007, it was found that 37% of workers were bullied, 13% currently and 24% previously (Workplace Mental Health Promotion, 2013). In addition, 40% of bullied individuals never tell their employers, and 62% of employers who are told ignore the problem, hoping that it will stop on its own, not knowing what to do, or normalizing this damaging behavior (Workplace Mental Health Promotion, 2013). Further, 45% of targets suffer stress-related health problems. Health care is identified as a high-risk area at 33% (Statistics Canada, 2007).

Health Care

The prevalence of workplace bullying in health care settings is gaining increased recognition that matches its rising trend. In an earlier study of workplace bullying, Sofield and Salmand (2003) found that 98% of all health care staff, consisting primarily of nurses, had witnessed bullying types of behavior. As found by Kusy and

Holloway (2009), 94% of all health care leaders "had to deal with a toxic person at work." Similarly, Johnson (2009) found that 80% of doctors are disrespectful to other health care staff, and 33% reported that this had occurred weekly.

As it pertains to workplace bullying, "there is a drastic increase in the severity of work-related issues, with workplace violence and work-related conflict contributing the greatest increases" (Warren Shepell, 2002). "Dr. Tehrani conducted a study of 165 professionals in the caring sector such as nurses and social workers. Dr. Tehrani found that 36% of the men and 42% of the women reported having experienced bullying" (Knight, 2004).

Nursing

Realistically, bullying in nursing has taken on a life of its own. As one Penn State University professor, Dr. Cheryl Dellasega, stated, "Nurses are really vicious to each other. ... It's not one hospital. It's not one type of nurse. It's the new nurse, it's the nurse from another floor, it's the ICU nurses feeling superior to the med-surg nurse ... it's endless." In essence, bullying in nursing knows no boundaries and does not discriminate who gets targeted, how, or why. In most cases it's a "free for all," and whoever is standing in the way, watch out, as you may be next.

The statistics that support the prevalence of bullying in nursing are phenomenal and troubling. As found by many, bullying in nursing is alive and well, but not well for the nurses on the receiving end. Nurse-against-nurse bullying is second only to physician-against-nurse bullying (Felblinger, 2009). As found by Quine (2001), 44% of community health nurses reported experiencing one or more types of bullying in the previous year, while 50% witnessed the bullying of others.

Bullying in nursing is suggested to be underreported. Many believe that bullying in nursing occurs more frequently than is reported. As found by Woelfle and McCaffrey (2007), for example, a positive correlation between sabotage efforts and increased work satisfaction seems somewhat paradoxical; however, it could be attempts by nurses to normalize their bullying experiences or their attempts to rationalize happiness in the workplace.

Nursing Students

For nursing students as well, the trend continues. At a point in their lives when nursing students have decided to become nurses as a career of choice, they are often dismayed by what they encounter on that journey. As found by Curtis, Bowen, and Reid (2007), more than 50% of nursing students experienced or witnessed bullying during their clinical placements. So significant was this experience that 51% of these students indicated that it would affect their future career and their choice of the facility where they would seek employment opportunities. Randle (2003) found that nursing students' "sense of self was greatly influenced by how they were treated by nurses in clinical areas," and the whole process of becoming a nurse was stressful and "psychologically damaging."

However, research further suggests that workplace bullying is so culturally integrated into the environment that nursing students can quickly learn to become bullies as well. Randle also noticed that so much did nursing students witness bullying of patients or their nursing colleagues that they began to incorporate bullying tactics into their own practices. For nursing students who are typically eager and willing to learn new ways of practice and thinking, it was like just another learned activity, only this time it enabled them to gain social control, a power over something or someone that became integral to their own self-esteem and confidence (Randle, 2003).

THE IRONY

From Florence Nightingale's time to today, nursing has been renowned for its compassionate approach to caring for patients. In fact, nursing has been defined as the "body of knowledge that is related to the study of caring in human health that encompasses both the science and art of nursing" (Monti & Tingen, 1999, p. 27). Jarrin (2007) further elaborates this notion and suggests, "The central focus of the profession of nursing is using the art and science of caring to improve the health of human beings within their environments." As is found in much of the nursing literature, the theme of caring is threaded through the nursing profession for as long as we can remember. The primary purpose of health care in general is to address patients' physical, emotional, physiological, and spiritual needs (Vonfrolio, 2005). Many of us went into nursing for very nonselfish, altruistic reasons underpinned by a philosophy that we wanted to do good for those who are in the unenviable position of battling illness or disability. The finding and witnessing of workplace bullying in the caring profession of nursing is ironic at best. As Rowell (2008) and many others ask, "Why do we find such a high prevalence in nursing if it is supposed to be synonymous with caring, altruism, and/or compassion?"

Caring in nursing symbolizes many actions and behaviors practiced as we endeavor to assist our patients on their road from illness to wellness and recovery. The nursing profession is distinctive in that aspects of the discipline remain deeply influenced by scientific knowledge while balanced with the art of caring. Caring, I believe, is a common thread in all aspects of nursing practice and the application of knowledge. One of the most crucial components of daily nursing practice is nurturing relationships and finding innovative and creative ways to maintain them over the long term. Further, it is characterized by much kindness, caring, compassion, and concern for others that have even been derived often from our own upbringing. As Kagan, Smith, Cowling, & Chinn (2009) suggest, caring is the "foundational knowledge and ethic for nursing that focuses on loving, valuing, and nurturing self and others" (p. 69). The caring theory of Watson (2013) suggests that effective caring promotes healing, health, individual/family growth, and a sense of wholeness, forgiveness, evolved consciousness, and inner peace. Nursing, as defined by Schim, Benkert, Bell, Walker, and Danford (2007), is a "learned humanistic art and science that focuses upon personalized individual and group care and a caring relationship" (p. 76). This is substantiated by the International Code of Ethics for Nurses (International Council of Nurses, 2006), which states that "inherent in nursing is safeguarding human rights ... the right to life and choice ... to be treated with respect ... unrestricted by a person's race, ethnicity, culture, political or spiritual beliefs, social or marital status, gender, sexual orientation, age, health status, place of origin, lifestyle, mental or physical ability or socioeconomic status" (p. 17).

However, somewhere along the way through the duration and trajectory of their nursing careers, many nurses lost the concept of caring. What were once a compassionate, caring profession and nurse have become replaced in some instances with negativity, evil innuendos, and tactics of intimidation and humiliation. Perhaps as a result of organizational change, political bureaucracies, decreased morale, threatened personhood, or generational cohort differences, among many others, the upbeat, altruistic demeanor and attitude of some nurses have deteriorated. This trajectory of change is thought to begin when nurses are students. As found by Randle (2003), during nursing students' clinical placements and learning experiences, where bullying of colleagues and patients were frequent occurrences, beliefs around nursing as a caring and supportive profession began to be questioned. Nursing students came to believe that patients were no longer integral to their nursing practice. This process of professional socialization for nursing students occurred as their previously kind, caring, and empathetic nature became quickly replaced by actions, words, behaviors, and attributes that perpetrated bullying antics.

A second irony is that bullying typically refers to children who tend to, as a result of immaturity, be cruel to one another. This is not something that would typically be expected from adults, who have lived through many of life's milestones and experienced challenges, and who are professionally educated and mature adults.

WHY DOES BULLYING OCCUR? THEORETICAL UNDERPINNINGS

Young Shin Kim, a professor at the Child Study Center at the Yale University School of Medicine, says there is no set reason why bullying among adults, like bullying among children, occurs. It can be what you are wearing, what you have achieved in life, a recent scholarship you have received as you work on your master's or doctoral degree in nursing, or even your hair color. Some triggers identified by Namie and Namie (2000), world experts in workplace bullying, are as follows:

- Fifty-eight percent are targeted because they stand up to unfair treatment by the bully.
- Fifty-six percent are mobbed because the bully envies the target's level of competence.
- Forty-nine percent are targeted simply because they are nice people.
- Forty-six percent are bullied because they are ethical.
- Thirty-nine percent are bullied because it was just their turn.

There are many theoretical underpinnings and triggers as to why workplace bullying occurs. From an organizational perspective, there are many factors that seem to encourage the development of a bullying culture. These are as follows (Dunn, 2003; Quine, 2001):

1. Male-dominated organizations
2. Leadership styles; being reprimanded in front of others was a common reason (Dunn, 2003) for a nurse to sabotage the efforts of another

3. Low level of job control
4. Role conflict; the expectation to do another's work often prompted workplace bullying (Dunn, 2003)
5. Lack of participation in the decision-making process. As found by Daiski (2004), managers often do not include nurses in the decision-making process
6. Lack of support from senior staff. As found by Daiski (2004), managers often show little if any respect for their nurses
7. Lack of reward and recognition. As found by Dunn (2003), when nurses were not being recognized for their own hard work, it often prompted them to sabotage the work of others. While nurses themselves often think their work is important, they feel it often goes unrecognized by their manager (Daiski, 2004)

From a general perspective, there are many other variables that contribute to workplace bullying among nurses. Antecedents to workplace bullying in nursing are the following (Embree & White, 2010):

- Lack of empowerment
- Authoritarian leadership
- Negative nursing culture
- Toxic work culture
- Low level of self-esteem
- Shrinking resources
- Conflict-avoiding culture
- Personal behaviors
- Manager's broad span of control
- Relationships
- Professional lack of cooperation
- Poor coping skills
- Previous abuse

In addition to organization variables, there are many underlying theoretical constructs to support why bullying occurs. A brief discussion of these theories follows.

Oppression

One such theory to help illustrate why workplace bullying occurs revolves around oppression. Oppression can occur as a symptom of patriarchal attitudes from physicians, management, and administration when a buildup of tension is accompanied by an inability to address and solve issues with the oppressor.

"Bullying occurs when oppressed groups/individuals internalize feelings such as anger and rage and then manifest these feelings through behaviors such as gossip, jealousy, putdowns, and blaming" (Griffin, 2004; Hutchinson, Vickers, Jackson, & Wilkes, 2006; Ratner, 2006). For many decades, we have heard about nurses eating their young, and yet it still occurs without being adequately addressed. Why do we as nurses feel so powerless, so demoralized, and have such low self-esteem that the only way we can lift ourselves up is by tearing our colleagues down? These are critical questions to ponder.

Learned Helplessness

Some groups unconsciously adopt submissive attitudes or learned helplessness. Dominant groups identify the norms and then enforce from power given by submissive individuals.

Displaced Aggression

Nurses are worked off their feet and as a result exert displaced stress and aggression on one another. As Thomas (2003) suggests, this occurs when there is a withholding of anger; then, as the anger seeps out, it expresses itself as either passive or aggressive tendencies and behaviors. Griffin (2004) adds that workplace bullying occurs because nurses either overtly or covertly redirect their anger and "dissatisfaction inwards toward each other, towards themselves and toward those less powerful than themselves." Another similar thought was suggested by Rowell (2008) that perhaps adults just let their stress levels build up and leave them unaddressed, so they fester within them to create increased aggression levels. These stress levels accumulate over time and can often become predictive of their negative behaviors. This having been said, workload- and acuity-originated stress is not something that develops over years. As we pointed out, bullying often occurs for up to 2 years before people get the courage to step forward and do something about it.

Gender Differences

In the year 2014, we don't want to seem as if we are taking a step back in time, but in reality, gender differences as well contribute to bullying. Gender issues have been rooted in bullying because women have not been socialized to appreciate themselves, the roles they play, or the value they bring to the table of their workplace, organization, and society (Rowell, 2008).

Novice Nurse Phenomenon

The relationship between workplace bullying and new or novice nurses has received much attention in recent years. We have often heard the phrase, "Many senior nurses expect new grads to hit the ground running." For lack of a better phrase, I will call this the "novice nurse phenomenon." Because these nurses are newly hired/ recruited, they are in the most vulnerable position possible vis-à-vis the more powerful leaders and seniors nurses for whom they will now work. Their newness and increased vulnerability make them easy targets for bullies in the workplace (Freshwater, 2000; Hamlin, 2000). This status differential or power imbalance between novice nurses and senior nurses is what contributes to and exacerbates bullying among nurses and often reflects dissension among the ranks. As Bartholomew (2006) found, this status differential that can often precipitate workplace bullying in nursing has been a rite of passage for novice nurses and one that has come to be accepted, tolerated, expected, and normalized in the current nursing culture. So accepted and expected is this rite that it is no longer questioned on the grounds of ethics or morals in the nursing profession (Hutchinson et al., 2006). As outlined by Woelfle and McCaffrey (2007), oppression occurs when a "powerful and dominant group controls and exploits a less influential group." As a result, a divided and discordant group is formed. Farrell (1997) adds that this long traditional hierarchal power structure is what targets and victimizes the young and less experienced.

McKenna, Smith, Poole, and Coverdale (2003) suggest that the overt and covert forms of bullying, or horizontal violence, as some call it, are widespread among all novice nurses in all settings. So much so is it spread among nurses that many of them consider leaving the nursing profession after just 1 year. O'Lynn (2008) adds that "it's a wonder that the profession isn't experiencing a hemorrhage of new nurses leaving the profession." As a nursing educator, O'Lynn (2008) speaks of feeling "heartbroken" when he hears about the "pockets of abuse" novice nurses have experienced—how new graduates were humiliated, angrily shut down, restricted from practicing techniques, and even isolated by managers.

Power Imbalances

The differentials of power become evident not only with novice nurses but also with any other colleagues and professions with whom nurses interact and within the nursing ranks as well. Similar to the differential between the novice nurse and the senior nurse, a status differential between other players has been well proven to trigger workplace bullying among nurses (Giddings, 2005; Namie & Namie, 2000). These power imbalances occur when individuals feel they have more knowledge, skill, and expertise than someone else who is perhaps performing the same or similar role. Even though that may well be the case, they make the other person aware of it through their commands, gestures, and interactions.

The divide between physicians and nurses as the nursing role evolved historically has been well known. As found by Felblinger (2009), physicians are most often the instigators of bullying, particularly against nurses. The shift from the long-standing medical model of health care delivery to a more patient-centered, collaborative team approach and an increased focus on transparency and accountability has prompted a similar shift in health care professionals' expectations (Holloway & Kusy, 2010). The traditionally valued characteristics of nurses, such as warmth, nurturance, and sensitivity, are viewed as less important or even negative next to physicians, who typically dominate the culture of health care delivery and may not be so inclined to give up this dominance (Woelfle & McCaffrey, 2007). Hence, what typically follows from this is that nurses often lack autonomy, accountability, and control over their profession, and increased displaced and self-destructive aggression within the group occurs, as well as "infighting and self-criticism" (p.124).

In today's health care climate, in which professional autonomy and independence are crucial, professionals are gaining increased momentum in the authority they have earned. This paradigm shift in health care has allowed many more hands into the pot of patient care delivery. As a result, increased power struggles and hierarchy differentials are expressed in opinion conflicts, differing attitudes, and varying practices and approaches in the fight to get fiscally restrained resources; team cohesion gets destroyed, and bullying occurs perhaps more often than previously.

Survival and Infection

In the culture of a busy, fast-paced, and sometimes critical work environment of caring for the health and lives of others, a unique culture all its own develops. Only this culture has forgotten about the "caring" in nursing and health care. From the perspective of survival, workplace bullying finds yet another root to spur its growth and propagation. As found by Kusy and Holloway (2009), "toxic behaviors spread in response to people's efforts to survive." As health care personnel try to oppose the perpetrator of the negative abuse, verbalizations, and gestures, they can quickly develop camaraderie with others to abolish the very behaviors that have infected them. This widespread hostility and emotional negativity spreads, and pretty soon the whole workplace culture becomes infected, a new norm surfaces, and workplace bullying rears its ugly, egregious head. Even among nursing students, Randle (2003) found that because they lacked the know-how, they began to adopt bullying tactics themselves, incorporating them into their own nursing practice. This would help them ensure that they would be able to continue in their nursing program of study.

Internal Conflict

Internal conflict is generated when conforming to structural pressures subdues the desire for autonomy. As found by Daiski (2004), a great deal of infighting was observed that was fueled by a lack of respect, poor intraprofessional relationships, interdisciplinary hierarchies, and mutual nonsupportiveness.

Nursing Curriculum Format and Approach

For many years, since university nursing programs began to gain increased attention, there has been a recognizable divide between nurses who do college RN programs and nurses who do university bachelor of nursing programs. As health care corporations and health care authorities give up their costly ownership of college schools, the colleges of nursing are fading away in many countries while university bachelor of nursing programs grow. Therefore, the divide between bachelor of nursing university nurses and college-prepared nurses is yet another bone of contention for both nursing students and novice nurses. O'Lynn (2008), in his recollections of talking to nursing students in particular, mentions those who were condemned and called "clueless" by senior college-gradated nurses because they were taught the "book way" and needed to learn the "real way" of doing nursing skills.

Inflated Attitudes

Groups of people in a workplace unconsciously adopt inflated feelings and attitudes of superiority (power trip). Overly inflated attitudes can compound the low self-esteem of submissive individuals; therefore, they perpetuate a cycle of domination interacting with passivity.

Coping Strategy

Bullying in nursing is also thought to arise as a result of trying to cope with being bullied. Dunn (2003) suggests that bullying occurs as a result of individuals trying to cope with stress. What occurs is a dysfunctional output of sabotage because individuals are so angry and frustrated and know of no other way to deal or cope with it.

How Does Workplace Bullying Occur in Nursing?

Workplace bullying in nursing is manifested in many different ways, shapes, and forms. The role of being a bully takes on many facets of expression. Bullies have been known to utilize any and all information they have access to in their attempts to undermine, ostracize, humiliate, and intimidate their targets of interest. They are acutely aware of picking up on any cues and information they can such that these cues and information can later be manipulated, all for the demise of the target. Bullies do not want to see others succeed and so will do anything and everything possible that they can to ensure that the success of others does not happen.There are many ways that bullies demonstrate their actions; communication is the primary medium though which they achieve their goals.

As was highlighted when we spoke about the value of communication, the manifestations of bullying are often displayed either overtly or covertly. As you read through this section, recall from our previous discussion that nonverbal communication constitutes approximately 93% of message being sent and received (Blake, 2014). Overtly, bullies do not make any attempt to hide their actions and remarks; they express them in a manner that is quite open and observable to others. These are intentional efforts being made. They make no efforts at trying to hide, conceal, or be secretive about what they are doing or saying. Overt bullying tactics usually take the form of name calling, bickering, nitpicking, fault finding, backstabbing, gossiping, rudeness, discouragement, criticizing, belittling, intimidation, shouting, verbal abuse, threats, blaming, and putdowns; they also include slurs and jokes based on race, sexual orientation, ethnicity, religion, or gender; abrupt and aggressive responses; raising eyebrows; and making obvious face changes (McKenna et al., 2003; Workplace Mental Health Promotion, 2013). Dunn (2003) adds that stopping the conversation when others enter the room and complaining out loud about others are sure signs of bullying.

Covertly, bullies are much more subtle, sly, and secretive about the bullying tactics they are employing. They are very shrewd at trying to hide what they are doing or saying and concealing their comments and actions in such a way that they do not become obvious to others who may be present. Some examples of covert bullying that are often practiced are sarcasm, discrete eye rolling, ignoring or freezing someone out, refusing to help or work with a colleague, sabotage, isolation, exclusion, ostracism, minimization, fabrication of stories, breaking confidences, making someone a scapegoat, lacking interest, withholding support or patient information, denying access to opportunity, failing to respect privacy, and humorous putdowns (McKenna et al., 2003).

Workplace bullying can be expressed in an overt, blatant fashion or covertly in a more insidious, subtle manner. Overtly, such actions and behaviors typically include the following:

- Humiliation, ridicule, or unwarranted criticism in public or private
- Sadistic or aggressive behavior over time
- Treating colleagues as children, not as adults
- Exclusion from meetings

- Communication styles (verbal)
- Belittling
- Intimidation

Covertly, the following are often witnessed or suspected of occurring:

- Unfair assignments
- Sarcasm
- Eye rolling
- Sighing
- Making faces
- Ignoring
- Fabrication of stories
- Isolation
- Exclusion
- Withholding information to deliberately affect a colleague's performance
- Communication styles (nonverbal)

Experts suggest that covert expressions are more damaging to a person than are overt expressions of bullying (Griffin, 2004). Common cues that workplace bullying is occurring are the following (Workplace Mental Health Promotion, 2013):

- Conversations stop when someone comes into the office.
- Someone is not invited to meetings in which he or she is normally included.
- Information essential to someone's job performance is withheld.
- During interactions with the person, coworkers are either hostile or passive–aggressive.

IMPACT OF BULLYING

The general costs affiliated with nurses' compromised mental health are clearly outlined in Chapter 3. However, as workplace bullying is of such magnitude in nursing, I felt it significant to cover its impact here as a separate entity. "Bullying not only affects those directly involved, but also affects bystanders, as they too experience higher levels of stress. A number of Canadian provinces currently have legislation to address such behaviours" (Guarding Minds @ Work [GM@W], 2012).

Individual Impact

You get up at 4 a.m. to get ready to go to work. This is much earlier than you are used to by about 2 hours, but you have been twisting and turning all night, so you didn't get much sleep. You have difficulty getting your feet to the floor and pulling yourself out of the bed. You manage to get to the washroom and prepare for your shower. Your mind is so preoccupied that you don't even realize how cool the water is, or the fact that there is only a sliver of soap left for you to use. As you get into the shower, it seems that your heart begins to beat faster and louder. Your focus becomes narrowed, and you forget if you washed your hair yet or not. You step out to dry yourself. Your heart continues to pound fast and loud, and you wonder if your husband, who is now shaving at the sink, can hear it. You seem to be experiencing difficulty drying yourself because now your body is sweating a great deal and even the palms of your hands, no matter how much you towel them, won't seem to dry. You know the individual you are working with today is a very difficult person who picks on you regularly and consistently. But it's not just you for being quiet and shy; she picks on other nurses' weaknesses as well.

Workplace bullying in the nursing profession results in many negative ramifications for the nurse as a person. Just as a drug exerts adverse effects on a patient, so too does bullying exert unwanted and undesired outcomes on nurses who fall victim to it. In each dimension of psychological, physical, emotional, and social, workplace bullying among nurses shows no remorse.

Each individual incident of workplace bullying may seem inconsequential, but over a period of time, it erodes the self-confidence and self-esteem of the employee (Workplace Mental Health Promotion, 2013). Bullying also increases the prevalence of various mental disorders among the nurses who either witnessed or were targeted by it. As Quine (2001) found, significantly higher levels of depression and anxiety occur. McKenna et al. (2003) add that the effects of workplace bullying closely resemble those of posttraumatic stress disorder.

In the study by Curtis et al. (2007), what nursing students experience in bullying resembles that of more senior, seasoned nurses. Humiliation, lack of respect, powerlessness, feeling invisible, and the awareness of working in a hierarchy were common themes pulled from this study.

Other personal attributes and demeanors also impact nurses. Low self-esteem is one such attribute (Embree & White, 2010; Nazarko, 2001). As defined by Randle (2003), self-esteem "refers to the individual's perception of [him- or herself]," hence it is a "major predictor of human behaviors and how people interact with others." Further, the aggressive and destructive behaviors of workplace bullying undermine the confidence of the nurse (Nazarko, 2001), decrease self-worth (Randle, 2003), make one feel undervalued (McKenna et al., 2003), create self-hatred (Embree & White, 2010), compromise mental well-being (Holloway & Kusy, 2010), and can cause depression (Embree & White, 2010; Rowell, 2008), acute anxiety (Rowell, 2008), and posttramatic stress disorder (Rowell, 2008). In addition, they can compromise physical well-being (Holloway & Kusy, 2010), create powerlessness (Embree & White, 2010), decrease motivation (Holloway & Kusy, 2010; Woelfle & McCaffrey, 2007), drain nurses of their energy and work ethic (Woelfle & McCaffrey, 2007), cause burnout (Thomas, 2003), and cause weight loss or gain (Rowell, 2008). Further, as many as 10% of suicides may be related to workplace traumatization (Harvey, 2002). Finally, workplace bullying can also create physical and/or physiological symptoms such as hypertension (Rowell, 2008), cardiac palpitations (Rowell, 2008), irritable bowel syndrome (Rowell, 2008), and aggression, psychosomatic complaints, and musculoskeletal health complaints (GM@W, 2012).

Professional Impact

Professionally, workplace bullying among nurses leaves many scars of negativity and dangerous outcomes. Some of the research indicators include decreased level of job satisfaction, poor or compromised patient care, and damaged relationships.

Job satisfaction among nurses was found to drop significantly as a result of bullying (Cortrina, Magley, Williams, & Langhout, 2001; Quine, 2001). Similarly, significantly more nurses experienced a greater propensity to leave their current positions (Quine, 2001). As supported by McKenna et al. (2003), as cited in Embree and White (2010), approximately 60% of new nurses leave their first place of employment within the first 6 months because of workplace bullying.

Negative patient outcomes. Generally, bullying among nurses compromises the standards of nursing practice (Randle, 2003) and jeopardizes patient safety and care (Embree & White, 2010; Holloway & Kusy, 2010). As Nazarko (2001) suggests, it is impossible to deliver compassionate, quality care if nurses are working in an atmosphere of fear, intimidation, and humiliation. As found by Felblinger (2008), as cited in Holloway and Kusy (2010), 25% of all health care workers believed that disruptive behavior was positively correlated with patient mortality, and another 49% stated that intimidation by another practitioner resulted in medication errors being made. Woelfle and McCaffrey (2007) state that "when tension is elevated in patient care areas, nursing staff are not likely to perform at their best and the result is often poor patient care" (p. 123). Farrell (1997) adds that "impaired personal relationships between nurses at work can cause errors, accidents, and poor work performance." As observed and often perpetrated by nursing students, bullying patients admittedly placed the already vulnerable patients in an even more vulnerable and helpless position (Randle, 2003).

Bullying is also viewed as a risk to patient safety because it interferes with teamwork, collaboration, and communication, the underpinnings of patient safety and all key essentials to the provision of accurate, timely, and efficient patient care. Intimidation can influence communication in health care, and failed communication threatens patient safety. Further, from a leadership perspective, workplace bullying often causes nurses to experience damaged relationships (Embree & White, 2010), negative supervisory relations (Tepper, 2007), poor cooperation (Embree & White, 2010), and poor communication among team members (Holloway & Kusy, 2010).

Organizational Impact

In an environment of contempt, the impact of bullying also permeates the organization in its entirety. For example, nurses became more critical of different aspects of the organizational climate, such as trust (Quine, 2001). Further, organizations suffer because they now have a workforce of nurses that lacks the initiative to do well in their job performance (Rowell, 2008). As was once stated, "It is not just the victim that is harmed by mobbing; the workplace also pays a price in a loss of loyalty and performance from the mobbed employee" (Workplace Mental Health Promotion, 2013). A toxic work environment (Embree & White, 2010) undermines an organization's efforts to create a respectful work environment and a contented, satisfied, and happy nursing workforce (Woelfle & McCaffrey, 2007). Increased malpractice suits (Holloway & Kusy, 2010) may also occur. In Randle's (2003) study of bullying involving nursing students, it was found that the students often witnessed the bullying of patients as well, where "nurses used their positions to humiliate, belittle or isolate patients." From a functional perspective for the organization, there are reports of increased absenteeism (Holloway & Kusy, 2010; McKenna et al.,

2003; Rowell, 2008; Tepper, 2007); decreased productivity (Holloway & Kusy, 2010; Tepper, 2007); recruitment and retention difficulties and increased staff turnover (Cortrina et al., 2001; Embree & White, 2010; Holloway & Kusy, 2010; Rowell, 2008); and increased patient and family complaints (Rowell, 2008).

HEALTH CARE SYSTEM OUTCOMES

We have now had a closer look at the impact of workplace bullying on individual nurses; the magnitude of such effects also impacts organizations at large. Just as a cancer invades and disables a person, so too do the effects of workplace bullying permeate an organization. While most of these effects involve financial bottom lines of an organization, others can exert a more critical degree of effect such as that impacting patient care, service delivery, staff morale, and general liability.

The financial implications of workplace bullying among nurses is immeasurable. Workplace bullying typically creates difficulties with recruitment and retention of nurses; however, there is a price tag that goes with that. According to Jones and Gates (2007), nurse turnover costs up to twice a nurse's salary and can range from $22,000 to $145,000 depending on the geographical location and subspecialty area.

STRATEGIES TO ADDRESS WORKPLACE BULLYING

We have learned a great deal about workplace bullying thus far—its ability to jeopardize the operations and goals of any health care organization and, most importantly, the impact it has on the lives of nurses as people and nurses as professionals. We are left to wonder, then, how does such a toxic work environment thrive and what can we do to address it? Like all other stressors that we face in the run of the day, workplace bullying is no different. Therefore, with a similar urgency, we have to address it, control it, cope with it, and lessen its impact somehow. What follows from here are various strategies that have been posited as being effective against the act and impact that bullying exerts.

First, in order to stop workplace bullying, nurses must first recognize what it is. They must recognize that workplace bullying is occurring or being witnessed by them and as a result is creating significant negative consequences (DeMarco & Roberts, 2003; Rowell, 2008). These bullying behaviors have to be recognized if any nurse is expected to overcome them, and this may very well involve some personal and professional reflection (DeMarco & Roberts, 2003).

There are some key measures that can often help address workplace bullying. These require the following documentation: frequency, regularity, and patterns; build your supports, rarely are you alone; policies and legislation; debriefing in a supportive environment; assertiveness training; and conflict resolution training (Curtis et al., 2007).

Further, a supportive workplace environment helps to mitigate the stress of bullying by acting as a coping strategy. As Quine (2001) found, "Support at work was able to protect nurses from some of the damaging effects of bullying."

Murray (2009) suggests that nurses should take a collaborative approach to bullying; nurses should "look out for each other" and support victims of bullying during and following an episode, including reporting the incident. Victims are encouraged to document incidents of bullying, including the date, time, site of occurrence, and witnesses. Dellasega (2009) has this advice for nurses who witness an episode of bullying: "Intervene quickly to prevent minor conflicts from escalating." Often, she continues, "a misperception or false assumption triggers behavior that spins out of control." Because bystanders usually outnumber bullies and victims, they can act together to alter the situation's dynamic and avert a bullying incident. "You can intervene on behalf of a coworker who is being bullied by asking her to help you with a task in another location, speaking up on her behalf, or simply standing beside her." Dellasega also cautions nurses about participating in gossip, which is another form of bullying.

Policy Development for Bullying

Organizational policies to address workplace bullying are a must (Rowell, 2008). "Sadly, bullying has long been tolerated in health care. Sometimes called nursing's 'silent epidemic,' bullying might even be tacitly accepted with 'a wink and a nod,' or subtly encouraged by a failure to acknowledge or take steps to end it. This can give rise to an attitude of indifference toward bullying in the workplace and unwillingness to address it, even on the part of victims" (Stokowski, 2010).

The Joint Commission formed by the U.S. Government mandated that effective January 1, 2009, all hospitals and health care organizations should have in place policies and procedures to address such disruptive, toxic, and inappropriate behaviors and that these policies should assume a zero-tolerance approach to workplace bullying (Joint Commission Resources, 2006, as cited in Holloway & Kusy, 2010). These policies need to protect staff and hold staff accountable for their actions or in some cases inactions for not reporting it (Woelfle & McCaffrey, 2007).

The fact that workplace bullying has been going on for so long and has not been addressed is "one reason that a 'zero-tolerance' organizational policy about workplace bullying is now the bedrock of bullying prevention recommendations" (Stokowski, 2010).

A bullying prevention policy should include a statement from top management to all workers stating that bullying is inappropriate and will not be tolerated, describe bullying and the types of behavior that constitute bullying, include a statement of risks to the organization and individuals, identify where complaints should go (e.g., human resources), encourage workers who experience or witness bullying to report it, clearly state that retaliation against or victimization of workers who report workplace bullying will not be tolerated, state the process that will be followed if a complaint is received, and state a commitment to prompt action if workplace bullying occurs (Workplace Mental Health Promotion, 2013).

Legislation

The United States is perhaps the most productive country in making inroads in recognizing and fighting against the acts of workplace bullying. From the perspective of addressing and dealing with acts of bullying, legislation has a significant role to play as well. Many provincial occupational health and safety acts have been expanded to include harm to psychological well-being in the definition of harassment. Managers should never tolerate any violent behavior, including aggression, harassment, or threats of violence. Violent or aggressive behavior hurts the mental health of everyone in the organization and creates a psychologically unsafe work environment filled with fear and anxiety (Workplace Mental Health Promotion, 2013).

The absence of laws against bullying leaves victims of bullying with little legal recourse. It appears that no legal definition of bullying exists. Bullying is often confused with harassment, which *does* have a definition in law, and for which a person *can* be sued. The first antibullying law in North America came into effect on June 1, 2004. Quebec had amended its Labour Standards Act to deal with psychological harassment in the workplace (Canada Safety Council, 2005). Over the past decade, workplace bullying has become an internationally recognized occupational health and safety issue, and various regulatory responses to the problem have been introduced in the following countries: France, Germany, Italy, Sweden, Spain, the Netherlands, Norway, Ireland, and Australia. A 1999 International Labour Organization report on workplace violence emphasized that physical and emotional violence is one of the most serious problems facing the workplace in the new millennium.

A jury in Indiana recently ordered a heart surgeon to pay $325,000 to a hospital employee who made a claim of workplace bullying. This rare case prompted many to ask the question, what legally constitutes workplace bullying? It is a question that the states are beginning to address. In March 2014, New York State became the ninth state in the U.S. to pass the Healthy Workplace Bill (Namie, 2014), a measure that would allow workers to sue for physical, psychological, or economic harm from abusive treatment at work. Now, workers in New York who can show that they were repeatedly subjected to malicious, hostile conduct, including bullying, can be awarded lost wages, medical expenses, compensation for emotional distress, and punitive damages. On February 6, 2014, Tennessee became the 26th state to introduce antibullying healthy workplace bills (Workplace Bullying Institute, 2014). Up to May 2014, 28 legislatures in the U.S. (26 states and 2 territories) have introduced healthy workplace bills to address the problem of workplace bullying (Namie, 2014).

Unfortunately, workplace policies against bullying are still largely unrecognized. In Canada, up to 2012, there was no jurisdiction that required employers to have a workplace violence prevention program in place. Canada also relies on its Canadian Human Rights Act (1976). In 2003, Bill C-451, the Workplace Psychological Harassment Prevention Act, to prevent psychological harassment in the workplace and to amend the Canada Labour Code, was initiated (House of Commons of Canada, 2003) but has since stalled under the current federal government. A recent Ontario Superior Court decision recognized that an employer owes a duty to its employees to provide a decent, civil, and respectful workplace (Canada Safety Council, 2010). As discussed in Chapter 2, it wasn't until January 2013 that the National Standard for Psychological Safety was introduced by the Mental Health Commission of Canada, a global precedent-setting move to address psychological harassment and bullying in the workplace.

Occupational health and safety acts of various states, provinces, and countries have undergone a slight shift in focus. Many provincial occupational health and safety acts have been expanded to include harm to psychological well-being. Organizations should not tolerate any violent behavior, including aggression, harassment, or threats of violence. Violent or aggressive behavior hurts the mental health of everyone in the organization and creates a psychologically unsafe work environment filled with fear and anxiety (Canadian Centre for Occupational Health and Safety, 2012). With the passage of Bill 168 into law in December 2009, Ontario took a first step toward declaring workplace violence unacceptable. Bill 168, an amendment to the Occupational Health and Safety Act, directly addresses workplace violence and harassment (Schwindt, 2010).

Whether intentionally or unintentionally, many coworkers actively participate or are complicit in workplace bullying, or mobbing as they call it, succumbing to the peer pressure more frequently associated with children and teens. Despite the fact that mobbing is far more prevalent than other destructive behavior, such as sexual harassment and racial discrimination, which are prohibited by legislation, in Canada only the province of Quebec has legislation to protect workers against mobbing (Workplace Mental Health Promotion, 2013).

Strategies for Organizations

"It is the legal duty of an employer to protect the mental and physical health of employees. That means protection from harassment, violence, and bullying. Across Canada, there has been a major push through legislative amendments to make employers more accountable for fostering mentally safe work environments. This push is backed by case law, which has found employers liable for exposing employees to unsafe work environments that have caused unnecessary psychological harm" (Workplace Mental Health Promotion, 2013). Nurse managers need to be educated to identify and take action to address workplace bullying among nurses (Thomas, 2003).

Organizations need to realize that their employees, particularly nurses in health care settings, are the backbone of their mission and of the delivery of services and patient care, so they require a great deal of attention that they often do not get (Farrell, 1997). "Previous strategies, sadly still popular, simply deal with the problem person in the form of reprimands, warnings, and coaching" (Holloway & Kusy, 2010). Each organization has the responsibility to develop processes for managing threatening and intimidating behaviors. Although no one-size-fits-all approach is likely to be successful for all bullies or all situations, most experts agree on the essential elements of a prevention and management approach to workplace bullying.

The root of the bullying culture in nursing could very well be an absence of respect in the workplace. In healthy workplaces, leaders promote and uphold a culture of respect, setting the example of harmony and collaboration for their staff. Taking the perspective that bullying is a safety issue, in 2008 the Joint Commission issued a standard on intimidating and disruptive behaviors at work, citing concerns about increased medical errors, poor patient satisfaction, adverse outcomes, higher costs, and loss of qualified staff. "Intimidating and disruptive behaviors are unprofessional and should not be tolerated." The Joint Commission's guidelines for the prevention of disruptive and inappropriate behavior are not specific to nurses because they also take into account physician behavior. However, many of these recommendations are clearly of value to any health care professional. Key recommendations include the following:

- Education of staff about professional and respectful behavior
- Holding individuals accountable for behavior
- Organizational policies that promise "zero tolerance" for intimidating or disruptive behaviors and protection for those who report these behaviors
- Leadership training for leaders who must model and uphold standards of behavior
- Surveillance and reporting systems for unprofessional behaviors
- The importance of documenting attempts to address bullying behaviors

In 2009, The Joint Commission added these leadership standards to further deter and mitigate workplace bullying: the hospital/organization should have a code of conduct that defines acceptable and disruptive and inappropriate behaviors, and leaders should create and implement a process for managing disruptive and inappropriate behaviors. "To combat mobbing in the workplace, organizations need to integrate their violence and harassment policy; provide education and training that ensures employees know how to recognize mobbing; and provide concrete ways for colleagues to recognize and talk about mental health issues in general. Managers in particular can contribute to a positive work environment if they have the skills and knowledge to identify and respond to issues before they escalate" (Workplace Mental Health Promotion, 2013). Policies can inform staff that they can request supports (accommodations), which can help employees with mental health issues thrive. Moreover, the organization protects itself from the legal liability of not meeting its duty to accommodate employees with disabilities. The following are examples of practical measures that employers can put in place to reduce the risk for workplace violence and harassment (Workplace Mental Health Promotion, 2013):

- Create written workplace violence and harassment policies and train employees on such policies.
- Include this element in the health and risk assessments done in the workplace to determine the possibility or prevalence of workplace violence or harassment.
- Disclose incidents of workplace violence and harassment to the health and safety committee.
- Provide ways for employees to report instances of or risks for workplace violence and harassment.
- Discipline employees for not following workplace violence and harassment policies or for committing workplace violence or harassment.
- If available to the organization, promote employee assistance program services so that employees who are subjected to workplace violence or harassment can talk to someone confidentially about the issues they are facing.

- Ensure that proper security measures are in place at the workplace to protect workers from members of the public or customers.
- Keep detailed records of any workplace violence or harassment, investigation, or work refusal.

Nurse-to-Nurse Collegial Strategies

Current practicing nurses need to recognize that nursing students and novice nurses are our nurses of tomorrow (O'Lynn, 2008), our future colleagues, and even perhaps the mentors of our own children and grandchildren who opt to study nursing as a profession. Professionally, they will be the nurses who some day care for you as a patient or will be your vacation relief when you wish to go on holiday in the midst of fiscal cutbacks, nursing shortages, and mandated overtime practices and policies.

On an individual level, Griffin (2004) found that the practice of cognitive rehearsal can help one cope with bullying. This requires cognitive thought processes and autonomic thoughts so that when information on bullying is received, it is processed but responded to differently than it would have been previously. The knowledge gained from learning about workplace bullying empowered and encouraged novice nurses to confront the perpetrator head-on. An enhanced understanding was found to enable them to perceive the bullying in a different and less threatening context.

Nursing students and novice nurses also need to be treated with respect and collegiality. As O'Lynn (2008) suggests, "Gently correct them when they are wrong, praise them when they do well, and be open to what they can teach you" (p. 7). Many also deem it essential to confront colleagues who abuse nursing students or novice nurses; they need to be told that this sort of abuse will not be tolerated (O'Lynn, 2008). Randle (2003) adds that the work environment needs to change, and nurses, nurse educators, and nurse managers can help this happen. Otherwise, each new generation of nurses will witness, experience, and adopt the nursing practices of workplace bullies and hence perpetuate the cycle of violence and discontent.

SUMMARY

Although the caring profession of nursing is not a typical place where you would expect to see bullying, sadly, bullying is alive and well there. Workplace bullying can destroy nurses and the work environment, and it jeopardizes patient care. While there are various degrees and forms of bullying, there are also many strategies to help address it. Because bullying can often make nurses feel demeaned, belittled, and ostracized, so much so that their own mental health becomes jeopardized, nurses need to rise beyond the deceit, the evils, and the negativities associated with bullying. However, to do so, a collaborated effort of the nursing leader and the organization, in addition to accompanying legislation, is needed for true success.

DISCUSSION QUESTIONS

1. Define workplace bullying and the various categories of bullying that can occur.
2. Why does workplace bullying occur?
3. Discuss the irony of bullying in a caring profession.
4. Identify and discuss the individual, professional, and organizational impact of workplace bullying.
5. Identify and discuss some key strategies that can be used to address workplace bullying.
6. Discuss how existing legislation in your jurisdiction can help to address workplace bullying.

REFERENCES

Adams, A. (1997). Bullying at work. *Journal of Community and Applied Social Psychology, 7,* 177–180.

Bartholomew, K. (2006). *Ending nurse to nurse hostility.* Marblehead, MA: HCPro.

Blake. (2014). *How much of communication is really nonverbal?* Retrieved from http://www.nonverbalgroup.com/2011/08/how-much-of-communication-is-really-nonverbal

Brunner, P. W., & Costello, M. L. (2003). *Advancing women in leadership: When the wrong woman wins: Building bullies and perpetuating patriarch.* Retrieved from http://www.advancingwomen.com/awl/spring2003/BRUNNE~1.HTML

Canada Safety Council. (2005). *Targeting workplace bullies.* Retrieved from http://www.safety-council.org/info/OSH/bully-law.html

Canada Safety Council. (2010). *Bullying in the workplace.* Retrieved from http://safety-council.org/workplace-safety/bullying-in-the-workplace

Canadian Centre for Occupational Health and Safety. (2012). *Violence in the workplace.* Retrieved from http://www.ccohs.ca/oshanswers/psychosocial/violence.html

Cortrina, L. M., Magley, V. J., Williams, J. H., & Langhout, R. D. (2001). Incivility in the workplace: Incidence and impact. *Journal of Occupational Health Psychology, 6,* 64–80.

Curtis, J., Bowen, I., & Reid, A. (2007). You have no credibility: Nursing students' experiences of horizontal violence. *Nurse Education in Practice, 7*(3), 156–163.

Daiski, I. (2004). Changing nurses' disempowering relationship patterns. *Journal of Advanced Nursing, 48*(1), 43–50.

Dellasega, C. A. (2009). Bullying among nurses. *American Journal of Nursing, 109*(1), 52–58.

DeMarco, R. F., & Roberts, S. J. (2003). Negative behaviors in nursing. *American Journal of Nursing, 103*(3), 115–116.

Dunn, H. (2003). Horizontal violence among nurses in the operating room. *American Operating Room Nursing Journal, 78*(6), 977–988.

Embree, J. L., & White, A. H. (2010). Concept analysis: Nurse-to-nurse lateral violence. *Nursing Forum, 45*(3), 166–173.

Farrell, G. A. (1997). Aggression in clinical settings: Nurses' views. *Journal of Advanced Nursing, 25*(3), 501–508.

Felblinger, D. M. (2009). Bullying, incivility, and disruptive behaviors in the healthcare setting: Identification, impact and intervention. *Frontiers of Health Services Management, 25*(4), 13–23.

Freshwater, D. (2000). Crosscurrents: Against cultural narration in nursing. *Journal of Advanced Nursing, 32*(2), 481–484.

Giddings, L. (2005). A theoretical model of social consciousness. *Advances in Nursing Science, 28*(3), 224–239.

Griffin, M. (2004). Teaching cognitive rehearsal as a shield for lateral violence: An intervention for newly licensed nurses. *The Journal of Continuing Education in Nursing, 35*(6), 257–262.

Guarding Minds @ Work. (2012). *The 13 psychosocial factors.* Retrieved from http://www.guardingmindsatwork.ca/info/risk_factors

Hamlin, L. (2000). Horizontal violence in the operating room. *British Journal of Perioperative Nursing, 10*(1), 34–42.

Harvey, J. (2002). Stereotypes and moral oversight in conflict resolution: What are we teaching? *Journal of Philosophy of Education, 36*(4), 513–528.

Holloway, E. L., & Kusy, M. E. (2010). Disruptive and toxic behaviors in healthcare: Zero tolerance, the bottom line and what to do about it. *The Journal of Medical Practice Management, 25*(6), 335–340.

Hutchinson, M., Vickers, M., Jackson, D., & Wilkes, L. (2006). Workplace bullying in nursing: Towards a more critical organizational perspective. *Nursing Inquiry, 13*(2), 118–126.

International Council of Nurses. (2006). *The ICN code of ethics for Nurses.* Geneva, Switzerland: International Council of Nurses. Retrieved from https://www.icn.ch/about-icn/code-of-ethics-for-nurses

Jarrin, O. F. (2007). An integral philosophy and definition of nursing. *Journal of Integral Theory and Practice, 2*(4), 84–89.

Johnson (2009). *Bad blood: Doctor-nurse behavior problems impact patient care.* Retrieved from http://www.ache.org/policy/doctornursebehavior.pdf

Jones, C. B., & Gates, M. (2007). The costs and benefits of nurse turnover: A business case for nurse retention. *The Online Journal of Issues in Nursing, 12*(3).

Kagan, P. N., Smith, M. C., Cowling, W. R., & Chinn, P. L. (2009). A nursing manifesto: An emancipatory call for knowledge development, conscience, and praxis. *Nursing Philosophy, 11,* 67–84. Retrieved from CINAHL Plus with full text database (Accession No. 2010509400).

Knight, J. (2004, August 17). *Bullied workers suffer 'battle stress.'* BBC News Online. Retrieved from http://news.bbc.co.uk/2/hi/business/3563450.stm

Kusy, M., & Holloway, E. (2009). *Developing healthcare leaders who really lead.* Keynote speaker address. VA Radiology Leadership Summit, Washington, DC.

McKenna, B. G., Smith, N. A., Poole, S. J., & Coverdale, J. H. (2003). Horizontal violence: Experiences of registered nurses in their first year of practice. *Journal of Advanced Nursing, 42*(1), 90–96.

Monti, E. J., & Tingen, M. S. (1999). Multiple paradigms of nursing science. In W. K. Cody (Ed.), *Philosophical and theoretical perspectives for advanced nursing practice* (pp. 27–41). Sudbury, MA: Jones & Bartlett.

Murray, J. S. (2009). Workplace bullying in nursing: A problem that can't be ignored. *MedSurg Nursing, 18,* 273–276.

Namie, G. (2009). *Workplace bullies.* Retrieved from http://www.workplace-bullies.com/2009/07/doctor-weighs-in-workplace-bullies-and.html

Namie, G. (2014). *2014 Legislative Session News.* Retrieved from http://www.healthyworkplacebill.org/states/ny/newyork.php

Namie, G., & Namie, R. (2000). *The bully at work.* Naperville, IL: Sourcebooks.

Nazarko, L. (2001). Bullying and harassment. *Nursing Management, 8*(1), 14–15.

O'Lynn, C. (2008). Handing off the novice nurse. *Interaction: Official Publication of the American Assembly of Men in Nursing, 26*(2), 1–7.

Pappas, S. (2010). *Behind bullying: Why kids are so cruel.* Retrieved from http://www.livescience.com/6325-bullying-kids-cruel.html

Quine, L. (2001). Workplace bullying in nurses. *Journal of Health Psychology, 6*(1), 73–84.

Randle, J. (2003). Bullying in the nursing profession. *Journal of Advanced Nursing, 43*(4), 395–401.

Ratner, T. (2006). Communication in the OR. *Nursing Spectrum, 23,* 10–11.

Rayner, C., & Hoel, H. (1997). A summary review of literature relating to workplace bullying. *Journal of Community and Applied Social Psychology, 7*, 181–191.

Rowell, P. (2008). *Lateral violence: Nurse against nurse.* Retrieved from http://nursingworld. org/mods/mod440/print_lateral.pdf

Schim, S. M., Benkert, R., Bell, S. E., Walker, D. S., & Danford, C. A. (2007). Social justice: Added metaparadigm concept for urban health nursing. *Public Health Nursing, 24*(1), 73–80.

Schwindt, R. (2010). Workplace bullying and mobbing as emerging issues for social workers in Ontario. *The Journal of the Ontario Association of Social Workers, 36*(1). Retrieved from http://newsmagazine.oasw.org/magazine.cfm?magazineid=7&articleid=129

Sofield, L., & Salmond, S. W. (2003). Workplace violence: A focus on verbal abuse and intent to leave the organization. *Orthopedic Nursing, 22*(4), 274–283.

Statistics Canada. (2007). *Criminal victimization in the workplace.* Retrieved from http://www. statcan.gc.ca/daily-quotidien/070216/dq070216a-eng.htm

Stokowski, L. A. (2010). *Approaches to bullying.* Retrieved from http://www.medscape.com/ viewarticle/729474_5

Tepper, B. J. (2007). Abusive supervision in work organizations: Review, synthesis, and research agenda. *Journal of Management, 33*, 261–289.

Thomas, S. P. (2003). Anger: The mismanaged emotion. *MedSurg Nursing, 12*(2), 103–110.

U.K. National Workplace Bullying Agency. (2009). *Those who can do, those who can't bully.* Retrieved from http://www.bullyonline.org/workbully/serial.htm

Vonfrolio, L. G. (2005). Get real: End horizontal violence. *Registered Nurse, 68*(2), 60.

Warren Shepell. (2002). *Workplace trends linked to mental health crisis in Canada. Research briefing puts stress, violence, conflict and harassment on the table.* Retrieved from https://www. shepellfgiservices.com/newsroom/pr-nov152002.asp

Watson, J. (2013). Nursing: The philosophy and science of caring. In M. C. Smith, M. C. Turkel, & Z. R. Wolf (Eds.), *Caring in nursing classics: An essential resource.* New York, NY: Springer.

Woelfle, C. Y., & McCaffrey, R. (2007). Nurse on nurse. *Nursing Forum, 42*(3), 123–131.

Workplace Bullying Institute. (2014). *Tennessee becomes 26th state to introduce anti-bullying healthy workplace bills.* Retrieved from http://www.workplacebullying.org/category/ workplace-bullying-laws

Workplace Mental Health Promotion. (2013). *Harassment, violence, bullying and mobbing.* Retrieved from http://wmhp.cmhaontario.ca/workplace-mental-health-core-concepts-issues/issues-in-the-workplace-that-affect-employee-mental-health/harassment-violence-bullying-and-mobbing

8

Violence at Work

Nothing good ever comes of violence.
—Martin Luther

LEARNING OBJECTIVES

By the end of this chapter, the learner will be able to:

1. Identify the seriousness of violence in the nursing profession and the epidemiological trends that have occurred.
2. Differentiate the various theories and causes of why violence may occur.
3. Discuss how the setting in nursing may have an impact on the prevalence of violence.
4. Be familiar with the various categories and forms of violence that can occur.
5. Discuss why the nonreporting of violence is a significant issue for nurse and patient safety.
6. Identify various interventions that the nurse, nurse leader, and organization can implement to help prevent or reduce violence.
7. Discuss the various indicators that can help nurses identify potential or impending violence.
8. Identify some of the adverse outcomes that can occur as a result of workplace violence in nursing.

Violence or the potential for violence is a real occurrence in the nursing profession. Whether it is violence among the nursing ranks at an intraprofessional or interprofessional level or violence directed at nurses by patients, families, or visitors, it can still exert the same negative impact and possibly compromise nurses' mental health. As nurses become more aware of it, they can be better prepared to deal with it when it does happen, but what really must happen is that nurses and managers have to begin talking about it and taking action against it. It is the purpose of this chapter to discuss violence with reference to the nursing profession, the different types of violence that exist, the factors that precipitate its occurrence, the impact it has on the nurses and organization, the characteristics of the perpetrators, and what can be done to identify, prevent, and address it personally, professionally, and organizationally.

THE MAGNITUDE, CHARACTER, AND SCOPE
OF WORKPLACE VIOLENCE IN HEALTH CARE

Violence has penetrated workplaces for decades. In the United States, 1.7 million injuries occur per year as a result of workplace violence; almost 50% of these occur in health care settings, and they account for approximately 20% of all violent crime in the United States. In 1990, homicide became the second-leading cause of death at the workplace (Centers for Disease Control and Prevention [CDC], 1998). When work environments become unsafe and individuals think they must protect and defend themselves, the entire organization suffers.

The Employee Assistance Trade Association has seen a growing need to develop solutions for employers with regard to appropriate response to the problem of workplace violence—and with good reason. Although there has been a noticeable 50% decrease in workplace violence, attributed primarily to staff training and policy development, corporate America spends about $4.2 billion to $6.4 billion a year in the aftermath of workplace violence situations by responding to the approximately two million violent incidents in the workplace annually. Canada, on the other hand, has 66% of its organizations reporting violence and spends $6.1 billion U.S. per year (Employee Assistance Trade Association, 2013).

Furthermore, two million physical attacks occur in the U.S. workplace per year and around six million are threatened, with approximately 1,000 murders occurring as a result of workplace violence per year at an average of three per day, leaving murder to be the third-leading cause of occupational death after motor vehicle accidents and machinery accidents (Bowman, 2012; Duhart, 2001). In Australia, Canada, and the United States, health care is noted to be one of the most violent industries (WorkSafeBC, 2009; Canadian Centre for Occupational Health Safety [CCOHS], 2012).

VIOLENCE IN NURSING

Acts of violence represent a reality in the nursing profession. Sources of violence in nursing often include colleagues (nurses or other disciplinary team members) and patients, families, or visitors. Many of us view our workplace as a place of safety and one that is healthy, but violence in nursing represents a significant occupational hazard and an infringement on that safety. Workplace violence is defined by the National Institute for Occupational Safety and Health (NIOSH; 2002) as "ranging from offensive or threatening language to homicide"; it is "violent acts (including physical assaults and threats of assaults) directed toward persons at work or on duty." Although much violence can occur, it does not mean it is an acceptable part of the job (Chapman & Styles, 2006). Nothing is more terrifying than being victimized through violence, when you work so hard to provide "care" for the vulnerable patients you serve and to achieve collegiality with your coworkers. While violence is rooted in inequality or the imbalance of power and control between two people or groups of people, the act of violence against someone is a choice that people make for one reason or another.

To be able to work in an occupationally safe and healthy work environment is the undeniable right of every nurse and is presented in many countries as a human right and freedom mandate. A safe and healthy workplace environment not only fosters a sense of respect, dignity, and support; just as importantly, it helps to ensure the delivery of safe, quality, and competent nursing care. Ironically, health care is identified as one of the highest-risk occupations and work areas in which violence occurs, with nursing particularly vulnerable (CCOHS, 2012; NIOSH, 2002). Paradoxically, the profession that is tasked with providing care, giving of oneself for the betterment of others, nurturance, and promoting good health has one of the highest risks of workplace violence (MacEwan & Dumpel, 2012), with nurses one of the most assaulted group of workers in the American workforce. Nurses often face the everyday reality and the terrifying possibility of experiencing violence and aggression at work (Chapman & Styles, 2006) while "caring" for their patients. Although health care organizations, just like other businesses, are obligated by law to provide occupationally safe and healthy workplaces, the occurrence of violence not only violates such laws and legislative acts but also impacts significantly an individual's mental health.

The various definitions of violence make it difficult to determine the prevalence of violence (Hasketh et al., 2003). Typically, while bullying can be positively correlated with acts of violence, it does not necessarily always involve violence. Workplace bullying, as a potential form of violence, seems to have taken on a life of its own in how it affects nurses and the nursing profession, so it was covered as its own entity in Chapter 7 and will be omitted from this chapter, in which the primary focus is on physical violence.

In a U.S. nationwide survey of nurses, the American Nurses Association found that 17% of all nurses had been physically assaulted in the past year and that 56.6% of those had been threatened or had experienced verbal abuse during that time (American Psychiatric Nurses Association, 2008). In the same study, 25% of nurses stated that one of their key sources of stress at work was fear of sustaining an assault while working. Further, 20.1% of nurses had experienced more than one type of violence; however, this figure is believed to be a gross underestimation (Hasketh et al., 2003). Gacki-Smith et al. (2009) add that 25% of emergency department nurses experienced violence more than 20 times in the previous 3 years of their study and that 20% reported verbal abuse more than 200 times during the same 3 years. The Federal Bureau of Investigation (2003) suggests that while all health care workers are at risk for violence, nurses are actually assaulted the most often. In Australia as well, the number of physical attacks on nurses by patients increased by 30% from 2005 to 2006 and that 35% to 80% of all hospital staff, inclusive of nurses, were physically assaulted at least once in their careers (Clements, DeRanieri, Clark, Manno, & Wolick Kuhn, 2005). For the safety of the patients and all staff, it is important to appropriately assess agitated and potentially violent individuals and rapidly intervene (Duong, 2010).

THEORETICAL UNDERPINNINGS OF VIOLENCE

The theoretical underpinnings of violence help to inform us of why the violence took place. Some of these will be discussed here. Ecological Theory is one such theory underpinning violence. It is based on the assumption that the interactions between different factors in the workplace are both complex and interactive. Many factors that arise at work related to the individual, family context, environment, and any external factors outside work can become interdependent; together, they create an escalation of violence and aggression (Duffy, Scott, & O'Leary-Kelly, 2005).

Learned Helplessness is another theory that helps explain violence. This is a mental state in which an organism that is forced to bear aversive or unpleasant stimuli becomes unable or unwilling to avoid subsequent encounters with those stimuli, even if they are "escapable," presumably because the organism has learned that it cannot control the situation (Nolen, 2014). From the roots of classical conditioning, introduced by Seligman at the University of Pennsylvania, it fosters a sense of low self-esteem, chronic failure, sadness, and physical illness and is associated with disorders and conditions such as depression, violence, aging, discrimination, drug abuse, and alcoholism (Boyd, 2014).

Frontier Justice Theory also helps to explain why violence may occur. Because what used to be handled as a grievance by one's union became stuck in binding arbitration, employees now seek to take matters into their own hands regarding any perceived injustices. Frontier Justice Theory depicts the lawlessness of shooters who retaliated because the legal system and industrial jurisprudence had failed them (Layden, 1999).

A fourth theory to help explain workplace violence is Transference of Domestic Problems. This theory uses various sources to identify how violence can be internally motivated. These include the following: internalized feelings of shame and humiliation leading to feelings of anger, hostility, and rage (Hale, 1994); Freudian systems of ego pathology and impaired object relationships in the development of sexuality or concerns about dominance, submission, and control as unresolved conflicts originating during the anal period of development; pathophysiological models such as "cognitive fracture," in which the amygdala is inhibited (Fried,1997); abnormal concentrations of trace metals (elevated serum copper and depressed plasma zinc) in the blood (Walsh, Isaacson, Rehman, & Hall, 1997); and general psychopathology models, such as those involving the American Psychiatric Association label of "conduct disorder," in which repetitive acts of patterned aggression toward animals and people are significant to the diagnosis (American Psychiatric Association, 2013; Barak, 2003, 2013).

The Frustration–Aggression Theory also helps to explain why workplace violence occurs. We experience frustration or a feeling of tension because our efforts to reach our goals, such as an expected pay raise that never comes, become blocked; hence, feelings of anger and even readiness for aggression can occur. This theory, however, does not justify the use of aggression and violence. Although this aggression can be enacted in the workplace, it can also be directed toward family members at home (Social Issues Research Center, 2012).

CAUSES OF VIOLENCE

In addition to the theoretical underpinnings of violence, it is important to investigate and be informed of other causes of violence. The Federal Bureau of Investigation (FBI) has noted several of these, such as the following: the increasing number of acute and chronically mentally ill patients being released from hospitals without follow-up care, who now have the right to refuse medicine and who can no longer be hospitalized involuntarily unless they pose an immediate threat to themselves or others; the availability of drugs or money at hospitals, clinics, and pharmacies; unrestricted movement of the public in clinics and hospitals; the presence of gang members, drug or alcohol abusers, trauma patients, and distraught family members and long waits in emergency or clinic areas, leading to frustration among patients and accompanying relatives or friends; and a lack of training of staff in recognizing and managing escalating hostile and assaultive behavior (FBI, 2003). Nurses in general may work with patients, in any hospital or community setting, who may be volatile or have a history of violence.

According to the FBI (2003), employers should adopt clear no-threats and no-violence policies and prevention plans. Policies and planning to prevent violence are instrumental for employers to help meet their legal and ethical obligations to provide a safe environment for their workers. Once plans are in place, organizations can also complete other tasks, such as communicate the policy to employees at all levels of the company; survey employees to get their ideas about the incidence of violence, possible risks, and suggested preventive measures; give support to violence prevention measures; provide violence prevention training for all employees on a regular basis; practice the plan; provide physically secure work spaces; adopt staffing policies that will help keep employees safe on the job; establish relations with police, social service and mental health providers, and other government and private agencies that can assist in threat assessment, threat management, and crisis management; put workplace violence prevention and training on the agenda of chambers of commerce, industry, and trade associations and other employer organizations; and evaluate the workplace violence prevention plan periodically or when workplace circumstances change or a violent event has occurred. A respectful, collegial, and trusting workplace needs to be created and should involve unions, governing bodies, and executive team members.

There are many precipitating factors that can increase the risk for violence to nurses. Nurses have two key sources of violence to be cognizant of: their patients and their colleagues. Although violence originating both from patients and families and from colleagues can occur at varying levels, with patient violence having a higher prevalence rate, the factors that can precipitate the act of violence often vary in number and magnitude.

The factors associated with nursing violence that originates from patients are many. Mentally and chemically impaired patients are a significant concern (Nurses Association of New Brunswick [NANB], 2002) because of the unpredictable nature of their thought processes. However, contrary to popular belief, individuals who have mental illness are not typically violent people (Kelen, Catlett, Kubit, & Yu-Hsiang, 2012). In fact, 95% to 97% of all violent incidents in the United States do not involve individuals with mental illness (Canadian Mental Health Association [CMHA], 2010; Monahan, 1996). Even when a person with mental illness exhibits behaviors of violence, the mental illness alone is typically not the cause. As Arboleda-Florez and Stuart (2001) found, people with mental illness are often the victims of violence and therefore are just as much in need of protection from workplace violence as any other person.

However, there are times when mentally ill patients experience acute exacerbations of their illness so that their level of confusion and disorientation becomes altered. For example, psychiatric nursing units have one of the highest rates of patient-to-nurse violence (Shields & Wilkins, 2009). This becomes more of a concern upon the admission of an acutely psychotic patient who may be aggressive, angry, and belligerent, particularly if this patient is certified as an involuntary admission and opposes such actions.

In addition, individuals under the influence of drugs or alcohol and those with addictions are a population to remain cognizant of. Those with addictions, in particular as they experience withdrawal, can often seek out any and all measures to obtain more drugs, and unfortunately this may include violence (Baltieri, 2014).

Nurses on surgery units can also be at increased risk for violence from patients. Patients who are admitted with head injuries, for example, can become confused and combative toward nurses because they are completely disoriented to their surroundings and have just recently experienced significant trauma (CCOHS, 2012).

Regardless of the cause or origin of the violence, all such episodes raise the volatility of emotions, levels of stress, and amount of aggravation and frustration in patients, families, and colleagues that can precipitate and result in acts of assault or abuse against nurses in the workplace by others (International Council of Nurses, 2006).

Patients and Families Experiencing Stress

Becoming acutely ill or being diagnosed with various diseases is traumatizing for most, if not all, of us, so much so that it can precipitate acts of violence (Grenyer et al., 2004). Also, the trauma sustained as a result of an accident significantly raises the level of distress for families. The stress, torment, and uncertainty of "what's next?" and facing life-changing events or modifications to one's daily routine can cause a great deal of turmoil for patients and their families. For example, being told about an inoperable brain tumor obviously raises one's level of anxiety and fear. As stress levels escalate, so too do frustration, anger, and the potential to lose control and strike out. For families experiencing caregiver burden, as well, similar behaviors and emotions can ensue to the point of losing one's control (NANB, 2002). Outside the issue of being given bad news, in the emergency department as well, the main perpetrators were patients or their families or friends (Lyneham, 2000).

Dealing With the Public

In some ways, nurses are in a position similar to that of salespersons, albeit at a more intellectual level, as they are regularly dealing with the public. However, for nurses, this point of contact is even more critical because members of the public are entrusting nurses with their lives and care or with the lives and care of their loved ones. People who seek health care services come to the health care setting with a variety of personalities, needs, expectations, demands, wishes, and previous experiences, most of which, if they have been problematic in the past, the nurse will not be privy to unless they were documented in the patient's chart or shared with the nurse somehow.

The Influence of Society

Nurses are abundantly on the front line of health care delivery and so are often the first ones to greet the people coming in to seek care. Generally, working with the public carries some degree for risk of harm to nurses (CCOHS, 2012). If something significant is occurring in society, or even catastrophic in nature, its effects can permeate a nurse's work environment. Increased levels of violence and frustration in society are positively correlated with nurses being assaulted in the workplace (NANB, 2002). Dealing with society's many different social and cultural behaviors is a great learning experience but may sometimes unintentionally percolate into misunderstandings (Grenyer et al., 2004).

Staff Shortages, High Patient Acuity, and Workload

Factors such as staffing, the acuity of patients, and the workload can filter into nurses' work environment. They can compromise patient safety and the quality of health care that becomes available (NANB, 2002). Chao and Henshaw (2003) add that particularly during times of increased activity, such as mealtimes and visiting times, staff levels are low, easing the way for violence to arise. Internal and rising levels of stress, frustrations, and short-temperedness exaggerated by poor leadership, poor collegial relationships, and patient demands all enrich the ground in which violence to germinate (CCOHS, 2012). As found by Hasketh et al. (2003), a shortage of human resources, as is commonly found, increases the risk for nurses to experience violence from patients, families, and coworkers, all frustrated because the quality of patient care is jeopardized (Hasketh et al, 2003). Finally, increased workloads, as well, are often generally concerning (Bowman, 2012).

From a general perspective, a nurse's low level of job satisfaction, if he or she feels unfairly treated, may precipitate actions of violence, as do a nurse's personal stressors, such as involvement in drugs, alcohol abuse, financial distress, and family or romantic difficulties, any of which can push a nurse over the edge (Bowman, 2012).

Working Alone

Nurses can work alone in many different circumstances. Regardless of where, the nurse or group of nurses is isolated from the security found in main health care centers. Many public health or community care nurses are alone or in isolation while transporting patients (CCOHS, 2013; Chao & Henshaw, 2003) or working in a mobile workplace environment, such as a mobile crisis response unit. Other isolating workplace environments can include a location adjacent to a high-crime area or next to empty, run-down buildings and structures that often attract people with bad intentions. These facilities are often small and typically do not have communication devices or alarm systems that can be used to call for help. Therefore, locations and isolated work environments such as these all carry an increased risk for violence (CCOHS, 2013; Chao & Henshaw, 2003). Chao and Henshaw add further that isolation may even occur during examinations, counseling sessions, and treatment, so caution should still be exercised, even in the confines of a main hospital or center.

Logistics of Nursing Practice

Even some of the logistics of nurses' work can predispose them to an element of violence. Nursing is one of the few occupations in which people work through the night during shift work; nurses may work late into the night and very early hours of the morning, when resources are at their lowest. Also late at night and in the early morning, security measures are at a minimum, while the public has free unrestricted access to the health care facility (CCOHS, 2013; Chao & Henshaw, 2003).

Poor Environmental Work Design

The design or layout of the workplace environment can also facilitate violence (CCOHS, 2013). Poorly lit corridors and dark entrances and side doors are rich areas for violence. Staff and nurses leave their units to go outside for a "smoke break," which they are forbidden to take within the confines of the smoke-free workplace, and often leave side doors open for reentry, providing a readily available way for perpetrators to enter. Finally, the large and dimly lit parking lots where nurses arrive at and leave work can be a breeding ground for stalkers and other perpetrators of violence for nurses in the workplace (Chao & Henshaw, 2003). As supported by Lyneham (2000), as cited in Chapman and Styles (2006), emergency department nurses in Australia were concerned about the physical layout of their department and about the presence of security personnel and equipment.

Patient Logistics

Patients enter hospitals on an outpatient basis to seek many different health care services. These services often include emergency departments, diagnostic imaging, laboratory services, and clinics. Rarely would patients enter an emergency department to be taken in immediately for triage and assessment unless they were transported by ambulance or showed visible signs of illness and distress, such as cardiac problems. When patients have appointments for blood work and x-rays, there can often be long waiting times (CCOHS, 2012; Chao & Henshaw, 2003; Grenyer et al., 2004 as cited in Chapman & Styles, 2006). When these lengthy waiting times are combined with overcrowded and uncomfortable waiting rooms (CCOHS, 2012; CDC, 2002 as cited in Gacki-Smith et al., 2009; Grenyer et al., 2004 as cited in Chapman & Styles, 2006), where others are perhaps sneezing and coughing repeatedly as a result of various illnesses, levels of frustration, stress, and agitation rise over the inability to receive services promptly (Chao & Henshaw, 2003). Further, patience becomes short, anger rises, and discontent lingers, possibly further precipitating an outburst directed toward clerical staff or nurses.

Nature of Nurses' Work

Other than the experience of dealing with a variety of personalities and expectations and the demands of the pubic, previously discussed, other key aspects of a nurse's work can also foster violence. These key aspects include that nurses have easy access to drug cupboards where narcotics and even alcohol are stored, perhaps in long-term care or residential settings. Further, nurses are often asked to store valuables for patients, particularly if jewelry is a health risk (e.g., chains) or someone is being prepared for surgery. Both drugs and valuables are enticing to potentially violent perpetrators, and nurses hold the key to both (CCOHS, 2012; Chao & Henshaw, 2003).

Professionally, nurses can engage in violence themselves, making for an unsafe workplace. First, as is covered in the chapter on addictions, nurses who do have drug or alcohol addiction issues are working with an altered state of mind and can resort to violence themselves, as well as be easy targets of violence. Second, receiving a performance appraisal that is not favorable or positive can be a critical turning point for a nurse to act out against the manager. Third, a nurse may often accompany a doctor who is delivering bad news to a patient or family. The bad news that someone's condition is terminal may elicit a negative reactive response in which the patient or family uses force on the nurse.

Organizational Change

Working during periods of intense organizational change, such as occurs during labor union disputes, downsizing, restructuring, and consolidation of services, can also set the stage for possible violence to occur. Anxiety is prevalent and runs high as people fear losing their jobs, having their hours reduced, and losing their security and benefits (CCOHS, 2012). Change comes with a great deal of uncertainty, and unless the lines of communication from hierarchal levels are clear, a great deal of animosity and "not knowing" can fester among front-line staff and nurses. As found by Hasketh et al. (2003), health services restructuring is a factor associated with increased vulnerability of organizations to violence. Further, downsizing can leave people feeling unfairly treated and seeking revenge, and rapid change as well can cause undue stress and explode in violence (Bowman, 2012).

Lack of Staff Training and Policies

Training and education of staff and supportive policies are needed for the identification, prevention, and management of crisis with potentially volatile patients (CCOHS, 2013). Nurses should receive some degree of training in recognizing and managing escalating hostile and assaultive behaviors in the workplace (Chao & Henshaw, 2003). In the absence of such training, nurses worry and can be left helpless as to what practices should be followed, hence allowing violence to escalate.

Access to Firearms

Some countries support the possession and ownership of firearms by public citizens, other than for the purposes of hunting for food or public safety. The United States is one such country; therefore, the prevalence of handguns and other weapons among patients, families, and friends is expected to be higher than you would typically find in other countries where rules against possession are more stringent. This easy access to firearms is particularly conducive to violence against nurses, considering that society is seeing a sharp rise in the number of gangs and alcohol and drug abusers, so often depicted through the media. As was found by

Kelen et al. (2012) in their analysis of U.S. hospital shootings, not all guns involved in the shootings are brought in by the perpetrator; in 25% of the emergency department shootings included in the study, a security officer's gun was taken and used (Kelen et al., 2012). Further, Australia emergency department nurses as well have noted an increase in the use of weapons such as guns, knives, needles, and syringes (Lyneham, 2000).

Police Utilization of Health Care Facilities

Increasingly, police and the criminal justice system are keeping criminals, the acutely disturbed, and violent individuals under the watchful eye of hospitals (Chao & Henshaw, 2003). This poses an added stress and potential threat of violence toward hospital staff, in particular the nurses who are typically working with these individuals.

Early Release of Patients

As pressures mount on today's health care systems, the demand for early patient discharges increases to unblock emergency department beds. However, an increasing number of acute and chronic potentially violent patients are being discharged from the hospital without follow-up care (Chao & Henshaw, 2003). These patients very well may be traumatically injured patients, patients with varying stages of dementia or altered cognitive thought processes, and acutely unwell patients with mental illness who have not yet been stabilized despite hospitalization efforts. In addition, these are often the same patients who can refuse any further medical treatment and can no longer be hospitalized involuntarily unless they pose an immediate danger to themselves, others, or property.

CATEGORIES OF VIOLENCE

Violence in the workplace comes in three different categories, as outlined well by Bowman (2012). These different types are categorized as type I, type II, and type III. Type I violence represents an outsider who has no relationship with the organization or workplace and who enters for the sole purpose of committing an act of violence. In a hospital setting, for example, a person who is posing as a visitor or delivery driver tries to physically harm a nurse.

Perhaps the largest historical example of type I violence involving nurses actually involved nursing students who trained and worked for a South Chicago community hospital in 1966. Mass murderer Richard Franklin Speck broke into a townhouse that functioned as a dormitory and tortured, raped, and murdered eight student nurses. Using a knife, he brutally stabbed or strangled them to death one at a time while one nursing student lay hidden under the bed. This was obviously not a targeted action as Speck and the nursing students were not known to each other. The randomness of this act is confirmed by the fact that he had planned only for a routine robbery at first while high on drugs and alcohol.

In a separate incident in Carthage, North Carolina, in 2009, a lone gunman burst into a nursing home and started shooting (Coleman, Chou, Bowens, & Heffernan,

2009). The shooter, Robert Stewart, known for his violent tendencies to his family members, had no known relationship to any of the patients or staff of the home. He shot and killed seven residents and one nurse and wounded others during the violent attack.

In the second category of violence, type II, the perpetrator has an identified relationship with the organization, workplace, or employed nurse (Bowman, 2012). On a nursing unit, for example, a patient or family member returns some time after being discharged from the hospital because of anger about the poor nursing care he or she believes was given during admission to the unit. In the emergency department, patients and visitors are some of the main perpetrators of violence against nurses (Chapman & Styles, 2006; Gacki-Smith et al., 2009). Similarly, as found by Hasketh et al. (2003), patients were the main source of violence, particularly physical assaults and threats of assault against nurses, accounting for from 95.9% of episodes in the emergency department to 100% in psychiatric units. In perhaps the most common form of violence against nurses we have witnessed, the spouse of a nurse is often the culprit. In one particular case that occurred in the Eastern Cape Health Department in Johannesburg, South Africa, a nurse was shot dead while she was working in her office at a medical clinic. Based on the findings that the shooter was the nurse's husband, it was suspected that the primary motive resulted from a domestic dispute. The husband then turned the gun on himself. As the shooter was the husband, it was obviously a targeted hit on a personal, not professional, level (SAPA, 2012).

In a more recent case, although a connection is not yet proven, James Holmes massacred people attending a movie theatre in Colorado on July 20, 2012. The headline read, "Nurse who aided Dark Knight shooting massacre victims mysteriously drowns on vacation" (Goodhand, 2012). The nurse, Jennifer Gallaher, who played a very pivotal role in providing care to the injured theatergoers, mysteriously drowned while she was on vacation. Although there has not yet been shown any direct connection to the work she performed on the survivors of that massacre, there is much suspicion that the two events may have been related.

In an even more recent case, which occurred in October 2012 on the property of a nursing home in Lexington, Kentucky, the husband of a nurse who worked at the home was shot while in the parking lot of the home (Kocher, 2012a, 2012b). Again, this case was deemed to be domestically related, with a specific target in mind.

The final category of workplace violence, type III, is violence that originates from a colleague or coworker, such as a fellow nurse, physician, or manager. This is what Bowman (2012) refers to as type III violence, or violence that occurs between people or groups that have had a previously established working relationship. For example, a physician who sexually assaults a nurse or a nurse who physically assaults another nurse would be one such example. In light of these three categories of workplace violence, nurses are often found to be involved in type II and type III violence, from patients, families or visitors, and colleagues, respectively. In addition to these categories of workplace violence, defined by the presence or absence of a relationship between the nurse and the perpetrator, there exist different forms of violence. In Australia, for example, 20% of nurses surveyed identified tension at work as an issue leading to aggressive behavior with verbal abuse by nursing administration and medical staff (Lyneham, 2000). Similarly, Hasketh et al. (2003) found that although patients were the biggest perpetrators of violence, hospital staff such as nursing colleagues was the most frequent source of nonphysical violence and accounted for 56.7% of all emotional abuse and 53.6% of all verbal sexual harassment in the clinical care setting.

As alluded to previously, for type III violence to occur, the perpetrator and the nurse must already be known to each other. There is already established some form of work-related relationship. Closely linked to category III violence is the concept of "going postal." However, it is not something you typically think about in the nursing profession. Nurses being subjected to a colleague "going postal" have become a reality in today's society. Going postal is the ultimate, most horrific form of violence nurses can experience. Although it is a rarity, it can and does occur. Many cases have been documented globally in which a nurse was killed as a result of someone going postal. Kelen et al. (2012) did an analysis of hospital shootings from 2000 to 2011 and found that 59% (n = 91) of all hospital shootings occurred inside the hospital and 41% (n = 63) occurred outside on hospital grounds. Together, all shootings occurred in 40 states and left 235 people either dead or injured. They also found that the perpetrators were most often male, 29% of shootings occurred in emergency departments, 23% occurred in parking lots, and 19% occurred in patient rooms. The most common victim was the perpetrator (45%). Hospital employees comprised 20% of victims; physician (3%) and nurse (5%) victims were relatively infrequent. Primary motives for the shootings were a grudge of some kind against the victim (27%), to commit suicide (21%), to euthanize a patient who was a relative (14%), and a prisoner escaping custody (11%; Kelen et al., 2012). Finally, the shootings that occurred in the emergency department setting had a lower fatality rate (19%) than those occurring in other areas/ sites (73%; Kelen et al., 2012).

A well-documented case was one that occurred in Windsor, Ontario, Canada, in 2007. This case involved a nurse who began to develop an intimate relationship with a doctor. A nurse by the name of Lori Dupont was stabbed to death by her former lover, Dr. Marc Daniel, an anesthesiologist, while working at the Hotel-Dieu Grace Hospital. In this case, a working relationship grew into a more intimate relationship, so there would obviously have been many emotions involved. Hence, this would not have been a random act of violence, but instead a targeted action. Unfortunately, many warning signs were there, and nurses alerted others to the possibility of the doctor going postal, but no one took any action. One nurse coworker in particular, Ms. Porter, spoke about the doctor's "death stare," his "creepy" and "stalking" behaviors, his previous suicide attempt, his flat affect, and his previously exhibited harassing behavior, for which an outstanding grievance existed. She stated she was even "afraid of him." Written off by management that he was perhaps having some health or emotional issues of his own and was taking medications for it, nothing was done. The very nurse, Ms. Porter, who was afraid of this doctor and had requested accommodation to not work the same shift as his was ignored despite promises from management to address the problem, and she even called in sick 6 days before her colleague's stabbing so she wouldn't have to work with him (National Post, 2007).

A similar case occurred in Manila, the Philippines, in June 2012. The story concerns a woman who was a nurse, Krizzia Legasi, and her husband, Nathan Legasi, who was a policeman. Obviously, the nurse did have a previously established relationship with her murderer, and this act of violence did not occur at the victim's place of work and was a targeted action, not a random act, in which the nurse was shot in the eye with a bullet that exited the back of her head (Cabayan, 2012).

Another case occurred in Castleford, West Yorkshire, United Kingdom, in 1998. Again, a male doctor, Dr. Thomas Shanks, shot and killed his girlfriend nurse, Vicky Fletcher, after engaging in what was referred to as a "tempestuous" relationship. Dr. Shanks and Ms. Fletcher worked at Pontefract General Infirmary, where the nurse died of wounds to her back, arms, and legs. She was shot multiple times by the doctor in the parking lot of a pub before the doctor calmly got into his car and drove away (Bennetto, 1998).

As nursing students may be considered "potential" nursing colleagues, in the world of nursing academics, a similar theme rings through. You are perhaps familiar with the shooting that took place in the school of nursing at the University of Arizona in 2002. It was perpetrated by a student nurse who was at risk of not passing the program; he shot and killed three of his nursing professors while injuring many other nursing students (Holguin, 2002).

In Buffalo, New York, in June 2012, a nursing student once again fell victim to a doctor (Warren, 2012). After a nationwide manhunt, with the assistance of officials of the FBI, U.S. Customs and Border Protection, and the U.S. Marshals Service, Dr. Timothy Jorden was arrested for killing nursing student Jacqueline Wisniewski. After expressing a great degree of fear of this man, being stalked by him with a GPS tracking device strapped to the bottom of her car, and being held captive against her will for 1 1/2 days under the threat of a knife, sadly nurse Wisniewski met her demise with four gunshots in the stairwell of the hospital while working one morning. Again, this was not a random act of violence, but a very targeted act as a result of a previously established work relationship.

Another shooting involving nursing students occurred at Oikos University in Oakland, California, where on April 1, 2012, a no-longer-enrolled nursing student barged into a lecture room and started firing a gun, shooting and killing seven people and injuring many others before walking into a Safeway supermarket and announcing, "I just shot some people" (Prince, 2012).

The case of the Fort Hood 2009 shooting of medical personnel by a psychiatrist is another such example (Wikipedia, 2012). What resulted from this was that 13 people were killed, four of whom were nurses or nurse practitioners. At this point in history, the United States has identified this as an act of terrorism and perhaps the worst act of terrorism since the 9/11 horrific terrorist events. The psychiatrist who did the shooting in this case was later found to be linked to the terrorist group Al-Qaeda.

Although there have been many documented shootings occurring in hospitals and significantly involving nurses, Jay Wolfson, a researcher at the University of South Florida, believes that the risk for shootings occurring in hospitals is "extremely rare" (Pittman, 2012) and that people should not be overly concerned about gun violence in hospitals, as the rate at which it occurs in hospitals is much lower than the rate at other work sites. Kelen et al. (2012) believe that the shootings that do occur in hospitals are not random acts of violence but instead are directly targeted and involve a perpetrator with a grudge, a suicide, or someone "euthanizing" a sick relative. Kelen states, "The likelihood of being shot in a hospital is less than the likelihood of being struck by lightning."

On the flipside of type III violence are nurses committing acts of violence themselves. Nurses, for example, can equally commit acts of violence against their patients and their colleagues. Regardless, such an act still has significant potential to affect workplace mental health for all involved. Such was the case for nurse Verna Deann McClain in Houston, Texas, who had previously been providing health care nursing services to Kayla Marie Golden. McClain, a registered nurse, gunned down Golden and snatched her 3-day-old baby boy from his mother's arms as she was leaving the clinic. Leaving the mother to die on the ground, the nurse drove off with the baby, later to be found by the SWAT team with the baby unharmed (Daily Mail Reporter, 2012).

FORMS OF VIOLENCE IN NURSING

There are various forms of violence that can occur in nursing. For example, physical assault occurs when someone uses a body part or an object to control another person's actions, such as through hitting, shoving, pushing, throwing objects, kicking, or grabbing. It also includes the application of force by an act or gesture, whether or not an injury was sustained. Again, actions against patients were also significant, as they reflect the ease with which colleagues would take such action. For example, after an elderly patient was slapped twice in the face, grabbed by the neck, and pulled up onto his pillow, after the victim recoiled from him, a licensed practical nurse was charged (Sobol, 2012).

Verbal abuse or the statement of threats of harm to nurses by patients and others is a common occurrence in many areas in nursing. About one third of teaching hospital emergency departments report daily verbal threats, and one quarter restrain at least one patient per day (Duong, 2010).

Sexual assault, in which a person is forced to take part in a sexual activity or act, can also occur, as was reported by Dean (2012) of the *Huffington Post* when a 98-year-old patient, who was paralyzed after a stroke, was sexually violated by two San Diego home care nurses.

Verbal sexual harassment is a form of sexual harassment at work that creates an intimidating, hostile, or offensive work environment (McShane, 2001). As found by Hasketh et al. (2003), 42.9% of cases of sexual harassment violence occur in psychiatric settings, with 7.6% of registered nurses experiencing it and only 23.3% of them reporting it.

A threat or expression of intent to cause harm to someone can also take the form of threatening behaviors or actions, such as shaking one's fists and destroying property. In nursing, this often occurs when a family member or patient gets angry at a nurse. Financial violence occurs when someone controls or tries to exert control over another person's financial resources without the person's knowledge or consent; this can also exist in nursing, such as when a nurse is found guilty of stealing a patient's money or valuables (Anonymous, 2012). Finally, arson as a form of violence can be a reality for nurses. One such incident occurred in Wythenshawe, Manchester, United Kingdom, when a nurse received an anonymous threat that her house would be burnt down if she did not drop a filed complaint against a colleague. In this event, which became viral news on the Internet, a nurse, Jenny Fecitt, and two other nurses blew the whistle on an alleged unqualified nurse, Daniel Swift, who left Ms. Fecitt mentally scarred from repeated threats of arson on her house and family. Although numerous reports and complaints were lodged with the health organization, no action was taken (Telegraph Media Group Limited, 2009).

Homicide, of course, belongs in a class of its own as a form of violence and may or may not be related to a nurse's work. Domestic and spousal violence are two such presentations. For example, in 2008 in Fayetteville, North Carolina, a marine was charged with first-degree murder in the death of his wife, an army nurse who worked at the Womack Army Medical Center in Fort Bragg (Mims, Charbonneau, & Bowens, 2008).

Vandalism as a form of violence against nurses is another reality. In June 2012, a nursing home was vandalized by angry family members after a recently admitted loved one died in the nursing home. Three ambulances and a medical shop were also vandalized.

The issue of stealing is not so much about the nurse being victimized as it is about the nurse victimizing others, such as patients. In North Carolina in July 2012, a licensed practical nurse was arrested for stealing a patient's bank card and taking, without the patient's consent, $1,800 from the patient's bank account. However, nurses are also victims of theft, such as occurred in 2012 in the John F. Kennedy Hospital in Liberia (The New Republic Liberia, 2012). After nurses took pity on a frequent and known patient with a specific condition and raised funds to help him get treatment, he stole the very same funds from the nurses and inserted them in his anus to hide them.

The issue of abuse and neglect is also of concern. Nurses typically receive a great deal of abuse from patients on a daily basis that can really challenge their mental health. As found by Speroni, Fitch, Dawson, Dugan, and Atherton (2013), 76% of nurses experienced violence from patients or visitors. Of these, the most serious career violence incidents ($n = 595$, 78.1%) were physical (63.7%; 60.8% by patients and 2.9% by visitors), verbal (25.4%; 18.3% by patients and 7.1% by visitors), and threatened physical assault (10.9%; 6.9% by patients and 4.0% by visitors). Speroni et al. (2013) add that the perpetrators of such violence were primarily White men 26 to 35 years of age who were confused or influenced by alcohol or drugs, resulting in actions that accounted for costs of $94,156 ($78,924 for treatment and $15,232 for indemnity). Gacki-Smith et al. (2009) found rates of violence among emergency department nurses to be 25% for physical violence and 20% for verbal abuse; however, most "respondents who experienced frequent physical violence or frequent verbal abuse indicated fear of retaliation and lack of support from hospital administration and emergency department management as barriers to reporting workplace violence."

NURSING SETTING AND ENVIRONMENT

As nursing exists in many different settings of health care, violence against nurses can occur in a multitude of areas. However, some areas can carry slightly more risk than others, particularly in psychiatry (NIOSH, 2002), emergency (Hasketh et al., 2003; NIOSH, 2002), surgery and geriatric units (NIOSH, 2002), and even in waiting rooms (NIOSH, 2002) and admitting departments (FBI, 2003). However, all groups of nurses from various settings were less likely to report a violence incident if a coworker was the perpetrator (Hasketh et al., 2003).

There are some common features that mark a troubled work environment and its susceptibility to violence. According to the Employee Assistance Trade Association (2013), these can include chronic labor–management disputes; an extraordinary number of injury claims; frequent or increased employee grievances or complaints, particularly of harassment; understaffing or excessive demands for overtime; high worker stress; layoffs and a correspondingly increased workload for remaining employees; and an authoritarian leadership style.

Medical–surgical nurses have one of the highest rates of physical assaults (24.2%) and the highest incidence overall of all forms of violence (FBI, 2003; Hasketh et al., 2003). While nurses in critical care had the fewest incidents of violence (Hasketh et al., 2003), the FBI recognizes it as one the most dangerous (FBI, 2003). Further, 9.5% of general hospital nurses are assaulted in any one year (Bowers et al., 1999).

Both physical and verbal violence in emergency department nursing are a global problem (FBI, 2003; Keough, Schlomer, & Bollenburg, 2003; Lyneham, 2000; Fernandes et al., 2002; Rodgers, Hills, & Kristjanson, 2004). The emergency department has become known as a "distillery of human fear and anxiety" for becoming too closely acquainted with violence and aggression (Tyrrell, 2000). Some say it is like working "on the front line of a war zone" (Sweet, 1991).

Psychiatric nursing as well brings many potential challenges. Psychiatric/mental health nursing is known to be a high-risk area for violence from patients (FBI, 2003; Whittington, Shuttleworth, & Hill, 1996). Interestingly, psychiatric nurses are most likely to report a violent incident (Hasketh et al., 2003).

Geriatric units as well are sometimes considered a high-risk violent area for nurses (CDC, 2002). For example, older adults experiencing organic brain illnesses such as different kinds of dementias and deliriums may pose an increased risk of violence for nurses at work. Dementia, for example, is often characterized by disordered thought process, paranoia, and even periods of acute psychosis (American Psychiatric Association, 2014). As a result, older adults afflicted with such disorders can become combative, angry, and unpredictable without any relevant or obvious cause or event (CCOHS, 2012).

PROFILE OF THE POTENTIALLY VIOLENT PERPETRATOR

Identifying a potentially violent person and using supportive interventions can often help prevent or deter violence from occurring. This is why it is important for nurses to know what to look for (Table 8.1). Whether the perpetrator is a colleague, patient, family member, or friend, if the person is prone to violence, he or she often has a history of stormy personal relationships, resents authority figures, holds grudges, and has extremist views/opinions and a sense of entitlement; additionally, the individual is self-righteous, tardy, absent a lot, forgettable, disorganized, and doesn't welcome contact with others (Bowman, 2012). Further, this person can

TABLE 8.1   Pyschiatric Versus Organic Etiology of Violence

FEATURES SUGGEST PSYCHIATRIC ETIOLOGY	FEATURES SUGGEST ORGANIC ETIOLOGY
Oriented	Disoriented
Alert	Depressed level of consciousness
Gradual onset	Sudden onset
Psychiatric history	No psychiatric history
Normal vital signs	Abnormal vital signs
Normal physical examination	Abnormal physical examination
Age younger than 40 years	Age older than 40 years (without psychiatric history)
Auditory hallucinations	Visual hallucinations
Flattened affect	Emotional lability
Able to redirect	Unable to sustain attention

have violent outbursts, substance abuse problems, knowledge of or experience with weapons and explosives, few or no supports or relationships, and a migratory job history; frequently files grievances or lawsuits; has work performance problems; has been seen to behave aggressively in the past; is impulsive, depressed, withdrawn, suicidal, and paranoid; has frequent conversations about violence; fails to modify behaviors after reprimands (Bowman, 2012); and shows signs of anxiety (pacing, clenching of fists, pressured speech, angry speech), defensiveness, and verbal threats or yelling (Duong, 2010).

IDENTIFICATION OF IMPENDING VIOLENCE

The immediacy of impending and escalating violence has many identifying characteristics or attributes that can be recognized in the individual perpetrator. These are a display of anger, rapid speech, angry tone of voice, fidgetiness, demand for attention, paranoid or delusional comments, aggressive statements and treats, clenched fists, increased motor activity, pacing, and tense posture (Presley & Robinson, 2002; Tyrrell, 2000). This person also typically presents with acute agitation, yelling, psychosis, and violent behaviors, which are common presentations in emergency department patients. In fact, the emergency department is the most common setting in the hospital for employee assault (Duong, 2010). While this individual may present very insidiously, with no such obvious behaviors noticed, violent actions do not typically occur suddenly, as some form of warning signs often lead up to them before they occur (Duong, 2010).

According to the Employee Assistance Trade Association (2013), the initially concerning behavior of a troubled employee who may pose a potential threat of violence includes verbally abusive, objectifying, and dehumanizing language; noncompliance with policies and procedures; challenges to authority; frequent arguments; frequent complaints from customers; instigation and spread of lies and rumors;

excessive use of profanity; inappropriate and sexually explicit language woven into conversation and angry outbursts; and frequent signs of frustration. When these initial concerns grow to become more serious, you will typically observe behaviors such as verbal threats; conveying unwanted sexual attention or violent intentions by letter, voicemail, or e-mail; holding others responsible for the employee's own unacceptable behavior; arguing frequently with escalated intensity; blatantly disregarding organizational policy and procedures; setting traps for others with malicious intent; stealing from the company or other employees; and damaging company property. Finally, the ultimate warning signs of impending violence are characterized by a fascination/obsession with weapons or violence in the media, substance abuse, indications of severe stress, suicidal verbalizations ("I can't go on like this"), violent history, romantic obsession, evidence of domestic abuse, hostile or erratic behavior, change in personality or decrease in work performance, social isolation with avoidance of others at the workplace, declining and poor hygiene, an inability to get along with peers, and poor work relationships.

There are many pitfalls that nurses fall victim to when it involves assessing an agitated patient for potential violence in the workplace. Dr. David Duong (2010) of the University of California at San Francisco suggests that to avoid these potential pitfalls, nurses need to obtain a complete set of vital signs, have a high degree of suspicion for emergent causes of agitated behavior and assume a psychiatric cause, and obtain an adequate history and physical examination after the acute agitation episode subsides and the patient is able to engage in a conversation. They should not trivialize a patient's threat for violence or feel embarrassed to ask for help, and have an assessment and treatment plan after restraining an agitated patient.

UNDERREPORTING OF VIOLENCE

Although nurses are entitled to the same sense of dignity and respect as all other health care workers, this is often not the case. Violence in nursing is a reality of the nursing profession. Although it most often originates from either patients or colleagues, it often goes underreported (Lyneham, 2000; Fernandes et al., 1999). While the rate of violence is suspected to be much higher than is reported in the statistics, this underreporting of violence in nursing occurs for various reasons. The true measures and extent of violence that occurs in the nursing profession are hard to determine for many reasons related to underreporting (Chapman & Styles, 2006).

Violence in nursing is often underreported because there is still the perception in society and organizations that the receipt of assault is part of a nurse's job and goes hand in hand with all of the other responsibilities that nurses perform on a daily basis and are considered the norm (Chao & Henshaw, 2003; NANB, 2002; Grenyer et al., 2004; Jones & Lyneham, 2000; May & Grubbs, 2002). Other reasons for not reporting violence in the workplace include such things as lack of institutional reporting policies (Chao & Henshaw, 2003; Gacki-Smith et al., 2009), employee beliefs that reporting is of no benefit to them (Chao & Henshaw, 2003; May & Grubbs, 2002), and employees fear that employers will believe that assaults probably result from nurse negligence or poor job performance (Chao & Henshaw, 2003; Sofield & Salmond, 2003; U.S. Department of Labor, 2004). In other words, if the nurse had been doing his or her job correctly, appropriately, and perhaps in a timely manner, this act of violence from the patient would never have occurred. In addition, many nurses feel empathy for the anger expressed by the patient and family (May & Grubbs, 2002); they don't want to disrupt the sense of teamwork in the unit/setting, which is vital to the functioning of the unit/setting (Lowry, 2000); the paperwork to report violent incidents/occurrences is burdensome (Lowry, 2000); and the amount of time needed to complete the paperwork is not worth it (Mahoney, 1991). Other reasons include fear of retaliation (Gacki-Smith et al., 2009); perceived lack of organizational support (Gacki-Smith et al., 2009; Lowry, 2000); dissuasive, subtle arguments from coworkers, administration, and law enforcement officials (Lowry, 2000); emotional abuse is not always considered a form of abuse and therefore is not taken seriously (Campbell, 2001); and finally the lack of physical evidence of personal injury (May & Grubbs, 2002). As reported by May and Grubbs (2002), 50% of verbal and physical assaults are never reported in writing.

As found by Hasketh et al. (2003), nonreporting can be a result of who is involved in the violent or potentially violent situation. For example, when the patient was the source of verbal sexual harassment, 27.9% of nurses reported it, compared with a 25% reporting compliance when the source was a family member or visitor. To the contrary, when the source of harassment was a physician (13.2%) or a colleague (4.5%), nurses were not so inclined to report it. Similarly, for physical abuse, when patients were the source, 37.5% of nurses reported it. However, when family or visitors were the source, 62.5% of nurses reported it, while 66.6% reported it when physicians were the source. The threat of abuse uncovers some similar trends. When the patient was the source of a threat of abuse, 36.1% of nurses reported it, compared to rates of 52.1%, 70%, and 33.3% for family/visitors, physicians, and colleague nurses, respectively. Finally, for emotional abuse, nurses reported it at rates of 28.6% from patients, 40.3% from family/visitors, 29.1% from physicians, and only 19.7% from nurse colleagues.

IMPACT OF VIOLENCE IN THE WORKPLACE

Nurses suffer significantly as a result of the violence directed toward them. Physically, there can be minor physical injuries (NIOSH, 2002), serious physical injuries (NIOSH, 2002), temporary or permanent physical disability (NIOSH, 2002), and even death (NIOSH, 2002). Mentally, there is much psychological trauma (Bowman, 2012; NIOSH, 2002), negative effects on one's personal life, such as personal losses (Bowman, 2012), and the emotional effects of anger, anxiety, helplessness, sadness, and physical abuse (Bowman, 2012; Brennan, 2001; Grenyer et al., 2004).

Professionally, workplace violence for nurses is directly linked to decreased job satisfaction and job performance, increased absenteeism, and mental health issues (Fernandes et al., 1999; Hasketh et al., 2003; Manderino & Berkey, 1997; Whittington et al., 1996). For example, nurses who had not experienced workplace violence had the highest level of job satisfaction, while those who experienced both emotional abuse and at least one other form of violence had the lowest level of job satisfaction

(Hasketh et al., 2003). Further, it is "an important marker" of the quality of the practice environment in hospitals (Hasketh et al., 2003), decreases morale (51%), increases workload for peers (45%), deters recruitment and retention efforts, particularly back to the bedside, and accounts for 52% of performance errors (Chapman & Styles, 2006).

Violence to nurses on the front line results in far-reaching consequences and costs to the organization as well. Organizationally, workplace violence can be very detrimental to the operations and function of the organization. By lowering morale (NIOSH, 2002) and increasing job stress even more (NIOSH, 2002), it increases staff turnover (Chapman & Styles, 2006; NIOSH, 2002), decreases the sense of trust in and respect for management and colleagues (NIOSH, 2002), decreases productivity (Chapman & Styles, 2006), creates a hostile work environment (NIOSH, 2002), and increases financial costs such as higher use of sick leave (Chapman & Styles, 2006), costing U.S. organizations and businesses more than $4 billion per year and a further $30 billion per year in security systems equipment and resources (Bowman, 2012).

As nursing shortages loom globally, issues of violence and abuse need to be addressed in an expected manner because they may indirectly impact an organization's ability to recruit and retain all health care professionals, inclusive of nurses (Alberta Association of Registered Nurses, 2001; Canadian Medical Association, 2001). If violence in the workplace continues to be tolerated and is not addressed, the recruitment and retention nurses will be made even more challenging (Chapman & Styles, 2006). From a patient safety perspective as well, the impact that workplace violence has on the quality of patient care needs to be considered and addressed in an expedited manner (Hasketh et al., 2003).

PREVENTION AND INTERVENTION

In a perfect world, there is no violence; however, we do not live in a perfect world. If violence can be prevented, then this is what everyone would ideally aim to achieve. Although violence can often be nonpredictable (Abualrub & Al Khawaldeh, 2013; Ricciardi, 2014; Ward, 2011), there are many warning signs and even triggers that can be identified to indicate that it may be impending (O'Connor, 2013; Ricciardi, 2014; Ward, 2011). This is where the old cliché penny wise, pound foolish can often be recognized. As we have already seen, violence can come in many different forms and from three different categories of people, at least with respect to nurses. Regardless of the source, form, or setting, efforts to help prevent violence are vital to implement, monitor, and sustain. In this section, we will discover various measures that can be employed by the individual nurse, the nurse leader, and the organization to help prevent violence.

Role of Nurse

As front-line workers dealing with the public, nurses are often in the most pivotal position to detect signs of impending violence. It is important not to trivialize any threats of violence and not to be embarrassed to ask for help. Although some violence has been suggested to be unpredictable, as identified above, there are many things that can be done from a nurse's perspective to help prevent it (Ricciardi, 2014). From the nurse's perspective, there are numerous things that the nurse can do to help assist in the early identification and prevention of violence in the workplace. Nurses must be assertive and refuse to tolerate the violence (Nurses Association of New Brunswick, 2002). This can be achieved through ways that use communication, assessment, the buddy system, and involving the nursing leader.

Nurses must support other colleagues who have been abused. They can achieve this by taking individual and collective action in the workplace (NANB, 2002). A similar action and advocacy can be achieved through efforts of their governing bodies and associations as well. Nurses must be encouraged to report violence in the workplace and be treated with dignity, respect, and credibility during the reporting process. Professionally, nurses have a role to play in promoting, advocating, and lobbying for change in society's attitude toward violence in nursing. Involvement of the occupational health nurse as well is encouraged.

If for any reason the nurse is feeling uncomfortable, threatened, or uneasy, trust your instinct and be cognizant of and alert to the people around you, including your colleagues (Presley & Robinson, 2002). Simply, you need to "ACT," that is, assess quickly, contain behaviors, and treat specifically.

Professionally, all nurses strive to ensure the personal safety and security of themselves and their patients, and collaborative work is the key. To ensure the development of trust and respect, multiple disciplines work together to assess, plan, implement, and evaluate strategies to protect everyone in a health care environment from violent incidents. In the role of learner, advocate, and educator, nurses need to become of a constructive means of violence prevention and become involved in task forces, labor–management committees, and agreements obtained through collective bargaining. As health care reform, changing demographics, and health care pressures mount, nurses know that personal security is critical to best meet a person's health care needs and qualify to take the lead in violence prevention efforts (Worthington, 1993).

Communication is key in the event of violence in nursing. Nurses need to report immediately any suspected or actual violence tendencies or acts of any patient or colleague. They should also report any known violence in a patient's history. This reporting structure should occur among colleagues as well as to the manager, in confidence of course. This helps to increase the awareness of all nurses so that they may exercise caution when they are working with or around the patient/colleague. Sometimes, as in the case of an elderly patient who has dementia, many nurses consider it part of the patient's illness; however, it still needs to be reported and documented so that all other nursing colleagues will be aware of the patient's potential for volatility and aggression (Davidson, 2012).

Duong (2010) also suggests the following measures, particularly when nurses are taking care of an agitated patient. As a practice, some of these are what nurses are trained to do anyhow, but just for clarity, they include talking to the prehospital personnel; calling the patient's family, psychiatrist, or primary care provider to obtain more historical information; and listening to their gut instincts. If you feel endangered by the patient, leave immediately and make colleagues and staff aware of potential violence; consider a finger stick blood glucose, as their sugar may be creating some of these symptoms; look for signs of trauma, infection, and intoxication; and address agitated behavior and potential violence as soon as it is recognized.

Law authorities need to become involved in the case of a code white, a code that many hospitals use to alert that extreme danger and violence is occurring. As stated by Jim Hood (2001), attorney general of the state of Mississippi, a law enforcement officer needs to be involved in cases in which there are threats of violence against others or suicide; numerous conflicts with patients, coworkers, or supervisors with impending danger suspected; intimidating or harassing behavior; bringing weapons to the workplace; statements of approval of workplace violence; statements indicating extreme desperation over marital, family, or relationship difficulties; a fanatical fascination with knives, guns, explosives, or other weapons; an expressed hatred of government or other groups; extreme financial hardship; alcohol or drug abuse combined with other factors; and extreme changes in behavior.

The threat assessment is an important tool for detecting violence. If your organization does not have any protocol to follow for a threat assessment, then it needs to get one. A threat assessment is the process of determining the magnitude of a potentially violent or stressful situation and providing a means of intervention to diffuse the situation. Because of the uncertainty of whether a violent episode will take place, the organization should always treat threats in a serious manner and act as if the person is likely to carry out the threat (Hood, 2001). This process allows an informed judgment to be made as to whether the person articulating the threats is likely to carry out a violent act or homicide and whether the threat is immediate and the act is imminent. It also helps the employer decide how to effectively handle the situation so that violence does not occur (Hood, 2001). The threat assessment will help you analyze the exact nature and context of the threat or threatening behavior, the identified target (general or specific), the perpetrator's apparent motivation and intent to carry out the threat, the perpetrator's ability to carry out the threat, the appropriate intervention that will help the perpetrator and protect others, and the perpetrator's background, including work history, criminal record, mental health, history, military history, and past behavior on the job (FBI, 2000).

An environment assessment is also a must for nurses to be familiar with. Nurses should assess their work environment regularly, particularly when there is a violent patient on the unit, for any objects in the vicinity that can be potentially used as weapons. Assessing for such risks will help to reduce or eliminate potential injuries. An unpredictable patient can grab a television remote or any other small object nearby and use it as a blunt instrument against a staff member or fellow patient. These risks need to be foreseen as much as possible to avoid injury (Davidson, 2012).

The buddy system is also an important intervention nurses can use when violence is suspected. When a violent patient is identified on the unit, nurses are encouraged to visit and check on patients in pairs. This can be difficult, as many health care facilities may not have the staffing to accommodate pairings. However, any patient who has shown aggressive behavior needs to be visited or treated by more than one attendant in the interest of safety for all involved (Davidson, 2012).

When preparing to interview a patient who is suspected of or has a history of violence, always inform your colleagues about whom you are going to be with and where. When faced with an actual threat of violence directly, there are also many strategies you can implement to better protect yourself. First, if you are in a room alone with a patient and feel you are in danger at any point in time, leave the room immediately. Otherwise, make sure you are positioned in the room so you have an easy means to escape; you should be closest to the door. Also make sure that the exits are not obstructed and that you are able to get immediate assistance from the security staff. Although it is ideally the case that the patient may already be in a hospital gown preparing for an examination and away from any pockets that may hold weapons, this may not always be so. As part of the mental health assessment typically involves the investigation of possible harm, this question needs to be asked directly. Further, the speed of onset of symptoms and any preceding symptoms and behaviors; the patient's history of medical diseases, psychiatric diseases or violence, and recent trauma; the context of the agitated behavior; suicidal and homicidal ideation; and the presence of hallucinations and delusion should be assessed and are all important information to collect.

As a violent patient can often present as an agitated patient, it is a priority to identify and treat life-threatening diagnoses manifesting as agitated behavior. After assessing and securing respiratory and hemodynamic stability, the nurse's first steps are to obtain a more complete history and physical. Keep the focus on the patient's health and how you can help the patient. Obtaining pertinent collateral information from family, friends, witnesses, paramedics, and police is also critical.

Recognize the cycle of violence. Never get into a heated argument that may escalate aggression and violence with your patient. While there is a cycle of violence in which with each repetition of the cycle the abuse tends to become more severe (Samsel, 2013), this should not be something anticipated in a workplace setting, unless of course it occurs unreported and unknown to others between a nurse and another nurse, other colleagues, a patient, or a family/visitor. However, it is good information for nurses to know and detect if and once it occurs as a recognizable pattern. In the tension-building phase, there are minor incidents such as verbal and psychological abuse and even slapping where fear in the victim becomes established. Here, the victim tries to rationalize and minimize these actions or even deny them, avoids the aggressor, begins to withdraw, and even makes excuses for the aggressor. In the second-outburst phase, injury, death, or property damage occurs over a few minutes to 24 hours. The victim feels trapped and helpless, with a loss of control, and may or may not seek out help because of distrust of the authorities. In the final spent phase (or honeymoon phase), the perpetrator feels "spent" and begins to feel ironically closer to the victim, who remains cautious yet grateful for the promise of more self-control and the apology, although this apology is just giving the perpetrator the right "not" to make any substantial life changes; it is nothing more than a self-granted pardon. The victim is feeling almost empathetic and responsible for the perpetrator; a perceived closeness develops that is quickly followed by an irritating remark or argument to begin the cycle all over.

Role of the Nurse Leader

The nurse leader needs to become involved when there is a threat of violence or an impending or actual act of violence. Leaders can help implement many measures and checks so as to prevent or minimize the impact of violence. They need to be support persons, advocates, counselors, and educators for what they can do and say to help their nurses work through impending or actual violence or the aftermath. Davidson (2012) suggests that the nurse leader hold daily briefings or attend report turnover with staff nurses to discuss and highlight any high-risk, violent patients admitted to the unit/setting. Further, the nurse leader can help to ensure that no nurses who report concerns or incidents of workplace violence face reprisals. The U.S. Occupational Safety and Health Administration (OSHA) specifically includes this in its guidelines to prevent employees from being discouraged in any way from reporting concerns to management (Davidson, 2012).

Communication is also a valuable strategy for the nurse leader. The leader is the common denominator among all nurses regardless of the schedule they work, and the leader would be the one key person to ensure all are aware of and informed of any potential violence or actual occurrences. Further, the leader would most commonly be the medium through which senior management and the executive team are informed.

The leader should also, after learning of a potentially violent patient or colleague situation, take whatever measures are needed to closely monitor the situation. The nurse leader should support the buddy system of nurses pairing up to monitor and check on patients together when there has been a violent patient identified on the unit or in the facility. As many facilities may be lacking in staff numbers, aggressive patients need to be visited or treated by more than one nurse to ensure everyone's safety. In this sense, the nurse leader would advocate for sufficient resources. Further, the need to encourage nurses to report any knowledge or concerns they have of known histories and acts or potential acts of patients' violence. These nurses should receive no reprisal for following through on this. Although privacy of health information acts now flood the world, there is still a due diligence to be upheld where the safety of other patients and staff need to be considered. Situations like this now enter the legal–ethical world of health care. Finally, they need to keep an open forum for daily discussion or debriefing about any new patients with violent histories or tendencies. This forum helps to ensure a collaborative approach to maintain a safe and healthy workplace.

Verbal de-escalation is an important intervention for nurses to recognize and use if and when needed (Cowin et al., 2003; Nordstrom & Allen, 2013; Stevenson, 1991). The overarching theme in verbal de-escalation is to convey a professional concern for the well-being of the patient and regard for his or her respect. In general, speak to the agitated patient in a calm, empathetic, yet controlled voice and use a nonconfrontational approach (Nordstrom & Allen, 2013). Be mindful of your body language and avoid potentially threatening stances, such as crossing your arms or waving a finger. Give assurance that the patient will not be harmed. It is basically the talking down of the agitated person in such a manner as to not make the person more irritated, so that the threat of violence can be reduced or eliminated. You need to do your best to not participate in further escalating the nonsituation into a potentially violent situation. In many cases, not participating is all the de-escalation you will need. Remove yourself from the situation; if you actually wronged another human being, then apologize, but demanding or expecting an apology from someone else is not worth someone getting hurt. If you were wronged, then swallow your pride and move on, unless, of course, you were physically attacked and had to defend yourself. The two most ideal ways to de-escalate a situation are not yelling and not saying the first, second, and maybe even the third thing that come to mind. Clear, well-articulated, and direct communication is key to de-escalation. If possible and there is no immediate danger, evaluate the person's behavior before acting. Be sure to listen with empathy and try to understand where the person is coming from, so give the person your undivided attention, be nonjudgmental, focus on the person's feelings, not just the facts, allow silence, and use restatement to clarify messages. Further, develop a plan, use a team approach, use positive self-talk, and recognize your personal limits.

Role of the Organization

The entire process of identifying and addressing violence must be free from the threat of reprisal to the victim (NANB, 2002). Policies need to be developed to address workplace violence and need to be accompanied by training for nurses. There needs to be a clear process and procedure in place that can help to promote change, particularly when a colleague is the perpetrator. These policies further need to follow a zero-tolerance directive to be effective (Chao & Henshaw, 2003).

Policies and practices for workplace harassment and conflict resolution also need to be developed, if they aren't already. An organization's strategic plan needs to have a crisis management plan incorporated. This needs to be clear, concise, and in-depth in recognizing the hierarchy of reporting, any executive limitations needed, and the roles and responsibilities of individuals in addressing such crises as violence. Other actions organizations can engage in include conducting health/risk assessments to determine the possibility or prevalence of workplace violence or harassment; disclosing incidents of workplace violence and harassment to the health and safety committee; providing open, transparent, and acceptable ways for nurses to report instances or risks of workplace violence and harassment; disciplining employees for not following workplace violence and harassment policies or for committing workplace violence or harassment; providing and offering employee assistance program options so nurses can at least have a professional to confidentially talk to; ensuring that proper security measures are in place at the workplace to protect workers from members of the public or customers; and keeping detailed records of any workplace violence or harassment, investigation, or work refusal.

Employee tools and toolkits can also be developed to help an organization bring perspective and guidelines around workplace violence. For example, Australia had developed a Code of Practice: Violence, Aggression and Bullying at Work to provide direction on identifying and addressing violence (Government of Western Australia, 2010), and Canada has developed a workplace violence prevention guide (CCOHS, 2013).

It is incumbent on organizations through their responsibility and accountability frameworks to make sure policies and procedures are in place to address workplace violence. As many nursing theories have been borrowed from the discipline of sociology, so too can a theory relating to violence prevention. This theory is called the "Broken Windows Theory" (Wilson & Kelling, 1982). It can be used to help determine measures to prevent violence in the workplace, as it enforces a zero-tolerance approach to ensure that once acts or threatened acts of violence are identified they are addressed immediately. This sends the message that violence in the workplace will not be tolerated.

It is also the responsibility of the organization to adhere to and enforce any government legislation and statutes respecting actions of violence in the workplace. OSHA has done some of its job thus far in developing guidelines for preventing workplace violence for health care services. These guidelines include various policy recommendations as well as practical measures that can help address, prevent, and possibly reduce the incidence of workplace violence for health care providers (Gacki-Smith et al., 2009). However, there is just one major pitfall with these guidelines; they are voluntary, not mandatory. Therefore, any hospitals or health care organizations who do not wish to follow them don't have to. As a result, many of these health care organizations and hospitals are "not" required to even have any workplace violence programs, or if they do, they may not even be effective, as there is no monitoring or auditing or accreditation purposes. U.S. federal regulations are very much needed to provide direction to these health care organizations and hospitals. Health care organizations should embrace such guidelines to do what they possibly can to ensure safe and healthy workplaces for nurses at all times that are free from violence to any extent possible.

The installation of metal detectors is often not feasible for hospitals; safety resources could be better used for training hospital staff to calm down agitated guests and patients and improving security (Kelen et al., 2012). Further, hospitals need to convene a panel of experts after the violence incident to examine the series of events that unfolded, in which the detection of unusual behavior and de-escalation training of personnel is often useful.

Other organizational tactics that can be employed to prevent violence from occurring or escalating are practices of implementing pre-employment drug screening and background checks, a substance abuse policy, informed management, fair treatment of employees, counseling and employee assistance program services, appropriate levels of security, a threat assessment team, an industry/occupational risk assessment, and aftermath training/post-incident interventions (Employee Assistance Trade Association, 2013).

An organization also needs to support and provide for a debriefing session, particularly after a major incident occurs. Talking helps relieve stress and can initiate future planning steps for what could have been done better, what worked well, and how this response can be improved.

From an overarching government perspective, the FBI (2003) suggest that "clear, comprehensive, and uniform legal guidelines should be developed and widely distributed to inform employers how they can strengthen violence prevention measures within existing law, without infringing on due process, privacy, defamation laws, or other employee rights." They add that these "relevant laws and liability issues should be reviewed to see if there are ways to improve employee safety without jeopardizing individual rights. In particular, there should be a review of legal restrictions on exchanging information between employers or between law enforcement and private companies concerning past criminal convictions or violent behavior by an employee or job applicant."

LEGISLATION AND LEGAL LIABILITY

As mandated by many countries' occupational safety and health legislation, an organization is legally obligated to provide for its employees a safe and healthy workplace. Unfortunately, even organizations sensitive to potential violence-related problems in their workplace or with their employees are limited by a variety of legal issues in their ability to maintain a safe workplace. Potential liability under the law may increase an employer's difficulty in securing the workplace, but it also may increase an employer's responsibility to keep workers safe while they are at work. Legal consultation with the development and establishment of policies with regard to workplace violence is highly recommended (Employee Assistance Trade Association, 2013). Further, all licensed professionals, such as nurses, also have an ethical duty to report any known or suspected dangerous individuals so as to try to prevent acts of violence.

SUMMARY

The issue of violence is increasingly becoming a reality of the nursing profession. Nurses experience aggression and violence not only from their colleagues and other health care professionals but also from their patients, patients' families, and visitors. While many strategies exist that can help the nurse, the nurse leader, and the organization to prevent and address violence in the workplace, violence can still scar individual nurses for a long period of time and infringe on their good mental health. Its presence can also jeopardize the delivery of patient care and the organization's bottom line of safe, competent patient care; its mandate and values; and its profit margins in some cases. Hence, the experience and impact of violence for nurses has far-reaching effects; therefore, it is prudent for all involved to recognize and identify violence and strategically put into place actions, policies, and plans to address and decrease it.

DISCUSSION QUESTIONS

1. Why is violence in nursing a very serious issue to address in regard to how it impacts nurses' mental health?
2. What are some of the underlying theories and causes of violence?
3. How does the setting of nurses impact the prevalence of violence?
4. What are the various categories and forms of violence that occur?
5. Why is the nonreporting of violence a significant issue for nurse and patient safety?
6. What are some interventions that the nurse, nurse leader, and organization can implement to help prevent or reduce violence?
7. What are some of the various indicators that can help nurses identify potential or impending violence?
8. What are some of the adverse outcomes that can occur as a result of workplace violence in nursing that affect the nurse, the patient, and the organization?

REFERENCES

Abualrub, R. F., & Al Khawaldeh, A. T. (2013). Workplace physical violence among hospital nurses and physicians in underserved areas in Jordan. *Journal of Clinical Nursing, 12.* doi:10.1111/jocn.12473

Alberta Association of Registered Nurses.(2002). *New report confirms increasing shortage of registered nurses in Alberta* [media release]. Retrieved from http://www.nurses.ab.ca/newsrel/Ryten%20Report%20June%2002.html

American Psychiatric Association. (2013). *Diagnostic and statistical manual of mental disorders* (5th ed.). Retrieved from http://www.psych.org/practice/dsm

American Psychiatric Nurses Association.(2008). *Workplace violence: Position statement.* Retrieved from http://www.apna.org/files/public/APNA_Workplace_Violence_Position_Paper. pdf

Anonymous. (2012). *Nurse arrested for allegedly stealing from patient.* Retrieved from http://www.wwaytv3.com/2012/07/27/nurse-arrested-for-allegedly-stealing-from-patient

Arboleda-Florez, J. E., & Stuart, H. L. (2001). A public health perspective on violent offenses among persons with mental illness. *Psychiatric Services, 52,* 654–659.

Associated Press. (2012). *Nurse pleads no contest in Placerville nursing home death.* Retrieved from http://www.news10.net/news/article/215609/2/Nurse-pleads-no-contest-in-Placerville-nursing-home-death

Baltieri, D. A. (2014). Order of onset of drug use and criminal activities in a sample of drugabusing women convicted of violent crimes. *Drug and Alcohol Review, 1.* doi:10.1111/dar.12107

Barak, G. (2003). *Violence and nonviolence: Pathways to understanding.* Thousand Oaks, CA: Sage.

Barak, G. (2013). *Theories of violence.* Retrieved from http://www.greggbarak.com/custom3_2. html

Bennetto, J. (1998). *Police hunt doctor after nurse shot dead.* Retrieved from http://www.independent.co.uk/news/police-hunt-doctor-after-nurse-shot-dead-1160809.html

Bowers, L., Whittington, R., Almvik, R., Bergman, B., Oud, N., & Savio, M. (1999). A European perspective on psychiatric nursing and violent incidents: Management, education and service organisation. *International Journal of Nursing Studies, 36,* 217–222.

Bowman, D. (2012). *Your career is a business, so run it like one.* Retrieved from http://www.ttgconsultants.com/articles/careerbusiness.html

Boyd, N. (2014). *How Seligman's Learned Helplessness Theory applies to human depression and stress.* Retrieved from http://education-portal.com/academy/lesson/how-seligmanslearned-helplessness-theory-applies-to-human-depression-and-stress.html# lesson

Brennan, W. (2001). Dealing with verbal abuse. *Emergency Nurse, 9*(5), 15–17.

Cabayan, I. G. (2012). *Nurse shot dead by cop husband.* Retrieved from http://www.journal. com.ph/index.php/news/metro/31412-nurse-shot-dead-by-cop-husband

Campbell, J. C. (2001). A celebration of nursing research on violence. *Canadian Journal of Nursing Research, 32*(4), 3–10.

Canadian Centre for Occupational Health and Safety. (2012). *Violence in the workplace.* Retrieved from http://www.ccohs.ca/oshanswers/psychosocial/violence.html

Canadian Centre for Occupational Health and Safety. (2013). *Violence in the workplace prevention guide.* Retrieved from http://www.ccohs.ca/products/publications/violence.html

Canadian Medical Association. (2005). *Physician workforce executive summary 2001.* Retrieved from http://www.effectifsmedicaux.ca/reports/OccHRSummary-e.pdf

Canadian Mental Health Association. (2010). *Violence and mental illness fact sheet.* Retrieved from www.cmha.ca/bins/content_page.asp?cid=3-108&lang=1

Centers for Disease Control and Prevention. (1998). *Fatal occupational injuries—United States, 1980–1994.* Retrieved from http://www.cdc.gov/mmwr/preview/mmwrhtml/00052214.htm

Centers for Disease Control and Prevention. (2002). National Institute for Occupational Safety and Health. *Violence: Occupational hazards in hospitals.* Retrieved from http://www.cdc.gov/niosh/pdfs/2002-101.pdf

Chao, E. L., & Henshaw, J. L. (2003). *Guidelines for preventing workplace violence for health-care and social-service workers.* U. S. Department of Labor: Occupational Safety and Health Administration.

Chapman, R., & Styles, I. (2006). An epidemic of abuse and violence: Nurse on the front line. *Accident and Emergency Medicine, 14*(4), 245–249.

Clements, P. T., DeRanieri, J. T., Clark, K., Manno, M. S., & Wolick Kuhn, D. (2005). Workplace violence and corporate policy for health care settings. *Nursing Economics, 23*(3), 119–124.

Coleman, E., Chou, R., Bowens, D., & Heffernan, S. (2009). *Eight dead in Carthage nursing-home shooting.* Retrieved from http://www.wral.com/news/local/story/4837676

Cowin, L., Davies, R., Estall, G., Berlin, T., Fitzgerald, M., & Hoot, S. (2003). De-escalating aggression and violence in the mental health setting. *International Journal of Mental Health Nursing, 12*(1), 64–73.

Daily Mail Reporter. (2012). *Nurse who told relatives she was adopting baby 'gunned down new mother and ripped three-day-old son from her arms as she was leaving doctor's office.'* Retrieved from http://www.dailymail.co.uk/news/article-2131352/Verna-Deann-McClain-Nurse-shot-Kayla-Marie-Golden-ripped-baby-son-arms.html#ixzz2A8jqtzxy

Davidson, M. (2012). *Preventing workplace violence in nursing facilities.* Retrieved from http://www.ehow.com/how_6599732_preventing-workplace-violence-nursing-facilities.html#ixzz29a0 uERnz

Dean, J. (2012). *98-year-old patient sexually violated by San Diego home care nurses.* Retrieved from http://www.examiner.com/article/98-year-old-patient-sexually-violated-by-san-diego-home-care-nurses

Duffy, M., Scott, K., & O'Leary-Kelly, M. (2005). The radiating effects of intimate partner violence on occupational stress and well being. In P. Perrewé, J. Halbesleben, & C. Rosen (Eds.), *Research in occupational stress and well-being* (pp. 67–92). Bingley, UK: Emerald Group Publishing.

Duhart, D. T. (2001). *Violence in the workplace, 1993–99.* Retrieved from http://www.bjs.gov/content/pub/pdf/vw99.pdf

Duong, D. (2010). *The agitated patient.* Retrieved from http://www.cdemcurriculum.org/ssm/psych/agitated/agitated.php

Employee Assistance Trade Association. (2013). *Responding to workplace violence.* Retrieved from http://www.easna.org/2013/01/responding-to-workplace-violence

Federal Bureau of Investigation. (2003). *Workplace violence: Issues in response.* Retrieved from http://www.fbi.gov/stats-services/publications/workplace-violence

Fernandes, C., Bouthillette, F., Raboud, J., Bullock, L., Moore, C., Christenson, J., … Way, M. (1999). Violence in the emergency department: A survey of health care workers. *Canadian Medical Association Journal, 161*(10), 1245–1248.

Fernandes, C., Raboud, J., Christenson, J., Bouthillette, F., Bullock, L., Ouellet, L., & Moore, C. (2002). The effect of education program on violence in the emergency department. *Annals of Emergency Medicine, 39*(1), 47–55.

Fried, I. (1997). Syndrome E. *The Lancet, 350,* 1845–1847.

Gacki-Smith, J., Juarez, A. M., Boyett, L., Homeyer, C., Robinson, L., & MacLean, S. L. (2009). Violence against nurses working in US emergency departments. *Journal of Nursing Administration, 39*(7), 340–349. doi:10.1097/NNA.0b013e3181ae97db

Goodhand, A. (2012). *Nurse who aided dark knight shooting massacre victims mysteriously drowns on vacation.* Retrieved from http://radaronline.com/exclusives/2012/08/nurse-aided-dark-knight-shooting-victims-drowned-vacation-jennifer-galagher

Government of Western Australia. (2010). *Code of practice: Violence, aggression and bullying at work.* Retrieved from http://www.commerce.wa.gov.au/worksafe/PDF/Codes_of_Practice/Code_violence.pdf

Grenyer, B., Ilkiw-Lavalle, O., Biro, P., Middleby-Clements, J., Cominos, A., & Coleman, M. (2004). Safer at work: Development and evaluation of an aggression and violence minimization program. *Australian and New Zealand Journal of Psychiatry, 38,* 804–810.

Hale, R. (1994). The role of humiliation and embarrassment in serial murder. *Psychology: A Journal of Human Behavior, 31,* 17–23.

Hasketh, K. L., Duncan, S. M., Estabrooks, C. A., Reimer, M. A., Giovannetti, P., Hyndman, K., et al. (2003). Workplace violence in Alberta and British Columbia hospitals. *Health Policy, 63*(3), 311–321.

Holguin, J. (2002). *4 dead in University of Arizona shooting.* Retrieved from http://www.cbsnews.com/news/4-dead-in-univ-of-arizona-shooting

Hood, J. (2001). *Workplace violence prevention: A guide.* Retrieved from http://www.ago.state.ms.us/wp-content/uploads/2013/08/workplaceviolenceguide.pdf

International Council of Nurses. (2006). *Position statement: Abuse and violence against nursing personnel.* Retrieved from http://www.icn.ch/images/stories/documents/publications/position_statements/C01_Abuse_Violence_Nsg_Personnel.pdf

Jones, J., & Lyneham, J. (2000). Violence: Part of the job for Australian nurses? *Australian Journal of Advanced Nursing, 18*(2), 27–32.

Kelen, G. D., Catlett, C. L., Kubit, J. G., & Yu-Hsiang, H. (2012). *Hospital-based shootings in the United States: 2000 to 2011.* Presented, in part, at the annual meeting of the Society for Academic Emergency Medicine, May 2012, Chicago, IL.

Keough, V., Schlomer, R., & Bollenburg, B. (2003). Serendipitous findings from an Illinois ED nursing educational survey reflect a crisis in emergency nursing. *Journal of Emergency Nursing, 29*(1), 17–22.

Kocher, G. (2012a). *Man arrested in fatal shooting at nursing home.* Retrieved from http://www.knoxnews.com/news/2012/oct/16/man-arrested-in-fatal-shooting-at-nursing-home

Kocher, G. (2012b). *Second man charged in fatal shooting outside Lexington nursing home.* Retrieved from http://www.kentucky.com/2012/12/13/2442399/second-man-charged-in-fatal-shooting.html

Layden, D. R. (1999). *Law and culture: Workplace violence: Frontier justice on the job.* Retrieved from https://litigation-essentials.lexisnexis.com/webcd/app?action=DocumentDisplay&crawlid=1&doctype=cite&docid=23+Legal+Stud.+Forum+479&srctype=smi&srcid=3B15&key=f6334e3e7fc9903b865b7773ddfa0ee3

Lowry, K. (2000). Abuse unacceptable [letter to the editor]. *Canadian Nurse, 96,* 6.

Lyneham, J. (2000). Violence in New South Wales emergency departments. *Australian Journal of Advanced Nursing, 18*(2), 8–17.

MacEwan, D., & Dumpel, H. (2012). Workplace violence assessing occupational hazards and identifying strategies for prevention, part 1. *National Nurse, 108*(1), 18–27.

Mahoney, B. (1991). The extent, nature and response to victimization of emergency nurses in Pennsylvania. *Journal of Emergency Nursing, 17*(5), 382–394.

Manderino, M. A., & Berkey, N. (1997). Verbal abuse of staff nurses by physicians. *Journal of Professional Nursing, 13*(1), 48–55.

May, D. D., & Grubbs, L. M. (2002). The extent, nature, and precipitating factors of nurse assault among three groups of registered nurses in a regional medical center. *Journal of Emergency Nursing, 28*(1), 11–17.

McShane, S. L. (2001). *Canadian organizational behavior* (4th ed.). Toronto, ON: McGraw-Hill.

Mims, B., Charbonneau, M., & Bowens, D. (2008). *Marine charged in death of Army nurse wife.* Retrieved from http://www.wral.com/news/local/story/3200960

Monahan, J. (1996). *Mental illness and violent crime. National Institute of Justice research preview.* Retrieved from http://www.ncjrs.org

National Institute for Occupational Safety and Health. (2002). *Violence. Occupational hazards in hospitals.* Retrieved from http://www.cdc.gov/niosh/docs/2002-101

National Post. (2007). *Nurse warned doctor 'was going to go postal.'* Retrieved from http://www.canada.com/story.html?id=652aaeb6-638a-464a-bdbb-317c84b0fd79

Nolen, J. L. (2014). *Learned helplessness.* Retrieved from http://www.britannica.com/EBchecked/topic/1380861/learned-helplessness

Nordstrom, K., & Allen, M. H. (2013). Alternative delivery systems for agents to treat acute agitation: Progress to date. *Drugs, 73*(16), 1783–1792.

Nurses Association of New Brunswick. (2002). *Position statement: Violence in the workplace.* Retrieved from http://www.nanb.nb.ca/PDF/position-statements/VIOLENCE_IN_THE_WORKPLACE_E_2k8.pdf

O'Connor, T. (2013). Emergency nursing: Detecting family violence. *Nursing New Zealand, 19*(10), 39.

Pittman, G. (2012). *Hospital shootings uncommon, unpredictable.* Retrieved from http://in.reuters.com/article/2012/09/21/us-hospital-shootings-uncommon-unpredict-idINBRE88K15I20120921

Presley, D., & Robinson, G. (2002). Violence in the emergency department. *Nursing Clinics of North America, 37*(1), 161–169.

Prince, R. (2012). *Oakland school shooting: Former nursing student arrested.* Retrieved from http://www.telegraph.co.uk/news/worldnews/northamerica/usa/9182343/Oakland-school-shooting-former-nursing-student-arrested.html

Ricciardi, R. (2014). Violence prevention: A nursing issue. *Journal of Pediatric Health Care, 28*(1), 4. doi:10.1016/j.pedhc.2013.07.014

Rodgers, M., Hills, J., & Kristjanson, L. (2004). A Delphi study on research priorities for emergency nurses in Western Australia. *Journal of Emergency Nursing, 30*(2), 117–125.

Samsel, M. (2013). *Cycle of violence.* Retrieved from http://www.abuseandrelationships.org/Content/Basics/cycle_of_violence.html

SAPA. (2012). *Nurse shot dead at Eastern Cape clinic.* Retrieved from http://www.news24.com/SouthAfrica/News/Nurse-shot-dead-at-Eastern-Cape-clinic-20120810

Shields, M., & Wilkins, K. (2009). Factors related to on-the-job abuse of nurses by patients. *Health Reports, 20*(2). Retrieved from http://www.statcan.gc.ca/pub/82-003-x/2009002/article/10835-eng.pdf

Sobol, R. R. (2012). *Illinois nursing assistant charged with battery to a senior.* Retrieved from http://www.nhmonitor.com/2012/11/illinois-nursing-assistant-charged-with-battery-to-a-senior

Social Issues Research Center. (2012). *Alcohol and violence.* Retrieved from http://www.sirc.org/publik/alcohol_and_violence_4.html

Sofield, L., & Salmond, S. W. (2003). A focus on verbal abuse and intent to leave the organization. *Orthopedic Nursing, 22*(4), 274–283.

Speroni, K. G., Fitch, T., Dawson, E., Dugan, L., & Atherton, M. (2013). Incidence and cost of nurse workplace violence perpetrated by hospital patients or patient visitors. *Journal of Emergency Nursing.* pii: S0099-1767(13)00216-X. doi:10.1016/j.jen.2013.05.014

Stevenson, S. (1991). Heading off violence with verbal de-escalation. *Journal of Psychosocial Nursing and Mental Health Services, 29*(9), 6–10.

Sweet, V. (1991). Violence in the emergency department: California's response to tragedy … the death of Deborah Burke. *Journal of Emergency Nursing, 17*(5), 273–274.

Telegraph Media Group Limited. (2009). *Whistleblower nurse threatened with arson attack after highlighting NHS concerns.* Retrieved from http://www.telegraph.co.uk/news/uknews/law-and-order/6219018/Whistleblower-nurse-threatened-with-arson-attack-after-highlighting-NHS-concerns.html

The New Republic Liberia. (2012). *Liberia: Sick patient arrested at JFK for stealing from nurse.* Retrieved from http://allafrica.com/stories/201210310619.html

Tyrrell, M. (2000). The prevention of aggression and violence in the accident and emergency department. *Nursing Review* (Ireland), *18*(1), 14–18.

U.S. Department of Labor, Occupational Safety and Health Administration. (2004). *Guidelines for preventing workplace violence for health care & social service workers.* Retrieved from http://www.osha.gov/Publications/OSHA3148/osha3148.html#text1

Walsh, W. J., Isaacson, H. R., Rehman, F., & Hall, A. (1997). Elevated blood copper-zinc ratios in assaultive young males. *Physiology and Behavior, 62*(2), 327–329.

Ward, L. (2011). Mental health nursing and stress: Maintaining balance. *International Journal of Mental Health Nursing, 20*(2), 77–85. doi:10.1111/j.1447-0349.2010.00715.x

Warren, L. (2012). *'She was deathly scared he would kill her': Friends reveal fears of hospital receptionist 'gunned down by prominent surgeon lover now on the run.'* Retrieved from http://www.dailymail.co.uk/news/article-2159247/Timothy-Jorden-Jackie-Wisniewski-deathly-scared-surgeon-lover-kill-her.html#ixzz2snbaIVJi

Whittington, R., Shuttleworth, S., & Hill, L. (1996). Violence to staff in a general hospital setting. *Journal of Advanced Nursing, 24,* 326–333.

Wikipedia. (2012). *Fort Hood shooting.* Retrieved from http: //en.wikipedia.org/wiki/Fort_Hood_shooting

Wilson, J. Q., & Kelling, G. (1982). The police and neighbourhood safety: Broken windows. *The Atlantic Monthly, 249*(3), 29–38.

Worthington, K. A. (1993). Violence in the health care environment: Strategies for prevention. *Nursing Dynamics, 2*(3), 17–20.

WorkSafeBC. (2009). *Update: Workplace violence.* Retrieved from http://www.heu.org/sites/default/files/uploads/MemberResources/fs5-violence.pdf

9

Addictions

Addiction isn't about using drugs. It's about what the drug does to your life.
—*Enock Maregesi*

LEARNING OBJECTIVES

By the end of this chapter, the learner will be able to:

1. Discuss the risk factors for substance abuse and addiction.
2. Understand the physiology behind an addiction.
3. Identify why nurses are at an increased risk for the development of an addiction.
4. Understand the legal, ethical, and professional ramifications of being, working with, or leading a nurse who has an addiction.
5. Identify what a nurse leader and organization can and should do in response to knowing that a nurse has an addiction.
6. Discuss the dangers of the code of silence.
7. Highlight the adverse outcomes that can potentially occur when a nurse has an addiction.

The use of both drugs and alcohol is historically rooted in society (Breier-Mackie, 2007). In the many different cultures and various ethnicities, the use of drugs and alcohol has come to be accepted or rejected to varying degrees. For most of us, the use of drugs typically has been for therapeutic reasons—to alleviate pain and suffering, to stabilize various symptoms and illnesses, and to promote one's quality of life, survival, and longevity (Breier-Mackie, 2007). However, drugs and alcohol can also be used for nontherapeutic means. When they start to be used repeatedly to achieve feelings of euphoria and increased energy, then their use stretches into the boundaries of overuse, misuse, and abuse. Hence, an addiction is formed.

The overuse, misuse, or abuse of drugs and alcohol, as people differentially call it, is what is now termed an addiction (herein referred to often as a substance addiction). An addiction has been defined most thoroughly by the World Health Organization (WHO; 2014) as the "repeated use of a psychoactive substance or substances, to the extent that the user (referred to as an addict) is periodically or chronically intoxicated, shows a compulsion to take the preferred substance (or substances), has great difficulty in voluntarily ceasing or modifying substance use, and exhibits determination to obtain psychoactive substances by almost any means. Typically, tolerance is prominent and a withdrawal syndrome frequently occurs when substance use is interrupted. The life of the addict may be dominated by substance use to the virtual exclusion of all other activities and responsibilities." The *Diagnostic and Statistical Manual of Mental Disorders, Fifth Edition* (*DSM-5*, 2013) includes some more specific descriptors, such as significant impairment to daily function in which one of the following is present during a 12-month period: "(1) recurrent use resulting in a failure to fulfill major obligations at work, school, or home; (2) recurrent use in situations which are physically hazardous (e.g., driving while intoxicated); (3) legal problems resulting from recurrent use; or (4) continued use despite significant social or interpersonal problems caused by the substance use" (American Psychiatric Association, 2013). As health care professionals are often entrusted with our health, well-being, and life, these are the last individuals who would typically be expected to develop an addiction. However, they are at just as much risk, or more so, as anyone else when it comes to developing an addiction (U.S. Department of Justice, 2012). However, when nurses resort to using drugs, their behavior is often explained as a means of trying to cope; only this type of coping mechanism, of course, is a destructive one (Chen, Lin, Wang, & Hou, 2009; Violante, Benso, Gerbaudo, & Violante, 2009).

PREVALENCE RATES

Substance addictions are a significant health and societal concern in the United States, Canada, Australia, Europe, and many other regions today. As a subculture of the population of health care professionals, even though nurses are known as hardworking, compassionate caregivers (Oldenburg, 2012), they were found to have the highest prevalence rate of substance addictions of all health care professionals. These rates vary. The American Nurses Association (ANA) suggests that 1 in 10, or 10%, of all nurses (approximately 300,000 nurses in the United States) are suspected of having a drug addiction of some kind (Wisconsin Nurses Association, 2001). These rates reached as high as 15% to 16% (Heacock, 2012; Lippman, 1992; Oldenburg, 2012; Peck, 2009), 20% (Monroe & Kenaga, 2010; Virden, 1992), and even 32% when the use of marijuana, alcohol, cocaine, prescription drugs, and nicotine were included (Trinkoff & Storr, 1998). A further 6% to 8% of these nurses experienced interference with their work and impairment of their professional judgment (Burger, 2012; Daprix, 2003; Ponech, 2000). In fact, more than 90% of disciplinary hearings for all nurses in the state of Kentucky were related to drug and alcohol abuse (Alexander & O'Quinn-Larson, 1990). In spite of its prevalence rates, substance abuse among nurses remains underreported and underresearched (Monroe & Kenaga, 2010). Given that the prevalence rates are quite diverse, they are most likely much higher than reported here. Only those nurses who have extreme substance abuse problems and who are reported to the regulatory bodies for unsafe practices are recorded as reliable data (Breier-Mackie, 2007), but they would omit those from surveys and interviews and those not reported.

Subspecialty Impact

Interestingly, many have found that certain subspecialties of nursing have a higher addiction rate than others. While the risk for addiction is not limited to any one specialty, the specialties with the highest prevalence of substance abuse are intensive care unit (ICU), emergency room (ER), operating room (OR), and anesthesia (Heacock, 2012; RealityRN, 2008). Other findings suggest that ER nurses are 3.5 times as likely to use substances as general practice or pediatric nurses, oncology or administrative nurses are 2 times as likely to binge drink, and psychiatric nurses are 2.5 times more likely than general practice nurses to smoke (Trinkoff & Storr, 1998). Oldenburg (2012) adds that the nursing specialties of oncology, psychiatry, anesthesia, and critical care have higher levels of substance abusers because of intense emotional and physical demands. Further, high-achieving nurse academics with advanced degrees are also at increased risk because they have demanding jobs, they are respected by colleagues and loved by patients, and they hold themselves to high expectations (RealityRN, 2008).

HISTORY

Although "addictions amongst nurses have been recognized by professionals in the field for over 100 years" (Heise, 2003), they were largely disregarded in American society until the late 1970s, when the ANA began efforts to assist impaired nurses (Torkelson, Anderson, & McDaniel, 1996). Addiction has a long history in our profession, and ignoring this reality has perpetuated fear, anxiety, poor outcomes for the nurse, and risk for patients, as well problems for the profession as a whole. Providing early intervention and assistance is essential in helping colleagues and students recover from an addictive disorder, and providing a confidential, nonpunitive atmosphere of support may well be a life-saving first step for nurse and those in their care (Monroe & Kenaga, 2010). While Trossman (2003) suggested an addiction is not considered a disease but instead a moral failure or lack of will power, this could not be farther from the truth.

RISK FACTORS FOR ADDICTIONS

Addictions don't just happen for any unknown reason. The individual who experiences an addiction has been exposed in some way or another to a number of precipitating factors that make him or her more susceptible to developing an addiction. Generally, the precipitators of addictions include biological factors, such as genetics, age, and gender; physical factors, such as existing medical and mental illnesses and the nature of the substance consumed; and psychosocial factors, such as loneliness, peer pressure, and stress. In the context of nursing, these factors and many more specific to nursing have been identified to increase the risk with which nurses may develop an addiction.

Biological Factors

Genetics, for example, is one of the most frequently cited causes or risk factors for drug addiction (Irles, 2007). Alcoholics are 6 times more likely than nonalcoholics to have blood relatives who are alcohol-dependent. Numerous researchers have found that both alcohol (Irles, 2007) and drug addictions have a hereditary component. For example, a lack of endorphins in the body is thought to be hereditary in nature and increases one's predisposition to becoming addicted (Nordqvist, 2012).

Under the umbrella of genetics, some findings prove interesting. For example, as found by the Mayo Clinic (as cited in Nordqvist, 2012), males are twice as likely as females to develop substance addictions. In addition, with age as a variable, Nordqvist (2012) found that the earlier in life one begins consuming drugs or alcohol, the greater the risk that an addiction to those substances may develop. Further, stress hormones have been linked to alcoholism (Nordqvist, 2012), as have family histories of similar illnesses (Burger, 2012). As suggested by Monahan (2003), "A major underlying reason for substance abuse in health care professionals is related to family histories that include emotional impairment, alcoholism, drug use, and/ or emotional abuse that result in low self-esteem, overachievement, and overwork." Alcoholism in helping professions such as nursing is often associated with a higher incidence of alcoholism in the nurses' families of origin (Fisk & Devoto, 1990; RealityRN, 2008), with 80% of nurses having an alcoholic family member (Stammer, 1988).

Physical Factors

Various physical factors as well have been proved to have a relationship to the development of an addiction. These factors include such things as comorbidities (e.g., preexisting diseases, illnesses, or injury) and the type of substance consumed. Nurses involved in shift work may begin to abuse medications that induce sleep (RealityRN, 2008). For some, this may even be how an addiction begins.

The chemistry of the substance consumed is also a physical factor of concern in nurses who develop substance addictions (Nordqvist, 2012). First, the development of tolerance to the drug is what begins the addiction process. Over time and based on the degree of consumption, the individual requires increasing amounts of the drug to achieve the same effect. Second, the nature of the substance itself can be a significant precipitating physical factor. For example, what are termed more powerful substances, such as "crack," heroin, and cocaine, will cause an addiction much more quickly than, for example, alcohol would (Nordqvist, 2012). In today's society, in the presence of crystal meth, bath salts, and "ecstasy," it may only take one episode of drug consumption to spark an addiction.

Psychosocial Factors

Many different psychosocial factors can increase the susceptibility to becoming addicted to drugs or alcohol. From stress, loneliness, and peer pressure to family behavior and mental illness, all significantly impact the risk for an individual's developing an addiction because of either psychological or social factors.

Stress or one's response to it is believed by many to be perhaps the number one precipitating cause of why an addiction can develop. When stress levels are high, people often seek ways to cope and respond to them. Everyone has a need to reduce pain, including emotional pain, and to fill a void in life. It can be done with such things as relationships, work, hobbies, and recreation, but maladaptively, it can also be done with alcohol, drugs, Internet use, gambling, and other potentially addictive behaviors (Canadian Mental Health Association [CMHA] Ontario, 2013). The use of drugs or alcohol helps one forget about or black out a stressful hardship that has been endured. Unfortunately, responding to stress by using drugs or alcohol is not a healthy, acceptable, or productive way of dealing with stress.

Peer pressure, or pressure to conform to others' behaviors and expectations in an effort to be accepted, is another identified source of why addictions occur. Some of these behaviors and expectations can often take the form of using potentially addictive substances and ultimately developing an addiction (Nordqvist, 2012). For young people in particular, this is unfortunately a common occurrence.

Past parenting practices or the lack thereof is also cited for increasing one's predisposition to the development of an addiction. Compared with individuals who have strong family ties and who had a childhood conducive to optimal growth and development, individuals who do not have strong family ties to their parents, siblings, or others or those who were frequently abused, neglected, and degraded by their parents and other family members are a high-risk group for developing substance addictions (Nordqvist, 2012).

Psychologically, the presence of a mental illness can also increasingly predispose an individual to the development of a substance addiction (Nordqvist, 2012). People with mental disorders related to mood, personality, anxiety, or stress and people with attention deficit hyperactivity have a higher risk of developing substance addictions compared with individuals who do not have preexisting mental disorders.

Socially, feelings of loneliness can also increase one's risk for the development of a substance addiction (Nordqvist, 2012). As a coping mechanism, people seek refuge by using drugs or alcohol to avoid feelings of being lonely and isolated. As well, it serves as a medium through which individuals can fit in and be able to interact socially with others who have a common interest or lifestyle behavior.

No one can predict who will become an addict, but many nurses become addicts at the time in their lives when their children are teenagers and their parents are elderly, and, in women, when menopause strikes. Often, dependence occurs in adult life after 11 to 17 years of service, when an increased risk for physical injury and emotional pain and fatigue prompt the use of benzodiazepines or alcohol (RealityRN, 2008).

Environmental Factors

The mere nature of the chosen profession places nurses at an increased risk for substance addictions for many different reasons. For all intents and purposes, this significant category will be identified as environmentally related. The nurses' employment setting, as well as their identified roles and responsibilities, all contribute to an increased predisposition to becoming addicted to drugs. An addiction among nurses is a significant mental health issue identified in the literature and for many a daily struggle. For example, in one study, titled "Substance Abuse Among Nurses: Differences Between Specialties," it was found that nurses who work in emergency departments are most likely to use cocaine or marijuana, while oncology nurses have the greatest tendency to binge drink (Burger, 2012).

PHYSIOLOGY OF ADDICTION

To better understand the topic of substance abuse and addiction, knowing the physiology of an addiction is a must. The basic premise is involvement of the brain, which regulates the pleasure–reward mechanism. Using a drug and stimulating the brain to experience pleasure and reward lead to further and more frequent use of the drug to keep getting that pleasure and reward. This is a mechanism that can even alter the structure of the brain and its neurons. As suggested by the National Institute of Drug Abuse (2010), drugs tap into the brain's main communication system and impact how neurons send, receive, and process information. Drugs such as marijuana and heroin have a structure similar to the brain's neurotransmitters and actually mimic the actions of the neurotransmitters, fooling receptor synapses to lock onto and activate the neurons, only this time in a way that disrupts normal neuronal transmission. In addition, stimulants such as amphetamines and cocaine cause neurons to release abnormally large amounts of natural neurotransmitters, such as dopamine, that amplify transmission to disrupt neuronal messaging even more.

The pleasure component of drug abuse comes from the involvement of the brain's reward center, the limbic system, with dopamine, a main neurotransmitter responsible for each of movement, emotion, cognition, motivation, and feelings of pleasure. The overstimulation of this system is what produces such pleasurable responses and hence euphoric effects, prompting one to use drugs more and more. Through the long-term use of addictive drugs, the impact of dopamine becomes less and less, resulting in reduced pleasure and so the development of a flat affect, lifelessness, and even depression. To pull oneself out of this slump, one must then resort to using the drugs again, only this time higher and higher amounts of drugs are required to restore the dopamine levels to normal, a condition known by many as tolerance. Over the long term, both dopamine and glutamate, another neurotransmitter related to pleasure, alter the brain's chemistry and impair cognitive function; chronic exposure disrupts the brain's circuitry and inhibitory controls, leading to an addiction and the erosion of one's self-control and causing one to use whatever means possible to seek out and take drugs compulsively. As stated by one nurse, the "addiction biologically hijacks this brain system into a controlling, dominant, and vigorous force that prevails over reason and intellect" (RealityRN, 2008).

SIGNS AND SYMPTOMS OF ADDICTION

There are numerous signs and symptoms of addiction. The symptomology may even vary depending on the individual with the addiction, the substance the person is addicted to, and his or her personal circumstances and family history (Nordqvist, 2012). However, for the purposes of this discussion, the symptomology of addiction will be categorized as behavioral symptoms, physiological signs and symptoms, social ramifications, and financial consequences, all of which have common underlying threads.

Behavioral Symptoms

Behaviorally, what is observed is often what addicted individuals are doing or how they are acting in an effort to conceal their addiction. They may experience, or friends and family may witness, frequent occurrences of moodiness, bad temper, anger, bitterness, and resentment toward others, and they can even engage in acts of violence (Nordqvist, 2012). They have an overwhelming desire, focus, and energy to spend excessive amounts of time trying to figure out the means by which they get their substance and use it. These actions then typically drive them into secrecy and isolation. Further, these people typify high risk takers. They may resort to stealing, offering sex for money or drugs, and engaging in risky activities such as driving fast. They have difficulty coping and "need" their substance to do so. They are also in complete denial that an addiction exists, and they are either not aware or refuse to acknowledge that they have an addiction problem. Other noticeable occurrences may include a lack of interest in their previously loved and enjoyed activities and hobbies and problems with lawful authorities.

Perhaps unknown to others, addicted individuals will typically have powerful cravings (Nordqvist, 2012). They may wish to quit the addiction and probably have attempted to do so, but they find it personally challenging without some outside help. They may find that they have poor focus and feel depressed, empty, and frustrated (Nordqvist, 2012). They change jobs frequently, miss 2 or more days of work in a month, have resigned voluntarily from a job in the past year, have been terminated by an employer in the past year (Dunn, 2005), or have been involved in a workplace accident in the past year (Bush & Autry, 2002).

Physiological Signs and Symptoms

Many physiologically related signs and symptoms typify individuals who have an addiction. They typically present with dilated pupils, body trembling, seizures, hallucinations, body sweats, sleepiness or insomnia, marked nervousness, increased appetite, gastrointestinal upset, and they can even develop constipation or diarrhea (Monroe & Kenaga, 2010; Nordqvist, 2012). The addicted individual can also present with signs of other ongoing health illnesses, such as a sore throat, nasal soreness, a persistent cough, and even a persistent runny nose (Monroe & Kenaga, 2010) but still chooses to use the substance instead of attending to these other health concerns (Nordqvist, 2012). Rather than acknowledge that the body is trying to tell the individual that there is a problem, the addicted individual continues to engage in excessive consumption of the substance and may begin to experience blackouts and have difficulty remembering events (Nordqvist, 2012).

Social Ramifications

Many social ramifications become observable as well when someone develops a substance addiction. These individuals are more prone to relationship difficulties, experience challenges with maintaining previously enjoyed friendships and company, and are more apt to turn down invitations for social gatherings, functions, and outdoor activities (Nordqvist, 2012).

Financial Consequences

Difficulties with financial matters can also be a sign that someone is experiencing an addiction. However, in the absence of a significant spouse or relative, a matter such as this is often not visible to others until there comes the time when one's private property is repossessed by financial institutions or one sells assets to acquire more money to support the substance addiction. For example, in an effort to ensure that one's substance supply is met, the electricity bill goes unpaid for many months, resulting in the electricity being turned off, something that then becomes noticeable to friends and neighbors dropping by for a visit.

SIGNS AND SYMPTOMS OF ADDICTIONS SPECIFIC TO NURSING

In the practice and profession of nursing, there are many signs and symptoms that can occur and be observed. These arise specifically from the nature of the nursing profession and the relevance of its roles and responsibilities that provide the opportunity for addictions. Categorically, this symptomology can be identified as knowledge, behaviors, personal demeanour, work performance, documentation, and motivation. It should be noted, however, that "caution should be exercised if only one sign is observed; this may not necessarily indicate a problem with drugs and/or alcohol," as typically, "the observance of multiple symptoms, especially occurring over an extended period of time, may be indicative of impairment" (Roche, 2007).

There are two perspectives that help to characterize nurses with a possible addiction: first, the knowledge that they feel they have about medications and drugs in general, and second, the slippage in knowledge that they exhibit through demands, errors of judgment, behaviors, practices, and documentation errors, which can be a significant indicators of a possible addiction. Also, in terms of knowledge slippage, nurses experiencing addictions are often at risk for exhibiting judgment errors, unusual behaviors, documentation errors, and poor work practice. However, as Burger (2012) points out, the subtle signs of addiction usually appear long before the nurse starts making charting errors and other mistakes.

Behaviorally, nurses addicted to drugs tend to manifest very similar aberrant behaviors, such as the following: irritability; frequently leaving the unit (Burger, 2012; Monroe & Kenaga, 2010); work absenteeism in the form of absences without notification and an excessive number of sick days used (U.S. Department of Justice, 2012); frequent disappearances from the work site and unexplained long absences; making improbable excuses and taking frequent or long trips to the bathroom or to the stockroom where drugs are kept (U.S. Department of Justice, 2012); personality changes and mood swings (Alexander & O'Quinn-Larson, 1990; Monroe & Kenaga, 2010); and anxiety, depression, lack of impulse control, and suicidal thoughts or gestures (U.S. Department of Justice, 2012). Further behavioral issues include patient and staff complaints about the health care provider's changing attitude/behavior (U.S. Department of Justice, 2012); frequent trips to the bathroom; poor memory recall; rigidity and inability to change plans; incoherent or irrelevant statements; lack of cooperation with staff and deteriorating relationships (Monroe & Kenaga, 2010); and finally, the most evident, coming to work intoxicated and smelling of alcohol, blackouts, frequent hangovers, slurred speech, increased anxiety, unsteady gait, and excessive use of gum or breath mints (Monroe & Kenaga, 2010).

From the perspective of personal demeanor as well, signs of addiction become noticeable. For example, there is a progressive deterioration in personal appearance and hygiene (U.S. Department of Justice, 2012); the wearing of long sleeves when inappropriate (Monroe & Kenaga, 2010; U.S. Department of Justice, 2012); increased personal and professional isolation (Monroe & Kenaga, 2010; RealityRN, 2008; U.S. Department of Justice, 2012); and inappropriate prescriptions for large doses of narcotics (U.S. Department of Justice, 2012). Interpersonal relations with colleagues, staff, and patients suffer. Further, the nurse rarely admits errors or accepts blame for errors or oversights (U.S. Department of Justice, 2012) and often appears unkempt, with evidence of poor hygiene, physical abuse, and drowsiness at work (Monroe & Kenaga, 2010).

The work performance of a nurse also suffers because of an addiction. For example, the nurse may experience periods of confusion, memory loss, and difficulty concentrating or recalling details and instructions. Further, ordinary tasks require greater effort and consume more time (U.S. Department of Justice, 2012); the nurse is unreliable in keeping appointments and meeting deadlines (U.S. Department of Justice, 2012); there is a noticeable heavy "wastage" of drugs (U.S. Department of Justice, 2012), with broken vials of narcotics (Monroe & Kenaga, 2010); and the nurse insists on personally administering injected narcotics to patients (U.S. Department of Justice, 2012). Work performance alternates between periods of high and low productivity and suffers from mistakes made because of inattention, poor judgment, and bad decisions (U.S. Department of Justice, 2012). Excessive time is needed for record keeping, and assignments require more effort and time to complete. In addition, the following are characteristic behaviors: difficulty recalling and understanding instructions, difficulty in assigning priorities, lack of interest in work, absentmindedness and forgetfulness, alternating periods of high and low activity, increasing inability to meet schedules, missing deadlines, frequent requests for assistance, carelessness, overreaction to criticism, and tendency to blame others, with complaints received regarding poor care. (Monroe & Kenaga, 2010). Sloppy recordkeeping, suspect ledger entries, and drug shortages (U.S. Department of Justice, 2012), and an uncharacteristic deterioration of handwriting and charting (U.S. Department of Justice, 2012) can also occur.

In terms of the nurse's attendance, there are many signs to observe. These include excessive sick calls, repeated absences with a pattern, tardiness, frequent accidents on the job, frequent physical complaints, peculiar or improbable excuses for absences, frequent absences from the clinical area, frequent trips to the bathroom or locker room, long coffee or lunch breaks, early arrival or late departure, presence in the clinical area during scheduled time off, confusion about the work schedule, and requests for assignments in a less supervised setting (Monroe & Kenaga, 2010).

The diversion of medication becomes a significantly noticeable problem for the nurse with an addiction. For example, the nurse "signs out more controlled substances than other providers, frequently breaks or spills drugs, waits to be alone before obtaining a controlled substance for assigned cases, discrepancies between patients' charts and narcotic records, patient complaining of pain out of proportion to medication charted, frequent mediation errors, defensive when questioned about medication errors, frequent disappearance immediately after signed out narcotics, unwitnessed or excessive waste of controlled drugs, tampering with drug vials or containers, and use of infrequently used drugs" (Monroe & Kenaga, 2010). The nurse will also spend excessive amounts of time near a drug supply and often show up for work when not scheduled to be there (U.S. Department of Justice, 2012).

A nurse who may be experiencing a substance addiction is often the nurse who seems most motivated, hardworking, and eager to achieve goals and get the work done, particularly in times of staff shortages. The nurses who are stealing or abusing drugs are often the same nurses who volunteer for overtime (U.S. Department of Justice, 2012) and who arrive early or stay late (Oldenburg, 2012). It is this very workaholic personality that leads to other addictions as well (Heacock, 2012). Burger (2012) adds that working extra hours gives the nurses increased access to drugs. They are "supernurses" and typically take on extra patient care assignments and work overtime more than others. They seem to have increased energy, but no one complains because they are a great help to other, very busy nurses (Alexander & O'Quinn-Larson, 1990).

INCREASED PREDISPOSITION FOR NURSES

There are many reasons, and much discussion has been put forward, as to why nurses may be at an increased risk for developing a substance addiction. While much emphasis seems to be placed on workload, demands, and stress management, there are other contributing factors as well that place nurses at an increased risk for developing an addiction. Some of these factors relate to accessibility, exposure, and knowledge.

Nurses are known as hardworking, compassionate caregivers who strive to fulfill many demands of the job. However, the long hours, the emotional and physical stress of the job, and easy access to drugs create an environment ripe for substance abuse (Burger, 2012; Heacock, 2012). Drug abuse among health care professionals can cause personal harm and put patients at risk, and it can also lead to the loss of a license (Oldenburg, 2012). As health care professionals, we may be more likely to develop substance abuse problems than members of the general population because of a high level of work-related stress (Peck, 2009). Further, because their work is stressful as well as physically strenuous, nurses tend to sustain a lot of work-related injuries and often use drugs initially to ease their pain (Renata, 2013). Heacock (2012) suggests that because of the demand and stressful nature of nursing, "many nurses have fallen in the traps of substance abuse." Earlier, we identified some subspecialty areas of nursing in which the stress levels experienced by nurses are high—those being critical and acute care settings. Similarly, these very settings are the ones with an increased prevalence of nurse substance abuse (Heacock, 2012). Addiction in nurses occurs for a variety of reasons. However, the underlying issues always come back to the well-being of the nurse. Whether it is the stress from work, life, or personal health, nurses who become addicted are not all that different from nurses who suffer burnout, retire early, or simply move from clinical care to a less physically and emotionally stressful arena, such as management or research, on the assertion that "nurses with addiction actually become so to remain functional in work, they do so in quiet suffering, and in order to sustain themselves as useful functioning members of a caring profession" (RealityRN, 2008).

From an accessibility perspective, nurses have the most immediate access to the drug supplies used to treat patients. As health care professionals, we may be more likely to develop substance abuse problems than members of the general population because of increased access to controlled substances (Peck, 2009). Given the mere nature of the nurse's job, drugs are readily available (Renata, 2013). As highlighted by Oldenburg (2012), nurses work with drugs every day, and sometimes leftovers become part of a nurse's addiction. In her 2009 book, *Impaired: A Nurse's Story of Addiction and Recovery*, registered nurse Patricia Holloran wrote of being introduced to the painkiller nasal spray butorphanol when her doctor changed her migraine prescription. This was also the powerful drug she would inject into women in labor. When there were leftovers, she would take them to help her sleep after a long shift at work. She became addicted and recounts in the book her struggle with drugs and getting treatment. Further, even though the vast majority of practitioners registered with the Drug Enforcement Administration (DEA) comply with the controlled substances law and regulations in a responsible and law-abiding manner, you should be cognizant of the fact that drug-impaired health professionals are one source of controlled substances diversion. Many have easy access to controlled substance medications, and some will divert and abuse these drugs for reasons such as relief from stress, self-medication, or improvement of work performance and alertness (Burger, 2012; Heacock, 2012; U.S. Department of Justice, 2012).

Self-medication by nurses, sometimes called "pharmacological optimism," is done by those nurses who have an excessive faith in drugs (RealityRN, 2008). In our everyday working life as nurses we see firsthand the power of drugs, and how a patient's misery and anguish can be relieved. With our "Pavlovian" response in hand, we too "reach for a pill or a shot to relieve our own pain and suffering, so we rationalize that this is the right thing to do for ourselves." It is, after all, what we were taught, what we see, and what we do. Only this time, nurses don't have to go through great hoops to get the drugs as they are right there in front of them. In addition, the journey from the narcotic cupboard to the patient's bedside can be a long one, leaving much potential for gaps and opportunities for the nurse to pocket some of the drug or not deliver the drug at all to the patient as documented. As for benzodiazepines being a possible drug of choice, they are not considered narcotics and are therefore are not often not locked up so rigidly.

The knowledge derived from a nursing curriculum and the bonus of the clinical and practical experience thereafter obtained often create a false sense of knowledge that nurses know a lot more about drugs and addictions than they actually do. Nurses may think their knowledge of drugs enables them to be in control of the medication (Oldenburg, 2012). Therefore, as health care professionals, they may be more likely to develop substance abuse problems than members of the general population because of their knowledge of drug effects (Peck, 2009). As Patricia Holloran, a registered nurse fighting an addiction experience, states, "I thought having knowledge of addiction protected me from developing an addiction. I thought I was immune" (RealityRN, 2008). Nurses' altruistic natures and tendencies to care for others while neglecting themselves (Burger, 2012) are also factors that contribute to substance abuse in this profession. This is a phenomenon that leaves nurses to take care of others first and themselves last, thus leaving the addiction to "hide" personal needs (Heacock, 2012).

A nurse's susceptibility to being injured on the job (RealityRN, 2008) and perhaps the daily experience of witnessing trauma, death, and abuse can all cause mental distress to nurses. They are the front-line responders in times of crisis and need, and trauma contradicts what it is they set out to achieve. War veterans, although on a much more intense scale, often resort to using addictive substances to help them deal with trauma-induced posttraumatic stress disorder (PTSD; Addiction Search, 2013). Further, during and after the terrorist attacks on the World Trade Center and Pentagon on September 11th, 2001, rescue workers at the scene were significantly affected. This also speaks to the importance of secondary traumatic stress, or stress that occurs from the knowledge that a traumatic event happened to someone else (Addiction Search, 2013). Physical, sexual, and emotional forms of abuse also precipitate such tumultuous and traumatizing experiences.

For nurses with an addiction, criminal charges can also lie pending. In their attempts to obtain drugs to satisfy their addiction by any means necessary, nurses can be caught and charged with theft, which frequently occurs. For example, headlines reading "Nurse accused of stealing prescription drugs," "Rogue nurse attacks and steals from patients," "Nurse accused of trafficking prescription pills fired," "Nurse suspended for stealing and taking drugs while on the job," "Medication stolen from nursing home," and "Nurse accused of stealing meds at Manchester facility" are frequently cited.

NURSES' LEGAL, ETHICAL, AND PROFESSIONAL RESPONSIBILITIES

As a nurse, you have a legal, ethical, and professional responsibility to report any known incidences of drug use or abuse by your colleagues while in the workplace. You have a legal and ethical responsibility to uphold the law and to help protect society from drug abuse (U.S. Department of Justice, 2012). If you are aware that drugs are being stolen from the workplace, such as from patient medication supply cupboards, it has to be reported. "Drug abuse and drug dealing are serious problems that should be handled by qualified professionals. If you suspect that a drug deal is in progress, do not intervene on your own. Contact security or notify the police" (U.S. Department of Justice, 2012). According to the ANA, a nurse who is impaired by drugs while on the job is in violation of the code of ethics and can put patients at great risk (Renata, 2013). The ANA policy regarding impaired nurses is based firmly on the ethical principle stated in Provision 3 of its Code of Ethics for Nurses: "The nurse promotes, advocates for, and strives to protect the health, safety, and rights of the patient" (Breier-Mackie, 2007). Further, "the ethic of advocacy and protection must go beyond our patients and into the realm of advocating for and protecting ourselves and our colleagues as well" (Breier-Mackie, 2007). In response to the growing demand and concern about addicted nurses, in 2002 the ANA developed "The Profession's Response to the Problems of Addictions and Psychiatric Disorders in Nursing," which helps to identify "ways to help addicted nurses engage in recovery and salvage their careers" (Breier-Mackie, 2007).

DISCIPLINARY RECOMMENDATIONS

When a nurse has an addiction or is aware that a colleague has an addiction that involves work as a source of the drugs, or whose addiction is jeopardizing safe patient care, action is needed. Whether that action takes the form of a punishment or an alternate dispute resolution with a goal of rehabilitation, it has to be taken.

You have a personal responsibility to protect your practice from becoming an easy target for drug diversion. You must become aware of the potential situations in which drug diversion can occur and safeguards can be enacted to prevent this diversion (U.S. Department of Justice, 2012). If you are a nurse who suspects that a colleague is addicted to drugs or alcohol, Heacock (2012) indicates that you must act. You cannot just sit idly by and do nothing, as the consequences of not reporting the addicted nurse can be far worse than those of reporting the issue (Dunn, 2005). Keep in mind that any direct approach to the nurse will likely meet with resistance and denial, so it is best to report your suspicions to your nurse leader or manager. Being aware, the nurse leader is in the best position to help the nurse obtain treatment and rehabilitation and get on the road to recovery. Given that most organizations offer drug and alcohol treatment programs, this may be a very real possibility.

An employer would rather treat a nurse and get him or her back to work than be compelled to invest in and train a new nurse. Heacock (2012) adds that you should not feel guilty about reporting your suspicions because if you are indeed correct, you have helped a fellow nurse get his or her life back on track, have enhanced patient safety, and have promoted the positives of the nursing profession. As a licensed practicing professional, you owe it to your patients and the public to help protect them in any way, and reporting an impaired colleague is a critical step to take.

If you are a nurse and you have a strong suspicion that you may be addicted to drugs or alcohol, you have already taken the first step and have recognized it as a possibility. Heacock (2012) highlights that you need to ask for help because an addiction is an illness, not a moral failure, and the earlier you seek help, the better the rehabilitation and recovery you experience will be. There are many people out there who can help you, but you need to ask for or seek this help. Don't let your addiction get to the point at which you steal, cheat, or lie to get your fix of drugs. You will be much more respected for your early efforts to seek help. It is critical to remember that your license to practice as a nurse is your income, your source of living and survival that puts a roof over your head at night, so the protection of your license is a sure must. You don't want to lose everything you have worked so hard to achieve. For recovering nurses, you know where you have been and what you have experienced, so use this newfound energy and lesson in survival to be an advocate for others who are battling the same issue.

The incidence of disciplinary actions taken against nurses has increased dramatically in recent years (Breier-Mackie, 2007). Nurses should be encouraged to embrace the ethic of advocacy and to inform their employers of impaired colleagues without any fear of retribution. Whistle-blowing is intended to facilitate the disclosure of unprofessional conduct and is in the public's best interest, although many negative ideas are still associated with it (Breier-Mackie, 2007). The public and society depend on skilled, responsible, reliable, trustworthy, knowledgeable nurses to render their care (Breier-Mackie, 2007).

Professionally practicing nurses should follow this same ethic of advocacy for their patients and should therefore intervene in order to protect the safety of the patients who are at risk for harm by an impaired colleague (Breier-Mackie, 2007). "If a nurse believes a colleague may be so impaired, a first step might involve having an honest discussion with the supervisor or professor during which the nurse emphasizes a desire to protect patients while assisting a fellow professional who may well be struggling with a serious disease" (Monroe & Kenaga, 2010). You have a professional responsibility to prescribe and dispense controlled substances appropriately, guarding against abuse while ensuring that patients have medication available when they need it (U.S. Department of Justice, 2012). According to Peck (2009), "The bottom line is that an impaired colleague is a danger to both [him- or herself] and [his or her] patients and needs intervention. If you suspect that a coworker is impaired, you need to connect with someone who can investigate and assess the situation or refer you to resources to do so. This could be your employer, the state board, or a representative from a Professional Recovery Network (PRN) or Caduceus group." Further, if you are aware that a colleague is impaired, that person needs to be relieved from duty immediately. But in order to fully do the right thing, you should also make an effort to connect the person with the support, advocacy, treatment, and recovery resources available. It may be best to shield yourself by giving the PRN the required information and letting the program initiate contact. It is not necessary for the affected individual to know who made the referral. In the United States, for example, it is through the PRN programs that many health care professionals are able to regain licensure and return to work while in recovery and subjected to practice restrictions, such as not being allowed to work unsupervised and not being able to work more than a specified number of hours per week. According to the ANA, fellow nurses are expected to take necessary action if they believe a peer is drug-impaired, in order to protect the safety of the patient. The nurse is also expected to function as an advocate, connecting the peer with help for the substance abuse (Renata, 2013). Further, this individual should be reported to the appropriate board or college of nursing (National Council of State Boards of Nursing, 2004; New Zealand Nurses Organization, 2007, as cited in Monroe & Kenaga, 2010). The American Nurses Association recognizes that a nurse's duty of compassion and caring extends to themselves and their colleagues as well as to their patients. Nurses who are challenged with substance abuse problems not only pose a potential threat to those for whom they care; they have neglected above all to care for themselves. That is why the American Nurses Association has developed the Impaired Nurse Resource Center, an online repository of information aimed at helping suffering nurses get help (ANA, 2014).

Although it is not a legal obligation in all states, the ANA encourages an "alternative to discipline" approach to helping nurses with substance abuse problems. These are programs that assist the nurse in a program of rehabilitation, with the eventual goal of returning to work (Renata, 2013).

ROLE OF PROFESSIONAL ASSOCIATIONS

Currently, up to 2014, 37 American states have enacted programs to guide impaired nurses to treatment, monitor their return to work, and prevent their licenses from being revoked or suspended (Thomas & Siela, 2011). "Protecting the public from unsafe practices and workers is the primary duty of each regulatory board or agency of nursing" (Monroe & Kenaga, 2010). "The American Nurses Association is a strong supporter of alternative or peer assistance programs that monitor and support safe rehabilitation and the eventual return to the professional workforce. While relapse is high, the goals for the substance-abusing nurse are to seek treatment, reach recovery, and re-enter the workforce" (Thomas & Siela, 2011). "The nursing profession should mandate workplace advocacy and the promotion of well-being" (Monroe & Kenaga, 2010). "Boards of nursing are charged with regulating nursing practice and protecting the public, and when a nurse or student is impaired, they must take action to see that such individuals are not in a position to do harm to patients" (Monroe & Kenaga, 2010). File a complaint with your state board of nursing if you believe that a nurse has a substance abuse problem. However, coworkers should report their suspicion to the nurse's supervisor first (Burger, 2012).

You need to remember that people do recover from drug addictions. For nurses, the "mere fact that their supervisor talks to them about their poor work performance is enough to help them change." However, for others "the problem may be more severe and require more drastic measures. The threat of losing a job may have more influence on a drug abuser than a spouse's threat to leave or a friend's decision to end a relationship. Many drug abusers will seek help for their problem if they believe their job is at stake, even though they have ignored such pleas from other people important in their life" (U.S. Department of Justice, 2012).

Encourage your coworker or employee to seek drug treatment assistance. Treatment programs range from self-help to formal recovery programs. A number of state licensing boards, employee assistance programs, state diversion programs, and peer assistance organizations will refer individuals and their families to appropriate counseling and treatment services. These services will maintain the confidentiality of those seeking assistance to the greatest extent possible (U.S. Department of Justice, 2012). "Alternative programs monitor and support the recovering nurse for safe practice. Strong recovery programs offer a comprehensive, bio-behavioral, individualized treatment plan. The phases include in-treatment or outpatient detoxification in a safe environment; education about the disease; group, individual, and family therapy; and most important a relapse prevention program. However, boards of nursing have a responsibility to safeguard the public, so they may suspend the nursing license of an identified impaired nurse if they suspect he or she may pose a danger to patients" (Thomas & Siela, 2011).

WHAT LEADERS AND ORGANIZATIONS CAN DO

There are many things a leader and an organization can do to assist a nurse who has an addiction. Leaders and organizations can promote open communication by discussing substance abuse in every work or school orientation, encourage an atmosphere more amenable for reporting by ensuring confidentiality, provide information about the signs and symptoms of impairment, conduct mock interventions to help allay fears or feelings of discomfort about confronting a coworker or fellow student about suspected chemical dependence, invite addiction experts to speak to the hospital or school administration and staff, and be sure to participate in scholarly forums about addiction among health care providers (Monroe & Kenaga, 2010).

For the nurse leader, recognition of the nurse's need for treatment is an important first step (Monroe & Kenaga, 2010). As suggested by Monroe and Kenaga (2010), "Providing early intervention and assistance is essential in helping colleagues' and students' recovery from an addictive disorder, and providing a nonpunitive atmosphere of support may be lifesaving for nurses and those in their care." Many countries now offer confidential, nonpunitive support for such nurses.

Alternative to discipline (ATD) or alternate dispute resolution (ADR) is best to use. "It will motivate nurses to voluntarily seek assistance for their dependency and will help a colleague in finding the help they need" (Monroe & Kenaga, 2010). Developed in the United States in the early 1980s, the ATD program has proven more successful than punitive measures for impaired nurses for four key reasons. Outlined by Monroe, Pearson, and Kenaga (2008), they are quoted as follows:

1. Assistance to colleagues and peers by advocating for rehabilitation is better than punitive regulatory discipline. Disciplinary approaches do not advocate for nurses, recovery, or return to work.
2. Self-regulation as a hallmark of a profession is preferable to regulatory intervention and professional discipline. Regulatory discipline results in recovering nurses being reported to the Office of the Inspector General, which insurance companies monitor, resulting in a nurse's exclusion from eligibility for liability or health insurance (Monroe et al., 2008).
3. Public health and welfare should be protected by preventing below-standard nursing practice. ATD programs have been shown to remove impaired nurses from practice within days to a few weeks (Monroe et al., 2008), while disciplinary approaches may take up to 3 years (Sullivan, Bissell, & Leffler, 1990).
4. Policy and action that promote safety and well-being in the workplace should be pursued through collective bargaining and workplace advocacy. Nurses suffering from addiction and who are willing and able to be rehabilitated should be treated with confidentiality and respect (Roche, 2007; Monroe, 2009) as they embrace this step forward in getting their lives back on track.

While many states in the United States have implemented ATD programs to assist impaired nurses (Monroe et al., 2008), there were no formal peer assistance programs for nurses in England (Boyjoonauth, 2003), Canada (Quinlan, 2003), or Australia (Bachman & Cusack, 2003). "Confidential programs, either wholly or in part, are now operating in Australia, New Zealand, and Canada" (Monroe & Kenaga, 2010). Such a program has been met with much success and a 75% decrease in the overall problem burden, which may help a nurse succeed in treatment and resist relapse (Geiger & Smith, 2003), helps to move nurses into treatment instead of facing punitive measures (Quinlan, 2003; National Council of State Boards of Nursing, 2004), helps to retain nurses when a shortage already exists (Haack & Yocom, 2002), and helps nurses return to work (Smith & Hughes, 1996). ATD programs help to "protect the public while advocating for nurses, which translates into better clinical care for clients, more support for nurses, and better outcomes for institutions" (Monroe & Kenaga, 2010).

In essence, as a nurse leader, it is your responsibility to follow a strategy or structured program. The following 10-step strategy for addressing addictions is just one example that requires you, the leader, to (1) understand substance abuse and addiction; (2) assess your workplace risks; (3) develop a wellness and substance-free workplace committee; (4) develop a substance-free workplace policy; (5) train other management; (6) educate your nurses; (7) respond to crisis; (8) help nurses get assistance; (9) get involved in the affected nurse's return to work; and (10) be sure to follow up with the affected nurse (Great-West Life Centre for Mental Health in the Workplace, 2013). Ensuring that managers and teams are supportive can be a key factor to finding success. Nurses need a supportive manager who will say, "We need your skills, we need you here, so tell me what you need from us." This makes a big difference. Organizations can also help employees build their self-esteem, confidence, and loyalty to the organization when they make employees feel valuable and valued.

Policy development is another critical step to take. "Poor or ineffective policies that mandate punitive action endanger the public by making it difficult for impaired nurses to seek help" (Monroe & Kenaga, 2010). So policies need to be clear, nonpunitive, and supportive for the nurse who faces disciplinary action for a drug addiction. These policies need to be very detailed (i.e., use of illicit drugs at work, alcohol consumption at work, inappropriate Internet use, etc.), and all employees must be made to be aware of them. Policies will provide a platform for managers and employers to talk to employees about their substance use. These policies let employees know that breaching the rules while at work can put their job security at risk (CMHA Ontario, 2013).

The use of random drug screens is also an option. However, this remains a hot topic of debate because the right of independent and autonomous nursing practice and the right of patients to know about a nurse's addiction and receive safe, quality care intersect. The theory behind random drug screens is that early detection and deterrents can significantly reduce the impact of the addiction. However, in the event that the organization has reasonable and just cause to believe a nurse is practicing under the influence, it can proceed to order and complete a urine drug screen. The purpose of the drug screen is twofold: to "safeguard the quality of patient care and to provide guidance and support for the nurse to obtain appropriate treatment and regain health" (Weber, 2011). Further, the privacy of the nurse would be maintained.

Nursing schools, as well as other health discipline schools and faculties, cover very little in their curriculum about dealing with occupational issues such as the development of an addiction (Maher-Brisen, 2007; Monroe, 2009; Peck, 2009). Therefore, those entering the professional practice of nursing are often not informed about such an issue. Further, nursing schools rarely develop and implement policies for nursing students at a very key starting point, entry into their lifelong career (Monroe et al., 2008). While addiction is a topic often covered under the umbrella of psychiatric and mental health nursing, the focus is on the patient and what you as a learning nurse can do for a patient who has a substance abuse problem. While aspiring nursing students can learn a great deal about addictions, interventions, and treatments from such a course and can incorporate this knowledge into their own lives and work, they would perhaps not often expect to see such an issue affect one of their colleagues, who can be held in high esteem with respect, collegiality, admiration, and competence. As an aside, Peck (2009) suggests that the course offered by the University of Utah School on Alcoholism and Other Drug Dependencies, now in its 58th year, helps students and professionals understand and cope with substance abuse. It can be viewed at http://uuhsc.utah.edu/uas.

ADVERSE OUTCOMES

The abuse of substances by nurses is most unfortunate, yet it continues to occur among many, regardless of the patient care delivery setting. Drug abuse among nurses is a dangerous and no-win situation for anyone, inclusive of the nurse with the addiction. Nurses who have substance addictions endanger not only their own well-being but also the health and safety of their patients (Breier-Mackie, 2007; Dunn, 2005; Monroe & Kenaga, 2010), for whom there is an increased risk for mistreatment, including incorrect care, errors in medication, and even death (Oldenburg, 2012). "Substance addictions can destabilize a nurse's physical, psychological, social, and professional performance" (Breier-Mackie, 2007).

Nurses can face serious professional consequences, including losing their licenses and jobs (Dunn, 2005; Monroe & Kenaga, 2010; Oldenburg, 2012) because the abuse of substances can alter their behavior, actions, clinical judgment, response times, cognitive thought processes, and even memory (Breier-Mackie, 2007).

For the nurse's family, friends, and colleagues, there are many short- and long-term emotional costs involved (Oldenburg, 2012), and these are just as important a part of the nurse's life and support system as is work.

From an organizational perspective, a nurse with an addiction is a concern. There is an increased risk of liability for unsatisfactory patient care, for which the organization is responsible, and there is also the threat of a damaged reputation (Dunn, 2005). For the profession, as well, there is a reputation to uphold, and a nurse with an addiction is viewed as anything but professional when a threat to the public exists (Dunn, 2005; Monroe & Kenaga, 2010).

The nurse's job may be terminated. However, employees struggling with substance use problems cannot simply be pushed out of the workplace; alcoholism, for example, is recognized under employment law as a disability, so employers cannot terminate an employee suffering from alcoholism without first trying to help (CMHA Ontario, 2013).

TREATMENT OF NURSES WITH ADDICTIONS

Treatment programs are necessary, not only for the sake of the health professional but also for the sake of the people whom these nurses have helped and have the potential to assist in the future (Addiction Search, 2013). "Organizations need to respond to the person, not the addiction, because addiction is often a mask that people in pain use to cope and disguise their mental health issues" (CMHA Ontario, 2013).

Further, they should look out for warning signs that indicate an employee may be struggling with substance abuse. Because nurses violate personal and professional codes of ethics when taking drugs, they may feel increased shame when their addictions come to light, such as is seen in the code of silence alluded to previously. Addicted nurses should enter an intervention program, not only for their health but also to save their jobs. By entering an intervention program, they commit to rehabilitation therapy, drug testing, and structured programs. A number of health care organizations offer such programs through their employee assistance programs (Oldenburg, 2012). Although recovery can be a lifelong process, when nurses find and embrace recovery, the denial will break and the healing will begin, so that they now have choices they can make instead of being driven by their addiction. These nurses, who once felt they were in a dark corner shrouded by their addiction, will become free and take responsibility for recovering (RealityRN, 2008). In the event that treatment is unsuccessful, the individual's nursing license can be permanently revoked. Severe cases can result in charges of malpractice (Burger, 2012).

THE CODE OF SILENCE

Substance abuse in nursing continues to be a taboo issue among many health care providers and nursing school faculty (Monroe & Kenaga, 2010). "Fear of punishment from the board of nursing or termination of employment keeps many nurses and those who would report them silent" (Maher-Brisen, 2007). The odds of a nurse not reporting an impaired colleague were 5 to 1 (odds ratio, 4.53; Beckstand, 2005). "This is alarming given the critical duties nurses perform for patients every day" (Monroe & Kenaga, 2010).

While the code of silence typically refers to how colleagues deal with knowing a nurse has a substance addiction, there is also a similar silence regarding how the addicted nurse deals with the matter. The stigma associated with a mental illness, the embarrassment, and the fear of disciplinary action and possible charges and other retributions for the nurse are identified in the literature and explain why nurses often do not come forward to seek help with their drug addiction. Everything they have ever worked for and their livelihood may potentially be on the line for them, so they would obviously be very apprehensive about coming forward to admit that they have compromised patient care and safety, breached their standards of practice and legislative obligations, and engaged in criminal activity—all to feed and hide their addiction to drugs. Additionally, most health professionals are smart people who are relatively good at hiding their problems (Peck, 2009).

The fear and shame a nurse experiences when confronted are strong, sometimes even causing the nurse to contemplate suicide (RealityRN, 2008). Those of us who do become addicted may be shielded from discovery by the trust of our patients and coworkers (Peck, 2009). Plus, we may work very hard to avoid discovery, fearing harsh professional, social, financial, and legal consequences (Dunn, 2005; Peck, 2009). It is important to remember that "the attitude held toward addiction interferes with the very spirit of nursing" (RealityRN, 2008). In addition, to the detriment of morale and patient safety, many employers or coworkers end up being "enablers" of health care practitioners whose professional competence has been impaired by drug abuse because they are given lighter work schedules, and excuses are made for their poor job performance. Excessive absences from the work site are often over-looked, so drug-impaired coworkers are protected from the consequences of their behavior, further enabling them to rationalize their addictive behavior or continue their denial that a problem even exists (U.S. Department of Justice, 2012).

Impaired nurses rarely speak up to admit they have an addiction problem (Breier-Mackie, 2007). As a result, many impaired nurses continue to practice (Clark, 2003). Other reasons for enforcing the code of silence for addictions in nurses include denial (RealityRN, 2008), rationalization that what they are doing is within their total control (RealityRN, 2008), established friendships, work history, loyalty, fear of confrontation, fear of jeopardizing a colleague's license to practice (Breier-Mackie, 2007; Dunn, 2005; Monroe & Kenaga, 2010; U.S. Department of Justice, 2012), fear of getting into trouble for not reporting the problem sooner (Monroe & Kenaga, 2010), and fear of retribution (U.S. Department of Justice, 2012). Further, "whistle-blowers continue to suffer from the myth of being vindictive 'informers' whenever they challenge the prevailing institutional and regulatory culture of secrecy and self-protection" (Breier-Mackie, 2007).

A nurse's failure to report an addicted colleague only exacerbates the problem for that colleague, as well as the facility and the patient on the receiving end of care (Breier-Mackie, 2007). Breier-Mackie (2007) state that "secrecy and self-protection have no place in the profession of nursing" and that nurses need to adhere to their responsibility of "duty to inform" and the "ethic to advocate" for patients when they suspect that a colleague may be impaired. You as a colleague need to become involved because in doing so you help someone who may be doing something illegal, and more importantly, your action can protect the safety and welfare of your addicted employee or coworker and those patients or members of the public who may come in contact with him or her (U.S. Department of Justice, 2012).

SUMMARY

Addictions in nursing are a significant issue, and the prevalence level of addiction is of much concern. As in any citizen of society, an addiction can develop in a nurse for a number of reasons: personal and professional stressors, genetics, and failed coping mechanisms. However, the nature of nursing and its environment, which offers easy accessibility to the very source of addictions, make addictions in nurses a unique concern. The substance-abusing nurse has many different levels of professional responsibility; the nurse is responsible and accountable to maintain an astute level of professionalism guided by adherence to the standards of nursing practice, and the nurse's colleagues, leader, and even the organization have roles to play as well. Given that an addicted nurse can jeopardize patient safety and care, as well as impact the nurse, the nurse's family and friends, the nursing profession, and the organization as a whole, the long-maintained code of silence is not an acceptable practice. As organizations and the nursing profession more readily accept that non-punitive measures focusing on rehabilitation are the best approach, more success should be anticipated in getting nurses on the road to recovery and diminishing risks to patient safety.

DISCUSSION QUESTIONS

1. From personal and professional perspectives, why does drug addiction in a nurse need to addressed?
2. What are some of the precipitating factors that can predispose nurses to the development of an addiction?
3. Discuss the code of silence and highlight why its presence can be dangerous.
4. What are some interventions the organization and the nursing leader or manager can and should provide to the nurse with an addiction?

REFERENCES

Addiction Search. (2013). *Substance abuse among healthcare professionals.* Retrieved from http://www.addictionsearch.com/treatment_articles/article/substance-abuse-among-health-care-professionals_49.html

Alexander, D., & O'Quinn-Larson, J. (1990). When nurses are addicted to drugs. Confronting an impaired co-worker. *Nursing, 20*(8), 54–58.

American Nurses Association. (2014). *Impaired nurse resource center.* Retrieved from http://www.nursingworld.org/MainMenuCategories/WorkplaceSafety/Healthy-Work-Environment/Work-Environment/ImpairedNurse

American Psychiatric Association. (2013). *Diagnostic and statistical manual of mental disorders* (5th ed.). Retrieved from http://www.psych.org/practice/dsm

Bachman, J., & Cusack, L. (2003). International perspectives: Australia. *Journal of Addictions Nursing, 14,* 157–158.

Beckstand, J. S. (2005). Reporting peer wrongdoing in the healthcare profession: The role of incompetence and substance abuse information. *International Journal of Nursing Studies, 42,* 325–331.

Boyjoonauth, R. (2003). International perspectives: United Kingdom. *Journal of Addictions Nursing, 14,* 157–158.

Breier-Mackie, S. (2007). Impaired nurses in the workplace. *Gastroenterology Nursing, 30*(3), 227–228.

Burger, J. (2012). *Substance abuse in the nursing profession.* Retrieved from http://www.ehow.com/facts_6752115_substance-abuse-nursing-profession.html#ixzz261Pw7TFe

Bush, D. M., & Autry, J. H. (2002). Substance abuse in the workplace: Epidemiology, effects, and industry response. *Occupational Medicine, 17,* 13–25.

Canadian Mental Health Association Ontario. (2013). *Substance use, misuse and abuse at work.* Retrieved from http://wmhp.cmhaontario.ca/workplace-mental-health-core-concepts-issues/issues-in-the-workplace-that-affect-employee-mental-health/substance-use-misuse-and-abuse-at-work

Chen, C. K., Lin, C., Wang, S. H., & Hou, T. H. (2009). A study of job stress, stress coping strategies, and job satisfaction for nurses working in middle-level hospital operating rooms. *Journal of Nursing Research, 17*(3), 199–211.

Clark, C. (2003). *A descriptive study of the impaired nurse in Idaho.* Retrieved from http://familystudies.boisestate.edu/pdf/Clark1.pdf

Daprix, J. (2003, September). The courage to care: Intervening with colleagues who demonstrate signs of impairment, *The Florida Nurse, 51,* 28.

Dunn, D. (2005). Home study program. Substance abuse among nurses—defining the issue. American operating room nurses. *Journal of Peri-Operative Registered Nurses, 82*(4), 573–596.

Fisk, N. B., & Devoto, D. A. (1990, December). The nurse employee who uses alcohol/other drugs. *Nurse Managers Bookshelf, 2,* 110–129.

Geiger, J., & Smith, L. (2003). Nurses in recovery: The burden of life problems and confidence to resist relapse. *Journal of Addictions Nursing, 14,* 133–137.

Great-West Life Centre for Mental Health in the Workplace. (2013). *Workplace strategies for mental health.* Retrieved from http://www.gwlcentreformentalhealth.com/english/display.asp?l1=7&l2=101&l3=102&l4=107&d =107

Haack, M., & Yocom, C. (2002). State policies and nurses with substance use disorders (profession and society). *Journal of Nursing Scholarship, 34,* 89–94.

Heacock, S. (2012). *Nurses and substance abuse.* Retrieved from http://www.nursetogether.com/DesktopModules/EngagePublish/printerfriendly.aspx?itemId=1515&PortalId=0&TabId=390

Heise, B. (2003). The historical context of addiction in the nursing profession. *Journal of Addictions Nursing, 14,* 117–124.

Irles, J. R. (2007). *Alcohol abuse is hereditary.* Retrieved from http://www.medicalnewstoday.com/releases/75738.php

Lippman, H. (1992). Addicted nurses: Tolerated, tormented or treated? *Registered Nurse, 55*(4), 36–41.

Maher-Brisen, P. (2007). Addiction an occupational health hazard in nursing. *American Journal of Nursing, 107,* 78–79.

Monahan, G. (2003, September–November). Drug use/misuse among health professionals. *Substance Use and Misuse, 38,* 1877–1881.

Monroe, T. (2009). Addressing substance abuse among nursing students: Development of a prototype alternative-to-dismissal policy. *Journal of Nursing Education, 49,* 272–278.

Monroe, T., & Kenaga, H. (2010). Don't ask don't tell: Substance abuse and addiction among nurses. *Journal of Clinical Nursing, 20,* 504–509. doi:10.1111/j.1365-2702.2010.03518.x

Monroe, T., Pearson, F., & Kenaga, H. (2008). Procedures for handling cases of substance abuse among nurses: A comparison of disciplinary and alternative programs. *Journal of Addictions Nursing, 19,* 156–161.

National Council of State Boards of Nursing. (2004). *Model nursing act and rules.* Retrieved from http://www.ncsbn.org

National Institute of Drug Abuse. (2010). *Drugs, brains, and behavior: The science of addiction.* Retrieved from http://www.drugabuse.gov/publications/drugs-brains-behavior-science-addiction/drugs-brain

Nordqvist, C. (2012). *What are the risk factors for addiction?* Retrieved from http://www.medicalnewstoday.com/info/addiction/risks-of-addiction.php

Oldenburg, A. (2012). *Nurses & drug addiction.* Retrieved from http://www.ehow.com/about_6393337_nurses-drug-addiction.html

Peck, A. (2009). *Substance abuse in the healthcare professions.* Retrieved from http://studentdoctor.net/2009/08/substance-abuse-in-the-healthcare-professions

Ponech, S. (2000, May). Telltale signs. *Nursing Management, 31,* 32–37.

Quinlan, D. S. (2003). Guest editorial: Impaired practice: Making progress towards advocacy. *Journal of Addictions Nursing, 14,* 115–116.

RealityRN. (2008). *How a nurse becomes an addict.* Retrieved from http://www.realityrn.com/more-articles/handling-stress/how-a-nurse-becomes-an-addict/296

Renata, R. (2013). *Nursing standards for drug abuse in nurses.* Retrieved from http://www.ehow.com/facts_7355000_nursing-standards-drug-abuse-nurses.html#ixzz261QLFvyw

Roche, B. (2007). *Substance abuse policies for anesthesia.* Winston-Salem, NC: All Anesthesia.

Sloan, A., & Vernarec, E. (2001). Impaired nurse: Reclaiming careers. *Registered Nurse, 64*(2), 58–62.

Smith, L., & Hughes, T. (1996). Re-entry: When a chemically dependent colleague returns to work. *American Journal of Nursing, 96,* 32–37.

Stammer, M. E. (1988, March). Understanding alcoholism and drug dependency in nurses. *Quality Review Bulletin, 14,* 75–80.

Sullivan, E., Bissell, L., & Leffler, D. (1990). Drug use and disciplinary actions among 300 nurses. *The International Journal of the Addictions, 25,* 375–391.

Thomas, C. M., & Siela, D. (2011). The impaired nurse: Would you know what to do if you suspected substance abuse? *American Nurse Today, 6*(8). Retrieved from http://www.americannursetoday.com/article.aspx?id=8114&fid=8078

Torkelson, D. J., Anderson, R. A., & McDaniel, R. E. (1996). Interventions in response to chemically dependent nurses: Effect of context and interpretation. *Research in Nursing and Health, 19,* 153–162.

Trinkoff, A. M., & Storr, C. L. (1998). Substance use among nurses: Differences between specialties. *American Journal of Public Health, 88,* 581–585.

Trossman, S. (2003, September). Nurses' addictions: Finding alternatives to discipline. *American Journal of Nursing, 103,* 27–28.

U.S. Department of Justice. (2012). *Drug addiction in healthcare professions.* Retrieved from http://www.deadiversion.usdoj.gov/pubs/brochures/drug_hc.htm

Violante, S., Benso, P. G., Gerbaudo, L., & Violante, B. (2009). Correlation between job satisfaction and stress factors, burn-out and psychosocial well-being among nurses working in different healthcare settings. *Giornale Italiano di Medicina del Lavoro ed Egonomia, 31*(1 Suppl. A), A36–A44.

Virden, J. (1992). Impaired nursing: The role of the nurse manager. *Paediatric Nursing, 18,* 137–141.

Weber, L. (2011). *The ethics of drug testing for medical professionals.* Retrieved from http://drug.addictionblog.org/the-ethics-of-drug-testing-medical-professionals

Wisconsin Nurses Association. (2001). The impaired nurse: How can we help? *Statistical Bulletin, 70*(2), 2–3.

World Health Organization. (2014). *Lexicon of alcohol and drug terms published by the World Health Organization.* Retrieved from http://www.who.int/substance_abuse/terminology/who_lexicon/en

10

Moral Distress and Ethics in the Workplace

Conscience protection is regarded as a matter of basic human and civil rights. It is a tradition in our country that must be protected.
Anonymous quote by the American Civil Liberties Union, 2009

LEARNING OBJECTIVES

By the end of this chapter, the learner will be able to:

1. Discuss the relevance of moral distress for how it may impact nurses' mental health.
2. Identify the factors and situations that can precipitate moral distress.
3. Discuss what causes moral distress.
4. Identify and discuss various strategies that can be used to minimize the impact of moral distress.
5. Provide an example from personal practice or experience of a morally distressing situation.

Often going unnoticed for how they may impact nurses' mental health are the numerous ethical situations in which they find themselves on a regular basis. What is accepted and experienced as part of a nurse's everyday work—caring for the dying, a patient in a coma and on life support because of a traumatic head injury, someone who is mentally unwell, a neglected or abused child or senior—is heart-wrenching and mind-challenging. Conflicting and ambiguous feelings are generated within the nurse—inner turmoil, torment, and anguish. This occurs across the continuum of life, from the young to the old, and across all nursing settings.

Although the concept of inner ethical conflict was identified and surfaced as an issue in the 1980s, awareness of such inner ethical conflict, often presented as either moral distress or a moral dilemma, is gaining increased momentum, particularly in the field of nursing. To provide clarity and differentiation, moral distress occurs when "one is unable to act on one's moral choices because of internal or external constraints" (Austin & Boyd, 2010, p. 91). Corley (2002) adds that moral distress occurs when a nurse's values and perceived professional obligations, practices, and duties are incompatible with the needs and prevailing views of the external work environment.

Moral dilemma along a similar dimension is a conflict "in which one feels a moral obligation to act but must choose between incompatible alternatives" (Austin & Boyd, 2010, p. 91). Moral distress is different from the classical ethical dilemma in which one recognizes that a problem exists, and that two or more ethically justifiable but mutually opposing actions can be taken. Often, in an ethical dilemma, there are significant downsides to each potential solution (Epstein & Delgado, 2010).

Moral distress is prevalent in nursing. For example, in one study from the United Kingdom, it was found that 70% of nurses "sometimes" left work feeling distressed, while 11% of them "always" left work feeling distressed (Royal College of Nursing, 2008).

As nurses and licensed practitioners, we have a moral and ethical obligation to adhere to our nursing standards of practice to maintain safe, competent, and quality patient care. However, when faced with the many different complexities of our patients, their beliefs, attitudes, and values, and the adversities that they sometimes face, nurses' moral obligations become challenged—all of which have to be respected. As so eloquently stated by Galvin (2010), "Nursing is a balance of the 'hand' (technical skills) and 'head' (protocols and evidence) with the heart (ethical and human dimensions)."

As moral distress is what is most commonly researched, this will be the primary focus of this chapter; however, please remain cognizant that any ethically challenging situation, whether it constitutes a dilemma or distress, can compromise a nurse's mental health.

UNDERSTANDING MORAL DISTRESS

Moral distress first became recognized and identified as such in 1984 by Andrew Jameton. He identified it as "a phenomenon in which one knows the right action to take, but is constrained from taking it" (Jameton, 1993). Moral distress in the nursing profession is well recognized, as stated by the American Nurses Association (ANA; 2014):

> *Nurses practicing in today's health care environment face increasingly complex ethical dilemmas. We encounter these dilemmas in situations where our ability to do the right thing is frequently hindered by conflicting values and beliefs of other health care providers. Some confront the ethical issues directly while others turn away. Upholding our commitment to patients requires significant moral courage. Moral courage helps us address ethical issues and take action when doing the right thing is not easy. Moral courage involves the willingness to speak out and do what is right in the face of forces that would lead us to act in some other way. Nurses who possess moral courage and advocate in the best interest of the patient may at times find themselves experiencing adverse outcomes. There is a need for all nurses in all roles across all settings to commit to working toward creating work environments that support moral courage.* (ANA, 2014)

This aspect of moral courage goes hand in hand with moral distress and moral dilemmas. Although moral distress is primarily discussed and was first recognized in the area of nursing, other health care disciplines are also susceptible to moral distress (Austin, Kagan, Rankel, & Bergum, 2008; Chen, 2009).

The nursing profession is constantly evolving. As a result, so are the many ethical decisions and situations that nurses face, given the complexities of the care they are increasingly required to provide. As stated by Ward (2012), "Maintaining the integrity of the profession requires consistent evaluation of recurrent situations" and further requires a "complete understanding of the American Nurses Association position statement" on such an issue as moral distress.

As briefly explained above, moral distress is pain and anguish that can impact the mind, body, spirit, and relationships with others. It is intricately tied to patient care, in which nurses are aware of a moral problem, acknowledge that they have a moral obligation to respond to it, and then make a moral judgment about what constitutes the best or most correct action (Nathaniel, 2002; Warren, 2008). As a result, nurses, in their effort to do what is best for their patients, participate in a perceived moral wrongdoing and so are not able to care appropriately for them.

While moral distress is very concerning and creates mentally challenging outcomes for nurses, the resulting moral residue can create an even longer-lasting negative impact.

RECOGNIZING MORAL DISTRESS

Like most forms of energy and challenges, ethically distressing events that nurses face provide the impetus for what they experience as moral distress or dilemmas. As suggested by Epstein and Delgado (2010), "Ethical debate in clinical settings can be productive and positive, a sign that health care providers are engaged in collaborative relationships and concerned about the quality of care for their patients. However, the presence of moral distress signals a different issue altogether."

Recognizing mental distress is important if nurses wish to maintain good mental health. Although you may visibly see such signs as crying, anger, and frustration on the outside (Elpern, Covert, & Kleinpell, 2005), it is often what you can't see on the inside that is most significant, particularly for how it can impact your mental health. It is these feelings of anguish, torment, and uncertainty that impact your moral integrity, your character, your attitude, and even your quality of life. Without getting into the impact too much here, because it is discussed in the next section, it is recognized that sometimes moral distress manifests as something recognizable to others to alert them that something is just not right.

IMPACT OF MORAL DISTRESS

Moral distress acts as a form of stress that can impact our bodies and our minds. Like all other forms of stress that we have talked about, it affects our patients and the organization for which we work. In addition, everyone responds differently to morally distressing situations, so what is perceived as morally distressing to one nurse may not be by another. For those entering the nursing profession, moral distress can be viewed by some as an inherent part or nature of the work, as you try to provide care for highly vulnerable patients while at the same time possibly experiencing obstacles that prevent you from providing that care or doing what you believe is ethically or morally just.

Physically, moral distress can cause headaches, gastrointestinal disturbances, shaking, neck pain, and even crying (Gallagher, 2010). Psychologically, moral distress can also lay the foundation for the development of mental health challenges. In fact, moral distress has often been referred to as a "psychological imbalance" (Anderson, 2013). This is manifested through anger, frustration, reduced job satisfaction, lowered self-esteem, and guilt (Warren, 2008). A nurse can even experience burnout, decreased self-worth, and social withdrawal as a result of moral distress that is not resolved and dealt with in a timely, effective manner (Gallagher, 2010; Warren, 2008). What happens is that the nurse begins to feel isolated, alone, powerless, demeaned, and even belittled, with devastating results for the nurse (Corley, 2002; Corley, Elswick, Gorman, & Clor, 2001). Jameton (1993) suggests that this occurs because of the constraints placed on nurses' behavior and their ability to fulfill the actions they feel need to be completed. These constraints can be manifested as fear of losing one's job, self-doubt, anxiety about creating conflict, or lack of confidence (Hamric, Davis, & Childress, 2006). Depression as well can set in (Anderson, 2013). In instances in which nurses feel that they are not able to provide the care needed for their patient, self-blaming and feelings of guilt can occur (Canadian Nurses Association [CNA], 2003).

Professionally, moral distress can devastate one's moral sensitivity to problematic clinical situations that is used daily to make clinical judgments about patients and their response to treatment, as well as decisions about one's career (Epstein & Delgado, 2010).

Organizationally, moral distress, particularly when it occurs repeatedly, also comes with a price. Absenteeism and staff turnover can increase because of rising stress levels and retention challenges, respectively. Nurses just generally find that they do not want to go to work (Anderson, 2013). As found by Corley (2002), moral distress can even prompt nurses to consider leaving the profession altogether. Most important perhaps is that patient care or the quality of patient care can become jeopardized as a result of moral distress and its residue (Anderson, 2013; Warren, 2008).

While moral distress exerts primarily a negative impact, it can have a positive impact as well. As found by Corley (2002), in the face of a distressing event, moral distress can increase nurses' awareness about the ethical problems they experience. They can reflect on the event; on how and what they feel about the event, and why; and consider it a lesson learned, a lesson that can strengthen them as persons and professionals with a greater integrity, insight, and character.

CAUSES OF MORAL DISTRESS

The causes of moral distress in nursing are many. They are not just the outstanding controversial issues, such as caring for a patient who is having an abortion or a Jehovah's Witness who cannot receive blood or blood products; also involved are many of the other idiosyncrasies of work life that are typically routine or part of everyday practice. In any event, moral distress is still very much fundamentally connected to the nurse's personal and professional integrity. Causes include such things as the use of resources (e.g., time, staff, equipment, space), increased technological and pharmacological advances, communication, and missing or forgetting important information (Warren, 2008). Further, moral distress can involve inadequate patient care or witnessing others providing inadequate care; providing care seen as "futile" or unwanted; the inability to effectively advocate for patients; values conflicts, such as conflicts with organizational values and other providers' values; a lack of knowledge, comfort level, or experience in dealing with ethical issues; uncertainty of ethics resources; power dynamics, such as being forced to execute decisions without providing input; being unable to address ethical issues in a team or organization and, from a team dynamic perspective, having values "trumped"; lack of managerial level support; ethical climate of the organization; moral sensitivity; and a heightened awareness of the ethical aspects of practice (Warren, 2008).

Further, as identified by Corley (2002), other examples are continued life support, even though it is not in the best interest of the patient; inadequate communication about end-of-life care between providers, patients, and families; inappropriate use of health care resources; inadequate staffing or staff who are not adequately trained to provide the required care; inadequate provision of pain relief to patients; and false hope given to patients and families.

As identified by Anderson (2013), nurses have "watched patients and families struggle with decisions" regarding whether quality or quantity of life is important. Another issue is obtaining informed consent, particularly if the patient declines to give consent, and it is the nurse's responsibility to make sure that the patient's right is respected (Ward, 2012). Telling the truth is another significant potentially distressing event, as nurses know that patients are entitled to have full disclosure about what their health condition is and any treatments possibly needed, whereas the physician may not fully disclose these matters (Ward, 2012). Similarly, in keeping with the theme of trust, nurses also know that patients trust them to be fully competent in the care they provide as well as keeping any patient information confidential (Ward, 2012).

STRATEGIES TO ADDRESS MORAL DISTRESS

When moral distress occurs, it is "a sign that ethical challenges are not being addressed adequately" (Epstein & Delgado, 2010). In order to move past morally distressing events and the impact it has on you, you need to address and resolve it, at least from your own mental health perspective. Failure to address moral distress can only set you up for failure, illness, or compromised mental health concerns, as we have just highlighted.

Given the rapid rise and concern about the moral distress nurses are experiencing, strategies to address moral distress are the focus of many discussions and research endeavors, although these are still very much in their infancy.

The American Association of Critical Care Nurses (AACN, 2005a) has identified moral distress as a priority area and has developed a 4A's approach to address and reduce it (AACN, 2005b; Rushton, 2006). Although designed initially for the critical care setting, the 4A's are adaptable and applicable in many non–critical care settings. The 4A's are Ask, Affirm, Assess, and Act (AACN, 2005b).

First, you need to ask appropriate questions. For example, are your colleagues exhibiting signs of moral distress as well? Am I feeling distressed or showing signs of suffering? Is the source of my distress work? Here, you need to determine if indeed moral distress is present, so it is best to review the definition and symptoms of moral distress and ask yourself if what you are feeling is indeed moral distress (AACN, 2005b; McCue, 2010).

Second, you need to affirm. Affirm your feelings about the issue. What aspect of your moral integrity is being threatened? What role could you (and should you) play? Here, you need to affirm your distress and your commitment to take care of yourself, and you can do this by validating your feelings and perceptions with others and affirm for yourself a professional obligation to act. The goal here is to make a commitment to addressing moral distress (AACN, 2005b; McCue, 2010).

Third, you need to assess. Begin to put some facts together, such as identifying the sources of your distress. Recognize that there is an issue but that you may be ambivalent about taking action to change it, and analyze the risks and benefits. What is the source of your moral distress? What do you think is the "right" action, and why is it so? The goal here is to be ready to make an action plan. What is being done currently, and why? Who are the players in this situation? Determine if you are ready to act (AACN, 2005b; McCue, 2010).

Finally, you need to act. Create a plan for action and implement it. Think about potential pitfalls and strategies to get around these pitfalls. Identify and implement some changes and strategies that you desire to enact this plan and be sure to maintain that desired change. The goal here is to "preserve your integrity and authenticity" (AACN, 2005b; McCue, 2010).

Many other strategies have been identified to help deal with moral distress in nursing (Epstein & Hamric, 2009; Hamric et al., 2006). For example, speaking up and voicing your opinion is good practice; if you don't express the way you feel, how will anyone know? Second, advocate for yourself; you need to find out who it is you need to speak to, so deliberately get out there and do it (Warren, 2008). Nurses should also seek out their nursing association, regulatory body, or union to provide guidance and support to them through this experience (CNA, 2003). Third, as you are a practicing professional, you are accountable for your actions; even when you feel you are in error, accept the consequences and know you tried your best. Fourth, build your social supports as your peers can be your main source. Make this issue known as you are probably not alone in this regard, but others may be hesitant to speak out. Talking to your fellow nursing colleagues can actually be empowering for you, and they also have the best understanding of what you may be going through because they perhaps have been there themselves (Anderson, 2013). Fifth, look at the big picture of the whole work environment, what you are assigned to do and be responsible for, and what you can change so you don't get too preoccupied with the one patient of concern. Sixth, enhance your education on this topic (Warren, 2008). Given that many nurses erroneously believe that moral distress is a "normal" occurrence, more education would prove beneficial (Anderson, 2013). Further, nurses who have experienced the signs and symptoms of moral distress in the past were greatly relieved once they were able to identify what it was they had. Next, build collaboration. Moral distress does not originate alone in the nurse or the nursing environment; the other disciplines with which you work are also affected, so get them involved and work to change the workplace environment.

Finding out the root causes also helps. Identifying and targeting those will help to isolate the root of your feeling so it can be addressed. Develop policies so that there is consistency of process and practice for others who are experiencing the same feelings. The development of policies and the identification of the need for a policy may initiate other changes as well. This will encourage open dialogue, build collaboration, and should involve the ethicist or ethics committee of your organization (Warren, 2008).

Nursing leaders can also engage in various strategies to assist their nurses. For example, leaders need to have a heightened awareness of and sensitivity to the possibility that moral distress can occur (Gallagher, 2010).

SUMMARY

In summary, moral distress in nursing is alive, but not well. Moral distress can act as a significant source of stress for nurses, so much so as to compromise their own mental health and precipitate mental disorders and symptamology. As it slithers its way into nurses' everyday activities and responsibilities, to the point that some nurses may not even realize what it is or what is happening to them, it should be addressed as soon as possible. Nurses themselves, as well as nurse leaders and organizations, all have a role to play in supporting nurses who are experiencing moral distress and moral residue. Nurses are, after all, the very backbone of the organizations that want to deliver on their promise of providing safe, competent, and quality care.

DISCUSSION QUESTIONS

1. What is the relevance of moral distress for how it may impact nurses' mental health?
2. What kinds of factors and situations can precipitate moral distress?
3. What causes moral distress?
4. Identify the various strategies that can be used to minimize the impact of moral distress.
5. What is an example from your own practice or experience that illustrates a morally distressing situation to you?

REFERENCES

American Association of Critical Care Nurses. (2005a). *AACN standards for establishing and sustaining healthy work environments.* Retrieved from www.aacn.org/WD/HWE/Content/hwehome.pcms?menu=Community
American Association of Critical Care Nurses. (2005b). *The 4A's to rise above moral distress.* Retrieved from www.aacn.org/WD/Practice/Docs/4As_to_Rise_Above_Moral_Distress.pdf
American Nurses Association. (2014). *Moral courage and distress.* Retrieved from http://www.nursingworld.org/MainMenuCategories/EthicsStandards/Courage-and-Distress
Anderson, L. (2013). *Addressing moral distress in your nursing career.* Retrieved from http://www.nursetogether.com/moral-distress-in-your-nursing-career

Austin, W., & Boyd, M. A. (2010). *Psychiatric and mental health nursing.* Philadelphia, PA: Lippincott Williams & Wilkins.

Austin, W. J., Kagan, L., Rankel, M., & Bergum, V. (2008). The balancing act: Psychiatrists' experience of moral distress. *Medicine, Health Care & Philosophy, 11*(1), 89–97.

Canadian Nurses Association. (2003). *Ethical distress in health care environments.* Retrieved from http://www.cna-aiic.ca/~/media/cna/page%20content/pdf%20en/ethics_pract_ethical_distress_oct_2003_e.pdf

Chen, P. (2009). *When nurses and doctors can't do the right thing.* Retrieved June 30, 2010, from www.nytimes.com/2009/02/06/health/05chen.html

Corley, M. C. (2002). Nurse moral distress: A proposed theory and research agenda. *Nursing Ethics, 9*(6), 636–650.

Corley, M. C., Elswick, R. K., Gorman, M., & Clor, T. (2001). Development and evaluation of a moral distress scale. *Journal of Advanced Nursing, 33*(2), 250–256.

Elpern, E. H., Covert, B., & Kleinpell, R. (2005). Moral distress of staff nurses in a medical intensive care unit. *American Journal of Critical Care, 14*(6), 523–530.

Epstein, E. G., & Delgado, S. (2010). *Understanding and addressing moral distress. OJIN: The Online Journal of Issues in Nursing, 15*(3). Retrieved from http://www.nursingworld.org/MainMenuCategories/EthicsStandards/Courage-and-Distress/Understanding-Moral-Distress.html. doi:10.3912/OJIN.Vol15No03Man01

Epstein, E. G., & Hamric, A. B. (2009). Moral distress, moral residue, and the crescendo effect. *Journal of Clinical Ethics, 20*(4), 330–342.

Gallagher, A. (2010). Moral distress and moral courage in everyday nursing practice. *OJIN: The Online Journal of Issues in Nursing, 16*(2).

Galvin, K. T. (2010). Revisiting caring science: Some integrative ideas for the 'head, hand, and heart' of critical care nursing practice. *Nursing in Critical Care, 15*(4), 168–175.

Hamric, A. B., Davis, W. S., & Childress, M. D. (2006). Moral distress in health care professionals. *Pharos, 69*(1), 16–23.

Jameton, A. (1993). Dilemmas of moral distress: Moral responsibility and nursing practice. *AWHONNS Clinical Issues in Perinatal & Women's Health Nursing, 4*(4), 542–551.

McCue, C. (2010). Using the AACN framework to alleviate moral distress. *OJIN: The Online Journal of Issues in Nursing, 16*(1).

Nathaniel, A. K. (2002). Moral distress in nursing. *ANA Center for Ethics and Human Rights Online Newsletter.*

Royal College of Nursing. (2008). *Defending dignity: Challenges and opportunities for nursing.* Author. Retrieved from http://www.rcn.org.uk/__data/assets/pdf_file/0011/166655/003257.pdf

Rushton, C. (2006). *Caregiver suffering in palliative care for infants, children & adolescents: A practical handbook.* Baltimore, MD: Johns Hopkins University Press.

Ward, J. (2012). *Ethics in nursing: Issues nurses face.* Retrieved from http://www.nursetogether.com/ethics-in-nursing-issues-nurses-face

Warren, M. (2008). *Everybody hurts: Addressing moral distress in health care practice.* Retrieved from http://www.nshen.ca/docs/Hurts/PP%20slides%20-%20moral%20distress.pdf

11

Working With Colleagues Who Have Mental Illness

*The difference between what we do and what we are capable of doing
would suffice to solve most of the world's problem.*
—*Mahatma Ghandi*

LEARNING OBJECTIVES

By the end of this chapter, the learner will be able to:

1. Discuss the presentation of various mental illnesses in nurses and the impact they can have.
2. Identify the obligations of nurse colleagues in supporting and working with other nurses who have mental illnesses.
3. Discuss the kinds of work accommodations needed for nurses who are working with a mental illness.
4. Discuss the implications of stigma and discrimination in the nurses' workplace.

The prevalence of mental illness varies across countries, counties, states, and provinces. In nursing as well, as we have learned throughout this book, the prevalence of mental illness can vary, often depending not only on individual nurses' genetic makeup and life experiences but also on their workplace environment and chosen coping strategies. Factors related to the workplace include stress levels and the many stressors nurses face on a daily basis, which range from a heavy workload and patient acuity to sometimes negative and derogatory relationships with colleagues and other health care professionals. Working with a mental illness can be challenging for obvious reasons; however, with supportive peers, leaders, and organizations in place, a nurse who has a mental illness can perform to the caliber expected of any nurse, perhaps even more so. If nurse colleagues and leaders are informed of the illness, they can be key players in helping to identify exacerbations and precipitating factors, as well as the behaviors that manifest as a result.

MENTAL ILLNESS DIAGNOSES IN PEERS, COLLEAGUES, AND EMPLOYEES

Just as we encounter individuals in society and provide care to patients who suffer from mental illnesses, so too can we work with people who experience and live with known mental disorders. Believe it or not, many people, with the help of treatment, can maintain employment and a productive value to society while enduring a chronic mental illness. As illustrated by the nonfictional story of John Nash, portrayed in the movie *A Beautiful Mind*, people with mental illness can succeed in all that they do and that their minds allow them to do. Some of the most intelligent, creative, and famous people in history—Albert Einstein, Buzz Aldrin, Ludwig van Beethoven, Delta Burke, Marlon Brando, Winston Churchill, Kurt Cobain, Calvin Coolidge, Diana Princess of Wales, Charles Dickens, Michelangelo, Abraham Lincoln, and Isaac Newton, to name a few—all suffered with mental illnesses.

As highlighted earlier, work serves a supportive and even a therapeutic role for many individuals who have mental illness. However, many mental disorders do cause symptomatology and behaviors that can negatively impact one's performance at work. In this chapter, we will learn how you can help promote the optimal functioning of a colleague who suffers with a mental illness. This is not meant to represent an additional work stressor for you, because much of what can be done consists of very simple, common sense tactics, knowledge, and activities that require understanding, support, and an appreciation for human life.

The prevalence and experience of mental illness are more widespread than many care to admit. At last check, 50% of all Americans at some time during their life will experience a mental illness and meet the criteria for a diagnosis of mental illness according to the *Diagnostic and Statistical Manual of Mental Disorders, Fifth Edition* (*DSM-5*; American Psychiatric Association, 2013; Kessler et al., 2005). However, the extent to which the mental illness will negatively impact their work performance depends on several factors, such as the stigma prevailing in the workplace and attitudes of employees, the context and nature of their work, the mental illness and its associated behaviors, the severity of the illness, and the established coping skills of the employee who has a mental illness. Openness of communication at work, the work atmosphere, which may or may not be based on a cohesive team, and the leadership style at the workplace are also factors impacting the integration, acceptance, and work performance of the employee with a mental disorder. Ronald Kessler, a professor of health care policy at Harvard University and lead author of a study conducted by the National Institute of Mental Health, cites data showing that 60% of Americans with a mental disorder get no treatment (Williams, 2012). Furthermore, 77% of Canadian workers now experiencing mental health problems suffer in silence because they are afraid or ashamed to disclose a mental illness (Gordon, 2013).

STIGMA AND DISCRIMINATION

The stigma associated with mental illness and discrimination against individuals with mental illness have permeated society for years. Although humankind and societies have made much progress in eliminating this prejudice, unfortunately it still shadows much of our everyday existence. In the days of barbaric treatment, including accusations of witchcraft and spiritual possession by Satan, individuals with mental illnesses were tortured, punished, and even killed for fear of the harm they could inflict on society. We have come a long way in recognizing mental illness as having identifiable sources and causes, as opposed to witches' spells, demonic possessions, and evil. However, even today individuals with mental illness are still often stigmatized, discriminated against, and ostracized by society. In the workplace in particular, attitudes toward mental health and mental illness make a big difference for all employees, especially for those experiencing mental health issues.

People with mental illness are often treated with disrespect and experience such behaviors as exclusion, bullying, aggression, ridicule, and devaluation, which often limit and pose barriers to many of life's opportunities (Higgins & Duxbury, 2013). The acts of stigmatizing and discriminating against colleagues with mental illnesses can negatively impact and create substantial health consequences for them (Storch, 2007). Sadly, some of the perpetrators responsible for perpetuating stigmatization are the very health care professionals who are supposed to help the mentally ill get better and become entirely healthy. For the purposes of our discussion, *stigmatization* is defined as being devalued by individuals or communities on the basis of one's real or perceived health status, while *discrimination* is defined as the legal, institutional, and procedural ways in which people are denied access to their rights because of their real or perceived health status (Gruskin & Ferguson, 2009). Further, stigmatization represents a personal attitude and belief that negatively labels a group of people, such as those with mental illness. Stigmatization creates fear and consequently results in discrimination, which discourages individuals from getting the help they need.

Although work should provide a nonjudgmental atmosphere and the utmost respect for one's human rights, not always does this occur. Stigmatization and discrimination at work can be very disabling for an employee who has a frequently targeted disorder. The person who experiences a mental disorder is already perhaps embarrassed, fearful, and uncomfortable admitting that he or she has a mental illness, for fear of how others may react. People who suffer from mental illness are afraid they are going to be treated differently—that they are not going to be as respected if they reveal that they have a problem. Some are even afraid of losing their jobs (Gordon, 2013).

In a work environment where there are already softly spoken or loudly expressed insults, slurs, jokes, and putdowns of people with mental illness, the employee with a mental illness will obviously be apprehensive about admitting to such. Nurses, in particular, have already found physicians who refuse to admit mentally ill patients to their case load because they are too complicated and absorb too much of their time (Lam, Lam, Lam, & Ku, 2013). As stated by Wallace (2012), "Stigma of mental illness thrives in the medical profession as a result of the culture of medicine and medical training, perceptions of physicians and their colleagues, and expectations and responses of health care systems and organizations." Otherwise, health care professionals from all walks of life, physicians and nurses, clearly admit that they do not know how to provide care to someone who has a mental illness. Aside from trying to get treatment for their own mental illness, nurses as well often stigmatize individuals with mental illness (Ross & Goldner, 2009), which can potentially compromise their relationships with the professionals with whom they work. As found by Ross and Goldner (2009), "Nurses do play the regrettable roles of the perpetuators and the recipients of stigma towards mental illness." Further, "Nurses who choose to work in psychiatry were themselves found to have negative attitudes and discriminatory behaviour towards segments of the MH/P (Mental health/Psychiatry) population (specifically BPD [bipolar disorder]), and to be more pessimistic about positive outcomes of psychiatric illnesses than were general nurses and the lay public. Stigma was also found to be turned inwards, and directed towards others within the nursing profession. This took the form of ostracizing and even shunning of nurses who have mental illness. As well, associative stigma was seen in the devaluing of psychiatric/mental health nurses' status within the profession" (Ross & Goldner, 2009). Again, we see much irony here, as the very health care providers who pride themselves on altruism, caring, and nurturing maintain damaging and judgmental stereotypes of their very own colleagues who suffer from illnesses, so much so that these nursing colleagues are frowned upon and are embarrassed to seek help when help is most needed.

This stigmatized tone has been set by society throughout the years; many have come to believe that you should avoid "weird" or "abnormal" people as if they are bad and even dangerous. In actual fact, people with mental illness are no more violent or aggressive than are the rest of the population in a society. The reverse of this is perpetrated in the media and in television shows, which inappropriately serve to reinforce the stigma of mental illness. Ironically, individuals with mental illness are more often the victims than the perpetrators of violence (Appleby, Mortensen, Dunn, & Hiroeh, 2001; Hiday et al., 1999; Institute of Medicine, 2006; University of Washington School of Social Work, 2014). The link between mental illness and violence is significantly exaggerated as a result of media propaganda, when in reality the number of individuals with mental illness who commit violent acts is very small (Institute of Medicine, 2006; Mulvey, 1994). Unequivocally, the vast majority of individuals who commit violent acts most often do not have a diagnosed mental illness (American Psychiatric Association, 1994).

Isn't it odd that we should even be having this discussion about stigma? After all, this is the 21st century. Unfortunately, the stigmatization of mental illness is alive and well. The very same issues that ostracized the mentally ill before the Common Era continue to condemn them thousands of years later. Obviously, society has not learned anything during this time.

Nurses who have preexisting mental illnesses know all too well what stigma and discrimination can do to them. The harmful effects of stigma and discrimination always seem to creep into the domain of one's work life as well. Stigma has been known to have some very negative consequences for the individual who already suffers with a mental illness. Some of these negative effects include the individual's typical reaction of fear and rejection, loss of self-esteem and self-worth, loss of trust, and alienation and difficulty making friends (Parle, 2012; Ross & Goldner, 2009). And yes, people with mental illnesses have even been denied employment opportunities and jobs too. All of these findings add cumulatively to who this person is today, the very nurse we have worked with for years. The stigmatizing and discriminatory reactions of others to those with mental illness have resulted in these individuals being even more reluctant, embarrassed, and ashamed to seek help for their mental illness for fear of what others may think, of being labeled "crazy." The reactions cause confusion for them and an increasing sense of denial of their illness. In the workplace, for example, negative reactions can translate into increased absenteeism, lost productivity, and increased corporate costs because mentally ill individuals are afraid to seek help. They continue to work under self-imposed duress without any therapeutic interventions or supports because they feel ashamed and embarrassed.

The impact of stigmatization and discrimination against colleagues with mental illness is debilitating. Most significantly, stigmatization has the power to prevent individuals from seeking help for their mental illness (Wrigley, Jackson, Judd, & Komiti, 2005). Further, it serves to decrease their self-esteem and self-efficacy (Link, 2001; Link, Mirotznik, & Cullen, 1991; Markowitz, 1998) and increase their risk for developing other mental illnesses, such as depression and anxiety, and it acts to "rob people of the opportunities that define a quality life: good jobs, safe housing, satisfactory health care, and affiliation with a diverse group of people" (Corrigan & Watson, 2002, p. 16). Lack of satisfaction with life and with self is also a negative outcome resulting from perceived stigma (Markowitz, 1998; Rosenfield, 1997). As found by Watson, Corrigan, Larson, and Sells (2007), "When individuals face the onset of a mental illness such as schizophrenia, these stereotypes become relevant to the self." It is this perspective and adoption of thought that cause individuals to limit their own social networks and interactional opportunities in anticipation of rejection due to stigma. As a result, they experience isolation, unemployment, and lowered income, not to mention increased stress and interference with their own recovery processes (Perlick et al., 2001; Sirey et al., 2001).

The ethical quandary for nurses as professionals in the realm of stigma and discrimination is the resolution of their own such feelings toward those with mental illness. Nurses should be able to recognize their own biases and beliefs and deal with them before they can effectively work with colleagues who have mental illness. Nurses who do not deal with their own stigmatization and stereotypical beliefs about mental illness have the potential to jeopardize professional working relationships, not to mention the care of the clients whom they serve. Nurses should at no point in their career have to stop and question why a colleague with a mental illness is deserving of any special consideration or accommodation. Many a seasoned nurse will recall cases where nurses mistreated their colleagues who had a mental illness through aggression, bullying, and disrespectful antics. Great strides and education are still needed for nurses in regard to how stigma and discrimination can impact the workplace, professional relationships, and nursing practice. Although many nurses struggle ethically with their own beliefs and values, they are in a valuable position to increase awareness, enhance understanding, educate others, and advocate against the disabling effects of stigma and discrimination on their colleagues with mental illness.

The impact of the stigmatization of mental illness is far-reaching. For example, as nurses who are suffering from mental health issues are being recruited and potentially hired, they are faced with the decision of disclosing their condition openly. While there is no legal obligation to do so, as identified above, many recruiters will tell you, although not always on the record, that an admission of mental health issues raises "red flags" and can be a factor in employer decision making (Williams, 2012). The stigmatization of a colleague with mental illness can wreak havoc in that person's life. It increases stress levels to a concerning degree, with the physical, physiological, and social ramifications discussed in Chapter 1, and also tends to discredit and isolate the individual psychologically, thus creating feelings of guilt, shame, fear, and inferiority. Negative workplace repercussions in particular can result in delayed access to treatment, which promotes disability, impedes recovery, weakens social supports, hinders social integration, prevents and obstructs the performance of social roles, reduces quality of life, diminishes self-esteem, and increases unemployment (Stuart, 2004).

While people do discriminate against those with mental illness, mental illness itself does not discriminate, and anyone can develop a mental illness or experience poor mental health. However, there is much that can be done to address the stigmatization of mental illness in the workplace. Some of these interventions include the following: increasing education and awareness through mental health literacy in the workplace; proactively implementing policies and programs that promote positive mental health in the nurses' workplace; supporting the early identification, treatment, and recovery of employees experiencing mental illness; speaking to them with dignity and respect; not patronizing and demeaning others; and focusing on their strengths, not their limitations.

The stigma of mental illness still alarms many. In 2008, the Canadian Medical Association found that only 50% of people would tell friends or coworkers that they had a family member with a mental illness, whereas 68% would disclose a family member's diagnosis of diabetes and 72% a diagnosis of cancer; only 12% of Canadians said they would hire a lawyer with a mental illness; 49% of Canadians said that they would socialize with a friend who had a serious mental illness; 46% of Canadians thought people used the term *mental illness* as an excuse for bad behavior; and 27% were fearful of being around people with a serious mental illness.

UNDERSTANDING BEHAVIORS, EXACERBATIONS, AND MENTAL DISORDERS

One of the most important things nurses can do for their colleagues who have a mental illness is better understand their mental illness, the behaviors that accompany that mental illness, the triggers that can exacerbate the illness, and how that exacerbation can impact their work performance. To do this, we will walk through the main diagnostic categories of mental illness that are often cited in the literature as set forth in the *DSM-5* (American Psychiatric Association, 2013) and how they are relevant for nurses.

Mood Disorders

Disorders such as depression, mania, and bipolar disorder can all impact one's performance at work. According to the *DSM-5*, mood disorders occur when there is disturbance in one's mood or an inappropriate, exaggerated, or limited range of feelings. "Everybody gets down sometimes, and everybody experiences a sense of excitement and emotional pleasure. To be diagnosed with a mood disorder, your feelings must be to the extreme. In other words, crying, and/or feeling depressed, suicidal frequently.

Or, the opposite extreme, having excessive energy where sleep is not needed for days at a time and during this time the decision making process in significantly hindered." As found by Ohler, Kerr, and Forbes (2010), nurses have a higher prevalence of depression than do other health care professionals. These levels reach about 10% and even 18% and occur for various reasons, but primarily as a result of job strain, role overload, and a lack of respect (Letvak, Ruhm, & McCoy, 2012; Ohler et al., 2010).

The treatment of mood disorders is also something that nurse colleagues can remain cognizant of in the workplace when working with nurses who have known mental disorders or mental health concerns. Lithium carbonate, for example, is a salt commonly used in the effective treatment of bipolar disorders and can affect the production of dopamine, epinephrine, and norepinephrine to stabilize moods, particularly to reduce manic episodes, exaggerated feelings of well-being, paranoia, aggressiveness, and irritability. However, the treatment of bipolar disorders and the use of lithium do not come without risks and side effects. For example, lithium toxicity is something nurse colleagues can be attuned to in the workplace because its narrow therapeutic range can create life-endangering outcomes. Lithium toxicity is characterized by symptoms of confusion, slurred speech, seizures, and coma.

The impact of depression, bipolar disorder, and mania on one's work performance has been clearly documented in the literature. To briefly reiterate, these disorders can lead to compromised patient safety and quality of care, poor job performance, and a sense of victimization that can lower morale and challenge the completion of needed tasks, further jeopardizing the health of the affected nurse (Letvak et al., 2012). However, mood disorders can be treated. For example, antidepressants can improve one's mood and quality of life; people treated with antidepressants may have fewer negative obsessive thoughts, be able to pause and consider their feelings and actions in a more balanced way, let go of negative thought patterns more easily, have more energy, sleep better, and even concentrate better.

Anxiety Disorders

We discussed anxiety and the different degrees of anxiety in Chapter 1, so here it will be covered from the perspective of how it impacts work for the nurse. Anxiety disorders comprise a large number of disorders whose primary feature is abnormal or inappropriate anxiety. In all likelihood, most people experience anxiety at some point in their life. Whether you were frightened by a sudden loud noise, watched a scary movie, or slammed on the brakes of your car when a dog was crossing the road unexpectedly, you most likely experienced an increased heart rate, tensed muscles, sweaty palms, and an acute sense of focus as you tried to determine the source. Once any medical cause is ruled out, an anxiety disorder may be the culprit (American Psychiatric Association, 2013). Welcome to the world of anxiety, and yes, anxiety occurs at work as well as in your private life.

The level of anxiety in nurses' workplaces is phenomenal. As found by Gao et al. (2012), anxiety among nurses has reached levels as high as 43.4%. The anxiety of nurses has far-reaching effects. It impacts them as people and as professionals, thus influencing their work performance, job satisfaction, and collegial interactions. As Gao et al. (2012) found, "Demographic factors (education, chronic disease, and life events), lifestyle factors (regular meals and physical exercise), work conditions (hospital grade, job rank, monthly salary, nurse–patient relationships, job satisfaction, and intention of leaving), job content (social support and decision latitude), effort–reward imbalance, and overcommitment were all significantly related to the anxiety symptoms."

Substance Use Disorders

Substance use disorders were discussed in Chapter 9. In this section, we consider abuse of or dependence on a substance. A substance can be anything that is ingested in order to produce a high, alter one's senses, or otherwise affect functioning. The substance most commonly thought of in this category is alcohol, although others, such as cocaine, marijuana, heroin, "ecstasy," "special-K," and "crack" are also included. Probably the most abused substances, caffeine and nicotine, are also included, although they are rarely thought of in this manner by laypersons (American Psychiatric Association, 2013). As outlined in Chapter 9, the prevalence of addictions among nurses is alarming, but there is much the nurse, the nurse's colleagues, the nursing leader, and the organization can do to abolish the addiction. Most important, in the area of addictions, is the damage that an addiction can create, not just to the nurse but also to the patients and workplace setting.

Impulse Control Disorders

"Disorders in this category include the failure or extreme difficulty in controlling impulses despite the negative consequences. This includes the failure to stop gambling even if you realize that losing would result in significant negative consequences. This failure to control impulses also refers to the impulse to engage in violent behavior (e.g., road rage), sexual behavior, fire starting, stealing, and self-abusive behaviors" (American Psychiatric Association, 2013). For example, gambling among nurses is one such impulse control disorder. Gambling has become an increasingly recognized trend in nurses and one that leads to compromised patient care, poor work performance, and even criminal charges, such as fraud (Rudan, 2010).

Psychotic Disorders

The major symptom of these disorders is psychosis, or delusions and hallucinations. Delusions are false beliefs that significantly hinder a person's ability to function—for example, believing that people are trying to hurt you when there is no evidence of this, or believing that you are somebody else, such as Jesus Christ or Cleopatra. Hallucinations are false perceptions. They can be visual (seeing things that aren't there), auditory (hearing), olfactory (smelling), tactile (sensing things on your skin that aren't really there, such as feeling that bugs are crawling on you), or taste (American Psychiatric Association, 2013). Although nurses with psychotic disorders are rare, one can find anecdotal accounts in the literature.

Somatoform Disorders

Disorders in the somatoform category include "those where the symptoms suggest a medical condition but where no medical condition can be found by a physician. In other words, a person with a somatoform disorder might experience significant pain without a medical or biological cause, or they may constantly experience minor aches and pains without any reason for these pains to exist" (American Psychiatric Association, 2013). While no research on somatoform disorders in nurses can be found in the literature, that is not to say they do not exist. As we highlighted earlier, the stigma that still exists often prevents nurses from seeking help (Wrigley et al., 2005).

Personality Disorders

Personality disorders are mental illnesses that share several unique qualities. They cause symptoms that are enduring and play a major role in most, if not all, aspects of the person's life. While many disorders vacillate in terms of the presence and intensity of symptoms, personality disorders typically remain relatively constant. To diagnose a disorder in this category, a psychiatrist or psychologist will look for the following criteria in a patient:

1. Symptoms have been present for an extended period of time, are inflexible and pervasive, and are not a result of alcohol or drugs or another psychiatric disorder. The history of symptoms can be traced back to adolescence or at least early adulthood.
2. The symptoms have caused and continue to cause significant distress or negative consequences in different aspects of the person's life.
3. Symptoms are seen in at least two of the following areas:
   - *Thoughts* (ways of looking at the world, thinking about self or others, and interacting)
   - *Emotions* (appropriateness, intensity, and range of emotional functioning)
   - *Interpersonal functioning* (relationships and interpersonal skills)
   - *Impulse control* (American Psychiatric Association, 2013)

Like those with psychotic disorders, nurses with personality disorders are infrequent in the literature. Again, anecdotal accounts of nurses being diagnosed with a personality disorder is often what you will find. The implications of a practicing nurse with a personality disorder reflects the very criteria that define the disorder. Hence, one can expect to see disordered thought processes, labile emotions, difficulty functioning, and impulse control concerns when patient care is delivered. In the case of nurse bullying, for example, increasing attention is now being given to the fact that nurse bullies may actually be manifesting a narcissistic personality disorder, as the characteristics of the two have an uncanny resemblance (Haselhuhn, 2005; Tim Field Foundation, 1996). However, it needs to be remembered that most mental illnesses can be effectively treated, so that the individual can lead a stabilized and fully functional life.

WHAT TO DO?

As clearly outlined in Chapter 6, there are numerous things that you as a person and a nurse can do to help yourself or someone else deal with stressors that threaten mental health, and maintaining your perspective is important when you are coping with stress. Do not get bogged down with detail as it can tend to escalate your stress even more, so it is best to learn to step back and take a deep breath and remember that you have to be realistic and that you cannot control everyone and everything all of the time. Also being good to yourself, patting yourself on the back, treating yourself well, and focusing on the positive things happening in your life can all help you or a colleague maintain positive mental health.

Remember the benefits of laughter; it can do wonders in preventative medicine and forces you to focus on the lighter side of life. Rather than let difficult or discontented managers and colleagues get a rise out of you, share a joke with a friend or coworker and try to see the humor in your predicament. A good chuckle is one of the best ways to reduce stress and put things in perspective.

Further, getting lots of exercise, proper nutrition, relaxing, volunteering, and building friendships and relationships with others can all support you through those difficult stressful times. Finally, enjoy time with your pet and your children, sit back, take it easy, and refocus.

As a colleague acting to support someone with a mental illness, there is also a great deal you can do. Identifying ways to address and become cognizant of discrimination and stigma is a great first step. Second, and perhaps most importantly, talk to the person about it; respect the importance of disclosure, confidentiality, and privacy; and identify the precipitating factors.

WORKING WITH PEOPLE WHO HAVE A MENTAL DISABILITY

The general rule of thumb for working with individuals who have disabilities such as mental disorders or mental health concerns remains the Golden Rule: "Do unto others as you would have them do unto you." Although some people make it a significant issue and overprepare themselves, this is not rocket science information. All it takes is a little sincerity, personal integrity, respect, compassion (you are nurses after all, correct?), and understanding. The person always comes first, and as you listen, observe, and act, you are interacting with the "person" and his or her skills, strengths, and character, not the disability, so be respectful of that. For example, listen carefully because many people who have a mental illness will not disclose this to their employer or coworkers for fear of stigma and discrimination. If you are aware of or suspect that a staff member is experiencing mental illness, the following steps might equip you to provide support (Australian Government, 2013):

1. Develop your own understanding about mental illness.
2. Use empathy to try to understand how the person may be feeling.
3. Ask the person about his or her health and well-being in general.
4. Be a nonjudgmental listener. If the person discloses having a mental illness and is willing to discuss it, encourage him or her to access workplace supports that are available.
5. Ask if there are particular stressors in the workplace that can be alleviated.
6. Encourage the use of stress-reduction strategies, such as accessing an employee assistance program, if one is available in your workplace.
7. Encourage the person to see a doctor to manage symptoms if appropriate.
8. Encourage the person to use sick leave if needed, as it is appropriate.
9. Offer your assistance, if the person seems receptive, by being an "advocate."

10. Help observe for any discriminatory remarks being made and address them directly.
11. As social events play a significant role in the workplace, help to ensure that the individual nurse is included.

Talking about your mental illness often seems too personal, too deep, and too complex. You might feel very happy to tell a colleague about a physical injury you've sustained, but when it comes to your mental health, where do you start? The answer is straightforward. Despite the fact that mental illness is very common—one in four of us will suffer mental health problems during our lives—we find it very difficult to talk about (Advisory, Conciliation, & Arbitration Service, 2012).

RIGHTS AND RESPONSIBILITIES OF EVERYONE INVOLVED

Everyone has a role to play in helping to ensure that the workplace is safe, respectful, fair, and free of discrimination, stigma, and prejudices. Whether you are a nurse, a nurse leader, or a nurse colleague, you are a practicing professional and so are accountable and responsible for taking actions to help ensure the workplace environment remains just that way. Whether it concerns areas of responsibility for safety, emergency procedures, discrimination, or disclosure, there is a great deal for the nurse, nurse colleague, and nurse leader to keep in mind.

In terms of safety, emergency procedures, and discrimination, all policies of an organization apply equally to all nurses. All nurses are held to the same level of accountability and responsibility and to the same code of ethical conduct regardless of whether or not they have a mental illness or concern.

Disclosure refers to the choice that people make about whether to tell others or the organization about their known or diagnosed disability. There is no legal obligation for workers to disclose information about their disability to colleagues or to their employer unless it is anticipated to affect their performance, ability to meet the requirements of the job, or ability to work safely and ensure the safety of colleagues and patients (Australian Government, 2013). While nurses do not need to disclose specific medical information about any disability they may have, they do have an obligation to help ensure that the essential requirements of the job are able to be carried out and the goals of the job achieved. In such cases, adjustments to the workload and tasks may be required. To achieve the goals of work, it would be most helpful for an affected nurse to disclose some medical information to the nurse leader and colleagues so that an understanding can be achieved and so that empathy, not conflict, will prevail.

The rights of nurses with a mental disability also need to be respected. These rights are (Australian Government, 2013):

1. The right to the confidential and respectful treatment of information about their disability
2. The right to access information about equity policies, practices, and strategies

3. The right to request information from the employer about the collection of personal and disability-related specific information and how it is used by the organization
4. The right to choose whether to disclose a disability at any point while looking for work or at work

If you are a coworker to whom a nurse has disclosed a medical condition, you are not permitted to share that information with anyone, unless, of course, the condition becomes a threat to others, property, and the nurse himself or herself.

NEW HIRES

Starting a job can be an anxious experience for any new employee. For a new nurse who has a mental disability, concerns about acceptance by coworkers can make the start of a job an especially stressful time. When a new coworker with a disability starts a new job in your workplace, ensure that you have a relaxed manner and work environment to help the new person settle in.

As with other coworkers, providing regular and ongoing feedback on work performance or other work-related behavior will provide direction and increased confidence and will make the settling-in period more successful. Providing feedback is also an effective technique to minimize stress at work. Stress does after all hold much potential to significantly impact one's work performance, concentration, memory, and cognitive thought processes.

WORK ACCOMMODATIONS

When nurses are either working or trying to return to work after being absent because of a mental illness, the nursing leader has an integral role to play. The nursing leader is in a position to support, accommodate, and even counsel and coordinate for the individual nurse and take whatever measures are needed so that the return to work is smooth, seamless, and not too overwhelming. A nurse leader is cognizant of what to look for when a nurse begins to show signs of deterioration. The leader can then engage in a series of actions in preparation to approach the nurse. You can never walk in another's shoes, but you can discuss with someone what will work best, as this is the life he or she has been living. As suggested by Rodwell and Martin (2013), "The contributions of informational and interpersonal justice, along with the main and interaction effects of supervisor support, highlight the centrality of the supervisor in addressing the impact of job demands." They add that psychosocial variables have utility beyond predicting stress outcomes to the work attitudes of nurses.

When a nurse is returning to work, contact him or her about 2 weeks before the expected return to work to find out if there is anything you can do to ease the transition. Take advantage of this contact and explore with the employee how you might, for example, adjust duties or schedule, increase motivation, and reduce absenteeism. This can be an ice breaker for the nurse to reinitiate contact with colleagues and develop a plan with the manager for how the return to work will unfold. As most nurses returning to work would like to be treated just as they were before leaving work, make this point known to other nurses. Take the time to welcome the nurse back to work, and in the following days and weeks, continue to pay particular attention to the nurse and to the nurse's performance and well-being.

Never make assumptions. Do not believe that the problems will resolve over time, and take preliminary action quickly while still respecting the autonomy and independence of the individual. Meet informally with the nurse and offer reassurance that confidentiality will be maintained. Share honestly and candidly what you have been observing in his or her behaviors and mood, use examples, and ask open-ended questions to be warm and inviting. You don't need to ask direct questions about a nurse's medical or mental condition; however, if he or she speaks about it, offer reassurance about the confidentiality of the matter.

Individuals may deny or avoid their mental health concerns, and they may not have a broad outlook regarding how their mental health is presenting itself, the treatment they can get, and the supports they need. Inform these nurses of your concern for them and encourage them to get help. Use your own discretion and clinical judgment when offering the services of an employee assistance program.

Keep the lines of communication open with other nurses in the workplace setting. You can help to address any prejudices and stigma that may exist among your team members. Don't be fooled that just because they are health care workers they understand mental illness, because not everyone does, and many still hold stigmatizing beliefs about individuals suffering with mental illnesses. Talk about this at your staff meetings and take the opportunity to educate your staff or hold information sessions with an invited speaker (Government of Canada, 2013). This education session may also take the form of disability awareness training. Disability awareness training can help you feel at ease when communicating and working with a new coworker who has a disability. It can also help a new coworker with a disability to feel supported by you when returning to work or commencing a new job.

Within an organization and assigned setting, the nurse leader can also be instrumental in creating policies and procedures on accommodating individuals with mental illness or mental health concerns.

SUMMARY

Nurses are among the ranks of so many other individuals who face a diagnosed mental illness. That does not mean that they are special, different, or indifferent; it simply means that you, as a colleague, need to know what you can do to help support them in the workplace as there may come times when their illness becomes exacerbated, so that confusion, anxiety, or unstructured thought processes interfere with the achievement of their goals. However, there is a great deal that can be done to help mentally ill nurses. Sometimes, it is just knowing what such persons experience and the treatment effects they endure. As colleagues of individuals who have a mental illness, we need to be supportive, respectful, and informed of what they are struggling with, for then and only then can we do our best to support and advocate for them.

DISCUSSION QUESTIONS

1. What can you do to help support a nursing colleague who has a mental illness?
2. Why is understanding stigma and discrimination important?
3. What can a nursing leader do to help assist and accommodate a mentally ill nurse in the workplace?
4. How can a mental illness impact a nurse's work performance?
5. Identify some of the rights of a mentally ill nurse who is working.

REFERENCES

Advisory, Conciliation, & Arbitration Service. (2012). *Promoting positive mental health at work.* Retrieved from http://www.acas.org.uk/media/pdf/j/2/Promoting-positive-mental-health-at-work-accessible-version.pdf

American Psychiatric Association. (1994). *Fact sheet: Violence and mental illness.* Washington, DC: Author.

American Psychiatric Association. (2013). *Diagnostic and statistical manual of mental disorders* (5th ed.). Retrieved from http://www.psych.org/practice/dsm

Appleby, L., Mortensen, P. B., Dunn, G., & Hiroeh, U. (2001). Death by homicide, suicide, and other unnatural causes in people with mental illness: A population-based study. *The Lancet, 358,* 2110–2112.

Australian Government. (2013). *Working with people with disability.* Retrieved from http://jobaccess.gov.au/content/how-work-people-disability

Corrigan, P. W., & Watson, A. C. (2002). Understanding the impact of stigma on people with mental illness. *World Psychiatry, 1*(1), 16–20.

Gao, Y. Q., Pan, B. C., Sun, W., Wu, H., Want, J. N., & Wang, L. (2012). Anxiety symptoms among Chinese nurses and the associated factors: A cross sectional study. *BMC Psychiatry, 12*(141). doi:10.1186/1471-244X-12-141

Gordon, A. (2013). *Canada launches workplace standards for mental health and safety.* Retrieved from http://www.thestar.com/news/world/2013/01/16/canada_launches_workplace_standards_for_mental_health_and_safety.html

Government of Canada. (2013). *Mental health first aid in the workplace.* Retrieved from http://managers-gestionnaires.gc.ca/tools-outils/mental-health_sante-mentale-eng.php#organization

Gruskin, S., & Ferguson, L. (2009). Using indicators to determine the contribution of human rights to public health efforts. *Bulletin of the World Health Organization, 87*(9), 714–719.

Haselhuhn, M. R. (2005). *Adult bullying within nursing workplaces: Strategies to address a significant occupational stressor.* Retrieved from http://www.minurses.org/files/files/Nursing%20Practice/bully032008.pdf

Hiday, V. A., Swartz, M. S., Swanson, J. W., et al. (1999). Criminal victimization of persons with severe mental illness. *Psychiatric Services, 50,* 62–68.

Higgins, C., & Duxbury, L. (2013). *The 2001 National Work-Life Conflict Study: Report one.* Health Canada, 2002. Retrieved from http://publications.gc.ca/collections/Collection/H72-21-186-2003E.pdf

Institute of Medicine. (2006). *Improving the quality of health care for mental and substance-use conditions.* Washington, DC: The National Academies Press.

Kessler, R. C., Berglund, P., Demler, O., Jin, R., Merikangas, K. R., & Walters, E. E. (2005). Lifetime prevalence and age-of-onset distributions of DSM-IV disorders in the National Comorbidity Survey Replication. *Archives of General Psychiatry, 62*(6), 593–602.

Lam, T. P., Lam, K. F., Lam, E. W., & Ku, Y. S. (2013). Attitudes of primary care physicians towards patients with mental illness in Hong Kong. *Asia-Pacific Psychiatry, 5*(1), E19–E28.

Letvak, S., Ruhm, C. J., & McCoy, T. (2012). Depression in hospital-employed nurses. *Clinical Nurse Specialist, 26*(3), 177–182. doi:10.1097/NUR.0b013e3182503ef0

Link, B. (2001). Stigma as a barrier to recovery: The consequences of stigma for the self-esteem of people with mental illness. *Psychiatric Services, 52,* 1621–1626.

Link, B., Mirotznik, J., & Cullen, F. (1991). The effectiveness of stigma coping orientations: Can negative consequences of mental illness labeling be avoided? *Journal of Health and Social Behavior, 32,* 302–320.

Markowitz, F. E. (1998). The effects of stigma on the psychological well-being and life satisfaction of persons with mental illness. *Journal of Health and Social Behaviors, 39,* 335–347.

Mulvey, E. P. (1994). Assessing the evidence of a link between mental illness and violence. *Hospital and Community Psychiatry, 45,* 663–668.

Ohler, M. C., Kerr, M. S., & Forbes, D. A. (2010). Depression in nurses. *Canadian Journal of Nursing Research, 42*(3), 66–82.

Parle, S. (2012). How does stigma affect people with mental illness? *Nursing Times, 108*(28), 12–14.

Perlick, D., Rosenheck, R., Clarkin, J., Sirey, J., Salahi, J., & Struening, E. (2001). Stigma as a barrier to recovery: Adverse effects of perceived stigma on social adaption of persons diagnosed with bipolar affective disorder. *Psychiatric Services, 52,* 1627–1632.

Rodwell, J., & Martin, A. (2013). The importance of the supervisor for the mental health and work attitudes of Australian aged care nurses. *International Psychogeriatrics, 25*(3), 382–389. doi:10.1017/S1041610212001883

Rosenfield, S. (1997). Labeling mental illness: The effects of received services and perceived stigma on life satisfaction. *American Sociological Reviews, 62,* 660–672.

Ross, C. A., & Goldner, E. M. (2009). Stigma, negative attitudes and discrimination towards mental illness within the nursing profession: A review of the literature. *Journal of Psychiatric and Mental Health Nursing, 16*(6), 558–567. doi:10.1111/j.1365-2850.2009.01399.x

Rudan, P. (2010). *Nurse's gambling addiction led to $32,000 fraud.* Retrieved from http://www.nsgamingfoundation.org/newsAnnouncementsView.aspx/816/Nurse%E2%80%99s-gambling-addiction-led-to-32,000-fraud

Sirey, J. A., Bruce, M. L., Alexopoulos, G. S., Perlick, D. A., Friedman, S. J., & Meyers, B. S. (2001). Stigma as a barrier to recovery: Perceived stigma and patient-related severity of illness as predictors of antidepressant drug adherence. *Psychiatric Services, 52,* 1615–1620.

Storch, J. (2007). Building moral communities in health care. *Nursing Ethics, 14*(5), 569–570.

Stuart, H. (2004). Stigma and work. *Healthcare Papers, 5,* 100.

Tim Field Foundation. (1996). *Narcissistic personality disorder: Narcissists, NPD and the serial bully.* Retrieved from http://www.bullyonline.org/workbully/npd.htm

University of Washington School of Social Work. (2014). *Facts about mental illness and violence.* Retrieved from http://depts.washington.edu/mhreport/facts_violence.php

Wallace, J. E. (2012). Mental health and stigma in the medical profession. *Health, 16*(1), 3–18. doi:10.1177/1363459310371080

Watson, A. C., Corrigan, P., Larson, J. E., & Sells, M. (2007). Self-stigma in people with mental illness. *Schizophrenia Bulletin, 33*(6), 1312–1318.

Williams, R. B. (2012). *The silent tsunami: Mental health in the workplace.* Retrieved from http://www.psychologytoday.com/blog/wired-success/201209/the-silent-tsunami-mental-health-in-the-workplace

Wrigley, S., Jackson, H., Judd, F., & Komiti, A. (2005). Role of stigma and attitudes toward help-seeking from a general practitioner for mental health problems in a rural town. *Australian New Zealand Journal of Psychiatry, 39,* 514–521.

12

Meeting the Mental Health Needs of Employees: A Personal Approach

God doesn't require us to succeed; He only requires that you try.
—*Mother Teresa*

LEARNING OBJECTIVES

By the end of this chapter, the learner will be able to:

1. Discuss some of the major interventions nurses can practice to help protect their own mental health at work.
2. Discuss how many different coping strategies may or may not fit into your lifestyle or belief framework.
3. Highlight the value of sleep for how it can help you deal with stress and challenges to your mental health.
4. Identify some commonalities of dealing with workplace negativity, workplace conflict, and backstabbing colleagues.
5. Discuss the value of the Golden Rule, talking to someone, eating right, and relaxing in strengthening your own mental health.

There is much truth to the old adage that "no one is going to look after you, only you." There are many personal directions that you, as a person, nurse, and colleague, can take to best promote and meet the mental health needs of your colleagues and yourself. If you recall what we highlighted earlier, you spend approximately 30% of your life at work, so you have to become instrumental in making the workplace one of respect, comfort, and collegiality, not only for your colleagues but for yourself as well. In essence, you have to be in control of your own attitudes, thoughts, decisions, and behaviors, as well as your desires and wishes. It is part of your own professional responsibility and moral obligation that you and all nurses just like you do your best to make your workplace a mentally healthy one. This chapter will highlight many different concepts and strategies that relate to your own mental health, what you can do to stay mentally healthy, and how you can address some of your most mentally taxing colleagues. To achieve such goals, you often need to look at your inner self and the lived experiences you have endured, and in doing so, you need to remember that no one will look after you as well as you will. Finding courage, strength, and motivation, you are in the driver's seat and in control to promote and maintain good mental health and to make your workplace a favorable environment for all.

WHAT YOU CAN DO

We have already talked about work–life balance and its role in preventing the development of mental health challenges among nurses. You need to enact this philosophy throughout your life and career trajectory at all times. As you face adversity, challenging patients, and disgruntled coworkers, you need to maintain your stance and balance so that none have increased leverage over what you can actually handle and deal with at any one time.

Always do your best. If you know you have tried your best and did not succeed then, you will just try again next time. Aim for quality of care delivery, so practice with honesty and integrity. You need to recognize that your own career is like a small business operation (Bowman, 2012), so recognize those boundaries at work, get to know your employer and patients, become involved in committees and interest groups, and show that you're interested. Be flexible, open, adaptable, and ready for change. Developmentally, you need to define who you are and what you can offer (self-awareness). You have a unique value, so recognize and use it, seek out continuing education and competency opportunities, and always practice a good work ethic. Also, you need to recognize the environment and how it can potentially impact your work area, so increase your awareness and understanding of issues pertaining to your area of work, media releases, and research, and become a self-professed expert.

TAKE CARE OF YOURSELF

Nurses are often really good at taking care of others and their patients, but they are not so great at taking care of themselves. As we highlighted earlier, their broad knowledge base has perhaps contributed to this problem. In essence, to continue being the good nurse that you are, you must also learn to listen to your own body and take care of yourself (Virginia, 2008). Taking care of yourself is more easily said than done for most of us. We are so used to taking care of others that our own health, thought processes, and stress levels go virtually unchecked.

Virginia (2008) suggests that the vast majority of nurses are still women, and women have been stereotyped by society to be the ones who are the "caretakers" and "nurturers," looking after and nurturing the needs of others as opposed to their own. The notion of nurses as handmaidens for doctors reinforces this stereotype (Hallam, 1998) and creates a ripe, fertile environment that causes nurses to end up "feeling conflicted, unappreciated, resentful, and burned out" (Virginia, 2008).

However, when it comes to tips about addressing the gap that nurses often experience blindly within themselves, both male and female nurses would be well advised to remain cognizant of the following recommendations from Virginia (2008): Take care of yourself; it allows you to better take care of others. Use your empathy and nurturing for yourself; care for and understand yourself with the same expertise you give your patients. Say no when you want to; if you have a hard time saying no, offer alternatives (I can't do that but I can do this); avoiding situations where you will be asked to do too much is really okay. Increase your self-awareness; unwind after work before you jump into your responsibilities at home (do not use alcohol to unwind). Do not base all your self-worth on your profession or your nurturing abilities; develop outside interests. If you volunteer, choose opportunities that have nothing to do with helping others! Don't identify with patients too much. Identify your feelings, and accept and allow them; this does not mean you have to act on them! Friendships where you can talk about your feelings are critical. Practice stress reduction techniques (exercise, relaxation, meditation, distraction); plan for regular breaks, days off, conferences, and vacations. Talk with colleagues to make plans for burnout prevention, take charge where you can, avoid chronic complainers, and know when to say "enough," or consider a transfer or a different area of practice if necessary.

For all of us, work is only one part of life's journey. Although we spend approximately 30% of our life working, we do have other lives and responsibilities outside work. These often take the form of family obligations, commitment to friends and personal activities, and interests of our own. Nurses are not just nurses; they are also sisters and brothers, mothers and fathers, daughters and sons, aunts and uncles, and granddaughters and grandsons. In addition, to increase the complexities of life, they may also be single parents, foster parents, widows, or caregivers to an elderly parent. From a societal perspective, nurses may also fulfill various roles, such as being a good friend and support, girl guide/scout leader, volunteer, or community leader/advocate.

When it comes to dealing with stress, there are many simple things you can do other than use the coping mechanisms identified later in this chapter. For example, simple things like becoming more organized, better managing your time, and making changes such as leaving your house earlier to avoid rush hour traffic all can help to lessen the amount of stress you experience. Further, plan ahead, and if you feel you are having trouble remembering things, write them down in your calendar or enter them into the scheduler of your smart phone, BlackBerry, or other personal electronic device.

THE GOLDEN RULE

No matter who you are, what you do or did and what you know, the Golden Rule will always apply. You need to treat others the way you would like to be treated yourself. As sometimes, what goes around comes around. As has been threaded through many of these chapters, treating others with respect and in the way you would like to be treated yourself can forestall many negative evils of the workplace, such as negative people, difficult personalities, condescending coworkers, and abusive patients. The Golden Rule will help you and the nurse leader to build commitment, respect, integrity, and a workplace that breeds positive mental health for all.

DON'T ASSUME ANYTHING

As identified in Chapter 6, you can never assume anything. At times, nurses can become distracted, preoccupied, and not really see the full picture as they are trying to multitask. Making assumptions can stress your own mental health for fear that you did or said something wrong unintentionally, and it also sets you up for failure and mistakes. Because assumptions can be predicated on gossip and rumors, avoid making assumptions at all costs and learn the facts first before passing judgment or being hard on yourself and others.

RECOGNIZE YOUR PROFESSIONAL AND LEGAL OBLIGATIONS

In Chapter 6, you learned how you as an individual can proactively prevent stress and your response to stress, and you also learned briefly of the standards of practice and the role that you play in providing ethical, legal, and safe patient care. Throughout the duration of your career, adhering to your standards of practice, your professionalism, and your common respect and courtesy will go far in helping you cope and deal with mentally challenging situations and people that you face in your daily work.

COPING

Nurses are often the most numerous health care professionals in a health care organization. Nurses are very astute at meeting the needs of their clients and others, but very little of their time and effort is devoted to caring for themselves and meeting their own health care needs. It is therefore perhaps even more important that nurses learn to recognize their stressors, their levels of stress, and the impact these can have on their bodies. Further, it is important to deal with workplace stress at the time, so that it doesn't lead to more serious symptoms.

In Chapter 1, we talked a lot about stress, different sources of stress, and the impact stress has on our bodies and minds. Now we are going to focus on how you as an individual can help yourself identify, deal with, and learn from stressful events, all of which help strengthen your own mental health and enhance the rigor with which you can respond successfully to other increasingly stressful events. However, you have to remember that people perceive, experience, and respond to stress in very different ways, so what works for your colleague may not necessarily work for you. Knowing your own body and the stressors that affect it is half the battle in responding productively to stress. For example, knowing the triggers of your stress can help better prepare you to respond to it once it does occur.

Effective interventions to combat stress in the workplace aim to develop the coping skills of employees and build a supportive environment. They can involve training in stress management and relaxation techniques, reducing noise, improving role clarity, managing conflict, and building healthy social relationships (Hosman & Jané-Llopis, 2005; Jané-Llopis, Barry, Hosman, & Patel, 2005). Individual interventions do not work as well as approaches that focus on system-level policy change. These should combine elements of both health promotion and illness prevention if they are to be effective at reducing job stress, such as policies to address workplace bullying and harassment (Keleher & Armstrong, 2005). Whether you're dealing with deadlines, boredom, bullies, or how company reorganization will affect your job, these tactics can help you manage workplace stress (Pfizer, 2014). Dealing with stress, particularly in the workplace, is not an easy task, and it can take a great amount of time. It is something you need to consciously be aware of and keep trying to achieve; in the end, it will be well worth the effort as it will provide you with effective coping strategies to help you deal with not just workplace stress but stress in other areas of your life as well. The following are some of the many tactics that exist to help you deal with stress and stressors and that act as an effective guide to help you achieve work–life balance (Canadian Mental Health Association [CMHA], 2014; Tomey, 2009; Yoder-Wise, 2011). It is important to deal with workplace stress now, so that it doesn't lead to more serious symptoms later. Learning to deal with stress takes time, but in the end you will develop coping strategies that will help you in many areas of your life—not just at work.

We all encounter different stressors, and we deal with those stressors in very different and individualized ways. There is no "one-size-fits-all" approach when it comes to dealing with stress. Helping others can be a very rewarding, self-fulfilling, and satisfying career, but it cannot come at the expense of our own health and mental well-being. As Virginia (2008) suggests, recognition of your own level of stress and needs for self-care is the first step to stress reduction and burnout prevention. We all need to "make self-care a priority." You are the agent of the change you want to see in the world. You are in control of your life, and this is the foundation of stress management, as "managing stress is all about taking charge of your thoughts, emotions, schedule, and the way you deal with problems" (Smith & Segal, 2013). While stress, anxiety, and compassion fatigue can be prevented, their mere presence and the fact that they have crept into our demeanor should be perceived as an indicator that something needs to be done to make a much-needed change to help restore our equilibrium.

Coping refers to "the thoughts and actions we use to deal with stress" (Kelly, 2010) and gives us strategies to best handle the stress presented to us, whether it is real or imagined. Although you may often feel at your wits' end—not knowing where to go, what to do, or where to turn—you have to remember that you are always in control. Acknowledgement of this control is what you need to remember to best control the stress (or should I say the "perception of stress") confronting you. Just as we all perceive and experience stress and stressors very differently, so too does our coping with stress and stressors become individualized. Only you, yourself, know if your coping strategies are working for you. Be aware of what triggers your stress and how you react. You may be able to avoid some of the triggers and learn to prepare for or manage others. Stress is a part of life and affects people in different ways. It becomes a problem only when it makes you feel uncomfortable or distressed. A balanced lifestyle can help you manage stress better. If you have trouble winding down, you may find that relaxation breathing, yoga, or meditation can help (Boyd et al., 2013).

Your perceptions, habits, attitudes, and excuses are also important to recognize, and as well as the fact that they may vary (Smith & Segal, 2013). For example, you cannot explain away stress as temporary. It is not part of your personality, and you cannot blame your stress on other people or outside events or view it as entirely normal and unexceptional. There are positive and negative coping strategies in life. Don't be afraid to ask for help. This can be as simple as asking a friend to babysit while you have some time out or speaking to your primary care physician about where to find a counselor or community mental health service. The perfect, worry-free life does not exist. Everyone's life journey has some bumpy terrain, and the people around you can help. If you don't get the help you need at first, keep asking until you do (Boyd et al., 2013).

Positive coping strategies would include things like exercising and eating better. The actual coping strategies used may very well be making the situation more stressful and worse for you than it already is (Smith & Segal, 2013). Positive coping strategies, such as relaxation techniques, visualization or imagery, and exercise, serve to relieve stress, improve sleep, promote positivism, and boost self-esteem and confidence. With your eye on being positive, it is helpful also to forget what you don't want and save your energy to focus on what you do want (Koffman, 2013), go for the gold, and succeed in what you want by committing yourself and staying motivated. Success is what gives you pleasure, but integrity in getting there is what will give you happiness. Meditation, acupuncture, massage therapy, eating spicy food, and breathing deeply—these all cause your body to produce endorphins naturally. Endorphins are the body's physiological brain-enhancing chemicals that promote positive mental health and elevated mood and reduce anxiety (Rattue, 2012).

However, *negative coping strategies* can include such things as overeating, smoking, drinking alcohol, and using drugs. Further, as found by Johansen (2012), conflict-avoidant management style was used to resolve conflicting priorities because emergency department nurses felt there was not enough time to address conflict, even though it could impact work stress and patient care. If your methods of coping with stress aren't contributing to your greater emotional and physical health, it's time to find healthier ones. Whichever option you choose, the four A's will assist you in this process (Smith & Segal, 2013):

1. **Avoid** unnecessary stress and address the stress you absolutely need to right here and now; don't waste your energy and brain power on stress you can't control. Learning how to say no can help you with this, so know your limits and stick to them. Surround yourself with calm, positive, and happy people as anxiousness can be contagious. Take control of your environment, and avoid controversial topics such as religion and politics. Prioritize what you need to do between the "shoulds" and the "musts."

2. **Alter** the stressor/situation if you can't avoid it. Figure out what you can do to change things so the problem doesn't present itself in the future. Express your feelings instead of bottling them up to avoid resentment. Compromise and deal with problems head on. Take a break to recharge your mind and body; rest, go ahead and read that book, or take that much-needed vacation.

3. **Adapt** to the stressor and change yourself, your values, or your attitudes if you can't change the stressor so that you still have some sense of control. Reframe your problems through a positive lens, pause, regroup your thoughts, and look at the big picture; is this worry really worth it? You may have to adjust your standards. Remember, no one is perfect, not even you!
4. **Accept** the stressor if you can't control any part of it, like the death of a loved one. Acceptance may be difficult. Look at what you can learn from it, share your feelings, and learn to forgive.

Managing your emotions, such as anger, fear, and frustration, is an important step as you try to cope with daily stressors. Identify those stress triggers, write them down (doing so decreases their power over you), pay attention to what works so that you keep on the right track, and talk to a friend. Take a break and go for a walk, find a quiet place to sit, or otherwise relax and refocus. Do not work through breaks and lunch when you are stressed, and of course don't forget to breathe so that the brain oxygen supplies remain adequate. As found by Ward (2011), the way in which nurses manage their stress is often intrinsically linked to their job satisfaction. Setting realistic goals, enjoying yourself and having fun, maintaining a healthy lifestyle, and talking also help to address stress in a healthy way (Mental Health Foundation, 2013). Finally, you need to accept who you are, or else you will never be happy or content with who you are and what you do.

A balance of work and life achieved with good coping skills enables you to better look outside the box to see more clearly what is making you distressed and uncomfortable. Seeing this then helps you to better manage stress. Boyd et al. (2013) in an open discussion suggest that you must know what coping mechanisms do and do not work for you. Some suggestions include:

1. Stay away from a state of "vegetation" or defensiveness. Use the coping skills.
2. Anger is a secondary emotion. If you are angry about something, there is an underlying primary reason for the anger.
3. Don't let any of the coping skills become addictive or controlling.
4. Think before you speak in order to say only positive or harmless words.
5. Keep your room, desktop, and workplace neat and organized; you will feel happier with organized thoughts.
6. Practice the five coping skills. They are a career (not necessarily your present job), positive support systems, exercise and health, a hobby, and spiritualism (Wong, 2013).
7. Use a journal to process emotions because writing things down helps put them into perspective.

Further activities to help you cope with stress do exist. These range from such things as yoga, massage, relaxation exercises, and visual imagery to mindfulness-based stress reduction (Marchand, 2013) and cognitive behavioral therapy.

Not all suggested coping strategies work. As I said before, no one size fits all. For example, emotional coping was not so helpful because it increased all outcomes of anxiety, depression, and somatic complaints (Adriaenssens, de Gucht, & Maes,

2012). Similarly, avoidance also served to increase the rate of somatic complaints; however, problem-focused coping did help to decrease psychological distress and perceived fatigue (Adriaenssens et al., 2012).

EXERCISE AND ACTIVITY

The value of exercise and physical activity in promoting good mental health is significant. Exercise not only helps you feel good about yourself physically but also enhances positive mental health.

Exercise promotes the release of many different chemicals and neurotransmitters in the brain that serve different purposes to promote good mental health. Endorphin is one neurotransmitter that is increasingly released by the brain when you exercise (Holmes, 2010). These natural opiates are chemically similar to morphine and boost activity in the brain's frontal lobes and hippocampus. Animal studies have found that exercise increases levels of other chemical neurotransmitters, such as serotonin, dopamine, and norepinephrine, that elevate mood (Holmes, 2010); increases levels of "brain-derived neurotrophic factor" (Rattue, 2012), which improves mood; promotes brain cell longevity, as seen in studies of dementia (Holmes, 2010); improves memory and learning; and even helps to control attention deficit hyperactivity disorder (ADHD) behaviors (Rattue, 2012). Further, it decreases the risk for depression (CMHA, 2014); decreases the abuse of drugs and alcohol (CMHA, 2013); reduces stress and anxiety (CMHA, 2013; Mental Health Foundation, 2013; Smith & Segal, 2013); elevates mood; decreases fatigue and anger (CMHA, 2013; Mental Health Foundation, 2013); and gets you out so that you interact with other people and make friends in social venues (CMHA, 2013).

Physically, exercise promotes a greater sense of self and body image; you look and feel really good about yourself. Hence, our levels of self-worth, confidence, and self-esteem rise (Mental Health Foundation, 2013). Even a hobby or passion can allow you to express your emotions and so can help to relax your mind, flush out the stress, and enable you to cope. Further, exercise helps to increase our attention and concentration, lift our mood, and prevent depression (Smith & Segal, 2013). Even taking the stairs as opposed to the elevator can increase your level of physical activity and keep the endorphins and serotonin flowing. Further, exercise promotes good sleep (Mental Health Foundation, 2013), clears the mind, improves blood circulation, and supplies the brain with more oxygen (Rattue, 2012); it also provides a natural energy boost, a sense of achievement, a focus in life and motivation, a healthy appetite, and a better social life to meet others (Mental Health Foundation, 2013).

It is important to recognize that you don't have to pay a lot of money and go to the gym to exercise when you can simply garden, vacuum, dance, and climb the stairs. Even shopping gets you moving around much more than just being sedentary at home watching TV. Combining physical activity with a balanced diet to nourish your body and mind keeps you feeling good inside and outside.

Taking your lunch break outside and including a brisk walk are ways to incorporate exercise into your busy schedule; nothing beats that natural high. A mere 30-minute session five times a week is not too much to ask to obtain such phenomenal benefits as exercise provides for our mental health.

SLEEP

Getting plenty of sleep, I am sure, is something many of you are so "tired" of hearing about. (Please pardon the pun.) Physically, sleep helps you feel refreshed, energized, and rejuvenated. The spinoffs of the physical benefits of sleep also merge to support and add to the mental health benefits of sleep. Hence, sleep plays a major role in promoting and maintaining good mental health (Karkoulias et al., 2013).

Although scientists at Harvard are still trying to tease apart all the mechanisms involved, sleep disruption affects levels of neurotransmitters and stress hormones; among other things, it wreaks havoc in the brain, impairing thinking and emotional regulation. In this way, insomnia may amplify the effects of psychiatric disorders. Studies report that REM sleep enhances learning and memory and contributes to emotional health in complex ways (Harvard Medical School, 2009). Even sleep-deprived patients who spent time in the intensive care unit (ICU) had impaired mental health scores following their transfer from that setting (McKinley et al., 2012).

Sleep serves many mental health purposes. It promotes good working memory (Kuriyama, Mishima, Suzuki, Aritake, & Uchiyama, 2008) and cognitive recognition (Schroder, 2010). In addition, it can prevent the onset of mental illnesses (Sloan, 2011), help the brain reorganize to adopt newly learned skills (Hitti, 2005), and even decrease hostility and aggression (Kamphuis, Meerlo, Koolhaas, & Lancel, 2012).

Sleep is a particularly important topic for nurses because many nurses work night shifts, which go against the circadian rhythm. Sleep has been found to increase the experience of happiness, concentration, the stability and strength of relationships, and energy levels; it makes one more receptive to positive emotions and decreases the risk for developing depression (Netdoctor, 2012). Dr. Robotham, senior researcher at the Mental Health Foundation, adds that "we use the phrase 'sleep on it' because sleep helps you process and assimilate new knowledge." If you're sleeping badly, you're more likely to make errors at work and lack your normal concentration, sharpness, and creativity. While everybody has the odd bad night, persistently poor sleep will leave you feeling mentally drained and inattentive, and your brain not functioning well.

You need to go to bed at a regular time each day and practice good habits to get better sleep and plenty of it. Sleep restores both your mind and your body. Allow yourself some unfocused time each day to refresh; for example, let your mind daydream. It's all right to add "do nothing" to your to-do list. Schedule into your calendar a blank space to do nothing. Jeff Weiner (2013), chief executive officer of LinkedIn, emphasizes the importance of scheduling nothing for yourself. Realistically, we know that for many front-line nurses this is often not possible except during their assigned scheduled breaks. Therefore, nurses working at the front line in all settings, particularly those in very busy acute emergency room (ER), medical–surgical, mental health, ICU, and critical care unit (CCU) settings, need to make sure they do just that, take their breaks from everything and view them as a short-term relief to catch their breath, talk light social talk, and sink into that comfy lounge chair. Taking breaks as scheduled time-out is the "best investment a person can make for [him- or herself]" (Weiner, 2013).

FOOD FOR THOUGHT

The old adage "you are what you eat" is just as true for health and well-being as it is for mental health. Nutrition is a new and rising area of research and discovery, and the selection of specific foods can actually strengthen the mind, as well as memory, perception, and concentration, and it can actually help ward off mental illnesses. Eating was the most frequently cited coping mechanism among nurses, followed by exercise (Nahm, Warren, Zhu, An, & Brown, 2012), so if you are going to eat to cope, let's do this proactively so you can enhance your own mental health physiologically as well. Omega-3 fatty acids, polyunsaturated fats, flavonoids, amino acids, vitamins (folate, B_6, B_{12}, C, E), minerals (zinc, magnesium, copper, selenium, iron), antioxidants, and glucose all act to enhance neurotransmitter effects and membrane function (Sathyanarayana Rao, Asha, Ramesh, & Jagannatha Rao, 2008).

From a mental health perspective, *vitamins* C and E exert an antioxidant effect and help to "clean" the brain. Vitamin deficiencies, in particular, can manifest as depression and cause mood swings, anxiety, and agitation (Mental Health Foundation, 2013).

Minerals, such as magnesium, along with the B-vitamin complex, help to decrease signs and symptoms of depression. Omega-3 fatty acids, such as those found in fish, nuts, herbs, spices, and olive oil, improve memory, recall, focus, and concentration (Holecko, 2013). Add the antioxidant power of nuts, in particular, and you also get increased mood stability and decreased insomnia.

Antioxidants, defined as "substances, found in foods, which inhibit oxidation in the body's cells" (oxidation is a chemical reaction that produces free radicals or molecules that damage DNA; Holecko, 2013), are found in omega-3 fatty acid foods. Dark berries, tomatoes, and citrus fruits contain a lot of antioxidants, which prevent oxidative brain cell damage and brain deterioration. By adding bananas to your diet, you can reduce fatigue and elevate your mood.

Flavonoids, found in black and green teas, bright-colored berries, and citrus fruits, help to maintain and improve memory, prevent damage to brain cells, and can even repair damaged cells, so that neurotransmission and neuromuscular function are not impaired or compromised.

Dairy products, such as milk and milk products, help to decrease fatigue, repair brain cell damage, stabilize mood, and promote feelings of general well-being.

Although many try to avoid carbohydrates for fear of weight gain, "good" carbohydrates in the form of brown rice, whole wheat products, oats, and quinoa stimulate the brain to increase its release of serotonin, which elevates mood and decreases the risk for depression.

Poultry products, including chicken, turkey, and eggs, contain various amino acids, such as tyrosine and tryptophan. These decrease stress levels; promote relaxation, restfulness, and tranquility; and elevate mood and decrease irritability, particularly when they interact with serotonin.

Dr. Felice Jacka and colleagues from Deakin University and the University of Melbourne, Australia, found that when women regularly consumed a diet of vegetables, fruit, whole grains, and high-quality meat and fish, their risk for anxiety disorders and major and chronic depression decreased by more than 30% (Cassels, 2011). Unequivocally, diets including excessive amounts of fat (particularly saturated and trans fats) and diets high in calories are associated with an increased risk for mental health conditions, so it is best to keep saturated fats (hydrogenated fat, animal fat, fat in processed meats, high-fat cheese and desserts) to a minimum if you want to enjoy good mental health. As highlighted by Cassels (2011), people who ate this "Western" type of diet had a 50% increased chance for depression and a greater risk for ADHD, Alzheimer's disease, and schizophrenia (Mental Health Foundation, 2013). Researchers add that trying to shortchange the brain also shortchanges the intellectual and emotional potential of the brain. Mental health professionals point out that good eating habits are vital for people wanting to optimize the effectiveness of medications used to treat mental illnesses and cope with their possible side effects.

In a simplistic approach to living, some other uncomplicated and inexpensive means of busting stress include simplifying your life by assessing your time management and setting your priorities, thinking positively, and trying to avoid negative thinking and overanalyzing what coworkers have said or done, as these can distort your perception and increase your stress levels. Also remember to laugh by sharing a joke with a colleague, curling up at home with a comedy on TV, and looking for the humor in every challenging situation. Developing new skills can also help as they can increase your assertiveness, ability to communicate, and professional etiquette and teach you how to say no (Pfizer, 2014).

LEARN TO RELAX

Take those well-deserved breaks. Nurses are so often "run off their feet" that they forget to take their break or feel they don't have time. Spending time away from your job can be the most positive thing you can do when you are feeling stressed. A week or so away can have a huge impact on your approach and attitude toward your work when you return. Try to make the most of time with family and friends who are not connected with your workplace. Your work is important, but it should not take over your life. Try to ensure that you have some other activities that stimulate a different part of your brain, such as making better use of time with your family, doing something creative like learning an instrument or starting a hobby, going for walks, exercising, or engaging in a sports activity.

Relaxation techniques are also a good practice to help you relax. For example, deep breathing, medication, mindfulness, and visual imagery can all help to relax your body, get you connected with reality, and improve your overall well-being, including your mental health.

Seeking help and making lifestyle changes can also prove beneficial. For example, eating healthier and exercising, as previously discussed, help to reduce tension, increase quality of sleep, and build self-esteem.

TALK TO SOMEONE

Talking to someone is perhaps one the best forms of therapy you can engage in to deal with stress and promote your good mental health. A friend, a spouse, a confidant, a coworker, or even a trained counselor can help you express your inner feelings, stress, and frustrations. Counseling or just talking serves to relieve stress and provides an outlet for negative energy, which can help you to see things from a better perspective, relieve some of the stress you were experiencing, and work optimally. Even talking to your organization through an employee assistance program can help, and yes, it is kept confidential.

ADDRESSING CONFLICT IN YOUR WORKPLACE

In Chapter 5, we talked about the role of the leader in preventing workplace conflict, and in Chapter 13, we will discuss how leaders can manage workplace conflict. However, there is much that you can do for yourself when faced with such a stress-provoking event as workplace conflict. Personality conflicts are perhaps by far most commonly experienced in organizations (Fredrickson, 2013), particularly in health care and nursing. These can compromise the quality of your work and personal life and destroy morale, and at toxic levels they can strain your mental health. Again, while you cannot change others' behaviors and actions, you can control your own behavior and reactions.

To help address and, it is hoped, resolve workplace conflict with others, Fredrickson (2013) suggests that you avoid discussing an issue with other colleagues because it can create "polarization" and "escalate the situation." Second, "never respond immediately to the person" who is bothering you; think your response through. Third, reflect on your own characteristics and what role you may be playing in this conflict, and "focus on what you can do differently." Next, you need to reframe the situation, step back, look at the broader picture, and not engage. Focusing on the other person's strength may also help you to acquire insight on how to get the problem resolved. "Use cooperative communication" to genuinely interact with the other person as you offer to work mutually with the person to end the conflict, and offer to listen to his or her ideas. Finally, document all interactions in a factual manner; you may need this documentation to help build your case later.

In general, nurses must address conflict rather than avoid or postpone it, and they must focus on the behaviors that created the conflict as opposed to the personal attributes of the colleague. Further, nurses should validate assumptions through open dialogue with colleagues rather than assume things, and they should collaborate with colleagues to identify the underlying cause of the conflict; a neutral party, such as a mediator, may also be used if needed.

DEALING WITH BACKSTABBING COLLEAGUES

Of late, backstabbing in the workplace has become a growing topic of concern in society and on various media platforms. Perhaps this is because we are living in a world where competition has significantly and noticeably increased.

As nurses engaging in a lot of teamwork and having close relations with your colleagues all day and all night, your colleagues should be your most valuable resource and mainstay of support. However, not every colleague is your ally or source of support (Phillips, 2012). When you work and interact with backstabbing individuals, you will always be watching your p's and q's for fear that they will take whatever you say or do and turn it against you to your detriment. Often at the very foundation of conflict, disrespect, bullying, and organizational politics and bureaucracies, backstabbing colleagues seek to sabotage your efforts. There are always people out there who will try to make themselves look good at the expense of making you look bad. As an individual who is battling a backstabbing colleague, you need courage, patience, charisma, and motivation, and once you realize the impact that the situation can have on you and your mental health, I am quite certain these driving traits will bring you to an area where you can deal with such a person.

You need first to deal with the issue, and do so immediately. As if you are taking a bull by the horns, you need to deal with the issue head on and let the colleague know you are not going to tolerate the backstabbing any further; if you do not, the individual will deem it successful and continue. However, be professional and discreet and genuinely ask the person "why" he or she is attacking you, so that it is known you will not be a pushover. Avoiding this encounter and pretending that the backstabbing did not occur may set you up for even more damage. As a professional and a genuine, caring person, you need to rise above such behaviors and let the colleague know you will not stoop to his or her level. Carry on with your duties and astute level of professionalism, even if you are still working side by side. Next, you need to use the proper channels and hierarchy of reporting, beginning with your immediate supervisor and reaching up to your human resources personnel. Bring your documented details with you as evidence. You also need to stay focused on the tasks of taking care of your patients because this person is just watching and waiting for you to make a mistake and to pounce. As a final option after exhausting all others, you can throw in the towel and move on; the risks to your own mental health are really not worth it. Keep your chin up and look for a brighter future (Phillips, 2012).

OVERCOMING WORKPLACE NEGATIVITY

Negative attitudes spread to the point where they eventually affect performance and decision making. That's the bad news. The good news is that enthusiasm and positive attitudes spread just as quickly and affect performance just as much—in the right direction. Negative attitudes are a lot like the common cold. It can start with just one employee, but soon everyone is feeling the effects, and morale and performance decline. However, unlike for the common cold, there's a cure. Enthusiasm and positive attitudes can spread just as quickly, improving performance and increasing productivity (Dale Carnegie, 2013).

To overcome workplace negativity, there are many strategies you can entertain. Barriers can be turned into opportunities, so "look at negative behaviors and attitudes as opportunities for improvement." Avoid the negative thoughts so as to not damper your self-esteem and self-confidence and create self-doubt and perceived failure. Second, replace negative self-talk with positive self-talk to produce positive actions and results. Third, build relationships based on trust, and do so with enthusiasm to influence positive change, increase comfort levels, and strengthen relationships. Fourth, win people to your way of thinking. "The only way to win an argument is to avoid it." View disagreements and debates as opportunities for positive change. "When disagreements arise, show respect for the opinions of others, never tell someone they are wrong, and try to see things from the other point of view" (Dale Carnegie, 2013). Finally, disagree agreeably so that you can keep the lines of communication open and try to see things from a different perspective. Take the time to really think about how the other person feels and why.

You can take action yourself. Regardless of the source of negativity, you can't control it, but you surely can help improve upon it and create a more positive atmosphere. However, if you can identify what is causing the negativity, it can help you to address it. If the negativity is impacting morale, you need to come right out and say it to your nurses—that you recognize that morale is suffering, but you would like to work with them to correct it. You need to implement any strategies at your earliest convenience and in so doing keep the lines of communication and your approach open.

Heathfield (2013) offers some tips you can use to manage ongoing workplace negativity. These include actions such as involving people and giving them the opportunity to participate in decision making, treating people with fairness and consistency, helping people to fit in, helping people to grow and develop supportively, and providing appropriate leadership, whether you are a mentor, a preceptor, a patient care coordinator, or a supervisor. You can be the very person who can begin to make all of the difference in the workplace and battle the low morale that is currently choking your unit.

Assertiveness can go a long way in eliminating negativity at work. For example, if you assertively deal with gossip, you will create a work culture and environment that do not support gossip (Heathfield, 2013). There are other things you can do to help reduce or eliminate workplace negativity. Identify aspects of the situation through which you can provide feedback to whoever needs to hear it. Next, you need to listen, listen, listen, so be visible and available to staff and schedule group discussion sessions. Challenge pessimistic thinking and negative beliefs, and provide the rationale and everything you know about a situation to build or reestablish trust.

If you are the one being targeted, inform the person about the negative impact he or she is having on you. Avoid becoming defensive, focus on creating solutions, focus on the person's positive aspects, and compliment the individual any time you hear a positive statement (Heathfield, 2013).

You actually may be part of the problem with workplace negativity, so recognize this. For example, you are only human and may oppose some work decisions. Not to be pessimistic but to be credible and trustworthy, know yourself and your own "hot buttons" well enough to recognize internally when you are becoming negative. Take a time-out or walk away by yourself when feeling stressed, spend time each day thinking about the positive aspects and your achievements, treat yourself with care, and don't beat yourself up or second-guess yourself; after all, you are only human. Finally, you need to focus on the big picture and not get bogged down in the day-to-day issues. Remember, you and only you are in charge of how you choose to reach out to stressful situations and people.

The expression "misery loves company" rings true when it comes to spreading negativity around the workplace (Rosenberg McKay, 2013) because those who have negative feelings will first seek out others who may feel the same way and then try to influence those who don't. Negativity, believe it or not, can actually be positive in the sense that "it can bring existing problems out of the darkness." Once out in the open, problems can then be dealt with and addressed. By making your criticism constructive, taking action, and not trying to fix what isn't broken, you can help to turn negativity into something positive and productive (Rosenberg McKay, 2013).

For yourself and your own physical and mental health, you need to deal with difficult people and coworkers. These difficult colleagues compete with you and undermine you and others for various things, such as power, privilege, and attention; therefore, how difficult it is for you to deal with this kind of person really depends on your own self-esteem, confidence, professional courage, coping skills, and practical know-how. Difficult people must be dealt with for various reasons, including that the situation will only get worse, not better, as it festers underneath and then explodes to the surface counterproductively at work. Also, after the shock of being treated unprofessionally and realizing what it meant, you can be angry, so it's better to address the difficult person while you can maintain some objectivity and emotional control. Further, if you are constantly complaining about someone's unprofessional and rude tactics, you will quickly "earn the title of a whiner or complainer." Finally, this series of events can turn against you and be blamed on you if not addressed in a timely manner because people then wonder why you aren't able to handle the situation like the mature professional you claim to be. Worse still is if your organization terminates you because it perceives you as a high-maintenance nurse.

To address the difficult coworker, you have many options. Whichever route you take, it is important for you to realize that at least you are doing something about the situation, and this is a strength of yours. For example, a first place you might visit would be your immediate superior or manager, who hopefully can take matters into his or her own hands and try to rectify the situation locally at first. Next, if nothing has been done or no action taken, you will move up the hierarchy to the director or vice president or to the human resources department. "Without making personal attacks, calmly state *the behavior* that's bothering you, and ask if something can be done" (Scott, 2012). Some human resources departments may even have outlined in their policies the use of an external mediator to help resolve this type of situation. Second, you need to address the offending person. You need to be assertive, to speak up politely but firmly and clearly that you do not appreciate the negative comments. Even if you get no response, at least you get to speak your mind and make the person aware of how you are being made to feel. Third, if these issues are only minor and don't bother you too much, just let them roll like water off a duck's back. You need to pick your battles and ask yourself if this one is worth fighting or using up your energy on. Finally, you can seek new employment. If you have done everything you can possibly do, you may opt to find another job or location. The aggravating stress that this individual can cause you is truly not worth your own mental health. Although it may seem as if the person is getting what he or she wanted, at least you may find a new home with more collegiality and, most importantly, a healthier you.

At perhaps one time or another, you will meet and work with people who are quite toxic. They are not toxic in any chemical sense, but in a social and interpersonal relationship sense. These are individuals who complain a lot, blame others for their wrongdoings, and overreact. They drain your energy because you are constantly trying to fend off their negativity or even boost their spirits. You may even sometimes "hate to see them coming towards you" or become angry at them because of how they make your feel after interactions (Paolino, 2013).

Just as a smile can be infectious, so too can negativity if you are subjected to it or witness it over a period of time. What happens is that you as well begin to experience sad or down moods, anxiety, and apprehension, thus leaving these individuals with an elevated mood because they have unintentionally transferred their negativity to you and brought you down to where they once were (Purse, 2012). These individuals can still be kind, generous, and compassionate and may not intentionally transfer their negativity to you; you just need to learn not to incorporate their negativity into your own demeanor. If you already have a mental illness of your own, such as depression, bipolar depression, or anxiety, you will especially want to avoid these toxic people because their negativity can play on your preexisting vulnerabilities.

"If you practice and make a conscious effort, in time you can transmute the energy of negativity. Instead of being affected by it, you can choose to send love to others who might be suffering. By protecting yourself from negativity you stay strong in your own energy; therefore, you have the ability to empower yourself and everyone around you" (Paolino, 2013). So whether it is a family member or a coworker, just try to make your interactions brief and move on, or try to tune the person out without coming across as being ignorant. Remember, you cannot change another's behavior, but you can surely change your own.

LOVING YOUR JOB

Hearing people say that they love their job is not a common event. However, because you spend so much time at work, you have the control and power to change your perspective of your job so that instead of negativity and disappointment about working, you experience happiness. According to human resources guru Derek Irvine (2012), identifying the 10 signs that you love your job will help you gain a fuller perspective, and perhaps you will come to enjoy your job that much more; after all, you do spend one-third of your life there. For example, you have friends at work who are people you can talk to and like and whose company you enjoy, you enjoy helping your colleagues, you find that time flies by very quickly because you are so engaged and absorbed in your tasks at hand, and you hate to be sick because you know others may be counting on you for a deliverable, such as patient care. Further, your weekends help you recharge for Monday, you look for ways to share credit with others because you know they are struggling to achieve goals, you go that extra mile to help out, office politics and annoyances do not bother you much, you look for solutions to problems, and you know and realize that what you do does matter and makes a big difference because the glass is always half full, not half empty.

SUMMARY

When you are faced with personal and professional adversity and cumulating stressors, your own mental health can become compromised. No one knows you better than you know yourself and your own body, but even then, you need clear recognition and effective coping strategies to do so. While workplace negativity, difficult colleagues, and workplace conflict can test your mental endurance, you need to maintain your sense of responsibility and accountability as well as use effective coping strategies instead of succumbing to the destruction that negative events can cause. While exercising, eating right, avoiding making assumptions, and taking care of yourself are effective, the extent of the stressor and the impact it can have on your mental health really depend on how you perceive it.

DISCUSSION QUESTIONS

1. Highlight why you have to be the primary source of initiative and motivation to maintaining good mental health.
2. Explain how the Golden Rule and avoiding assumptions can help you avoid a significant amount of stress and impact on your mental health.
3. Identify what would constitute effective coping mechanisms and why.
4. Discuss how you can help to address workplace conflict, backstabbing colleagues, and workplace negativity.
5. Integrating what you learned in Chapter 6, highlight why maintaining your sense of responsibility and accountability will better prepare you to maintain your legal and professional obligations as a nurse.

REFERENCES

Adriaenssens, J., de Gucht, V., & Maes, S. (2012). The impact of traumatic events on emergency room nurses: Findings from a questionnaire survey. *International Journal of Nursing Studies, 49*(11), 1411–1422. doi:10.1016/j.ijnurstu.2012.07.003

Bowman, D. (2012). *Your career is a business, so run it like one.* Retrieved from http://www.ttgconsultants.com/articles/careerbusiness.html

Boyd, R., Zack, Mussa, F., Daigneault, R., et al. (2013). *How to have good mental health.* Retrieved from http://www.wikihow.com/Have-Good-Mental-Health

Canadian Mental Health Association. (2014). *Take control of stress.* Retrieved from http://www.cmha.ca/mental_health/take-control-of-stress/#.UvWXp2JdX4s

Cassels, C. (2011). *More evidence confirms diet's link to mental health. Could an apple a day really keep depression and anxiety away?* Retrieved from http://www.medscape.com/viewarticle/751533

Dale Carnegie. (2013). *5 tips for overcoming workplace negativity with enthusiasm.* Retrieved from http://www.dalecarnegie.com/5_tips_for_overcoming_workplace_negativity_with_enthusiasm

Fredrickson, C. (2013). *7 steps to resolve personality conflicts.* Retrieved from http://www.businessknowhow.com/manage/persconflict.htm

Hallam, J. (1998). From angels to handmaidens: Changing constructions of nursing's public image in post-war Britain. *Nursing Inquiry, 5*(1), 32–42.

Harvard Medical School. (2009). *Sleep and mental health.* Retrieved from http://www.health.harvard.edu/newsletters/Harvard_Mental_Health_Letter/2009/July/Sleep-and-mental-health

Heathfield, S. M. (2013). *Tips for managing workplace negativity.* Retrieved from http://humanresources.about.com/od/workrelationships/a/negativity_2.htm

Hitti, M. (2005). *Sleep helps the brain learn. Learning a new skill? Sleep on it, say scientists.* Retrieved from http://www.webmd.com/brain/news/20050614/sleep-helps-brain-learn

Holecko, C. (2013). *Antioxidants.* Retrieved from http://familyfitness.about.com/od/fitnessvocabularyterms/g/antioxidants.htm

Holmes, L. (2010). *How does exercise improve mental health?* Retrieved from http://mental-health.about.com/od/depression/a/howexercise.htm

Hosman, C., & Jané-Llopis, E. (2005). The evidence of effective interventions for mental health promotion. In H. Herrman, S. Saxena, & R. Moodie (Eds.), *Promoting mental health: Concepts, emerging evidence, practice* (pp. 169–188). Geneva, Switzerland: World Health Organization.

Irvine, D. (2012). *10 signs you love your job (really).* Retrieved from http://www.recognizethis-blog.com/index.php/2012/10/10-signs-you-love-your-job-really

Jané-Llopis, E., Barry, M., Hosman, C., & Patel, V. (2005). Mental health promotion works: A review. *Promotion and Education, 2*, 9–25.

Johansen, M. L. (2012). Conflicting priorities: Emergency nurses' perceived disconnect between patient satisfaction and the delivery of quality patient care. *Journal of Emergency Nursing, 40*(1), 13–19. doi:10.1016/j.jen.2012.04.013

Kamphuis, J., Meerlo, P., Koolhaas, J. M., & Lancel, M. (2012). Poor sleep as a potential causal factor in aggression and violence. *Sleep Medicine, 13*(4), 327–334. doi:10.1016/j.sleep.2011.12.006

Karkoulias, K., Lykouras, D., Sampsonas, F., Karaivazoglou, K., Sargianou, M., Drakatos, P., et al. (2013). The impact of obstructive sleep apnea syndrome severity on physical performance and mental health. The use of SF-36 questionnaire in sleep apnea. *European Review for Medical and Pharmacological Sciences, 17*(4), 531–536.

Keleher, H., & Armstrong, R. (2005). *Evidence-based mental health promotion resource.* Report for the Victorian Government Department of Human Services and VicHealth, Melbourne, Victoria. Retrieved from http://www.gwhealth.asn.au/data/mental_health_resource.pdf

Kelly, O. (2010). *Coping.* Retrieved from http://ocd.about.com/od/glossary/g/Coping_Glossary.htm

Koffman, F. (2013). *Be a hero: Five steps to vanquish any problem.* Retrieved from http://www.linkedin.com/today/post/article/20130328120321-36052017-be-a-hero-five-steps-to-vanquish-any-problem?ref=email

Kuriyama, K., Mishima, K., Suzuki, H., Aritake, S., & Uchiyama, M. (2008). Sleep accelerates the improvement in working memory performance. *Journal of Neuroscience, 28*(40), 10145–10150. doi:10.1523/JNEUROSCI.2039-08.2008

Marchand, W. R. (2013). Mindfulness meditation practices as adjunctive treatments for psychiatric disorders. *Psychiatric Clinics of North America, 36*(1), 141–152. doi:10.1016/j.psc.2013.01.002

McKinley, S., Aitken, L. M., Alison, J. A., King, M., Leslie, G., Burmeister, E., et al. (2012). Sleep and other factors associated with mental health and psychological distress after intensive care for critical illness. *Intensive Care Medicine, 38*(4), 627–633. doi:10.1007/s00134-012-2477-4

Mental Health Foundation. (2013). *There are many reasons why physical activity is good for your body—having a healthy heart and supple joints are just two.* Retrieved from http://www.mentalhealth.org.uk/help-information/mental-health-a-z/E/exercise-mental-health

Nahm, E. S., Warren, J., Zhu, S., An, M., & Brown, J. (2012). Nurses' self-care behaviors related to weight and stress. *Nursing Outlook, 60*(5), e23–e31. doi:10.1016/j.outlook.2012.04.005

Netdoctor. (2012). *8 health benefits of sleep.* Retrieved from http://www.netdoctor.co.uk/interactive/gallery/main.php?g2_itemId=2484&g2_tab_id=

Paolino, K. (2013). *Protecting yourself from negativity.* Retrieved from http://www.netplaces. com/angels-guide/protection-from-the-angels/protecting-yourself-from-negativity. htm

Pfizer. (2014). *Stress-busting tactics for any workplace.* Retrieved from http://www. morethanmedication.ca/en/article/index/stress_busting_tactics

Phillips, C. (2012). *How to deal with a backstabbing co-worker.* Retrieved from http://www.ehow. com/how_4503892_deal-backstabbing-coworker.html

Purse, M. (2012). *Toxic people: What they are and why to avoid them.* Retrieved from http:// bipolar.about.com/od/support/a/070315_toxic.htm

Rattue, P. (2012). Exercise affects the brain. *Medical News Today.* Retrieved from http://www. medicalnewstoday.com/articles/245751.php

Rosenberg McKay, D. (2013). *Turning negativity into positive action.* Retrieved from http:// humanresources.about.com/od/workrelationships/a/negativitycause.htm

Sathyanarayana Rao, T. S., Asha, M. R., Ramesh, B. N., & Jagannatha Rao, K. S. (2008). Understanding nutrition, depression and mental illnesses. *Indian Journal of Psychiatry, 50*(2), 77–82. doi:10.4103/0019-5545.42391

Schroder, C. M. (2010). Sleep deprivation and emotion recognition. *Sleep, 33*(3), 281–282.

Scott, E. (2012). *How can I deal with a difficult co-worker?* Retrieved from http://stress.about. com/od/officepolitics/f/coworker.htm

Sloan, E. P. (2011). Sleep deprivation and postpartum mental health: Case report. *Archives of Women's Mental Health, 14*(6), 509–511. doi:10.1007/s00737-011-0247-x

Smith, M., & Segal, R. (2013). *Stress management.* Retrieved from http://www.helpguide.org/ mental/stress_management_relief_coping.htm

Tomey, A. M. (2009). *Guide to nursing management and leadership* (8th ed., Chapter 5). St. Louis, MO: Elsevier-Mosby.

Virginia, J. (2008). *Nurses must learn to take care of themselves.* Retrieved from http://allnurses/ com/general-articles-about/nurses-must-learn-300832.html

Ward, L. (2011). Mental health nursing and stress: Maintaining balance. *International Journal of Mental Health Nursing, 20*(2), 77–85. doi:10.1111/j.1447-0349.2010.00715.x.

Weiner, J. (2013). *The importance of scheduling nothing.* Retrieved from http://www.linkedin. com/today/post/article/20130403215758-22330283-the-importance-of-scheduling-nothing

Wong, T. P. (2013). *Spirituality and meaning at work.* Retrieved from http://www.meaning.ca/ archives/presidents_columns/pres_col_sep_2003_meaning-at-work.htm

Yoder-Wise, P. S. (2011). *Leading and managing nursing* (5th ed.). St. Louis, MO: Elsevier-Mosby.

13

Meeting the Mental Health Needs of Employees: A Professional Approach

Act in such a way that you always treat humanity, whether in your own person or in the person of any other, never simply as a means, but always at the same time as an end.

—*Immanuel Kant*

LEARNING OBJECTIVES

By the end of this chapter, the learner will be able to:

1. Identify and understand the various strategies a nurse leader can use to create a mentally healthy workplace.
2. Discuss the roles that duty to accommodate, workload management, conflict management, and change management can have in helping a leader to respond to nurses' stressors and foster a mentally healthy workplace.
3. Identify why it is important for nursing leaders to deal with problem and back-stabbing employees.
4. Discuss how complacency, politics, and different personalities can jeopardize the mental health of nurses at work.
5. Highlight why due diligence, stress debriefing, and sometimes the termination of a nurse are needed to maintain a mentally healthy workplace for nurses.

There are numerous strategies that nurse leaders can undertake, develop, promote, and implement to address threats to the mental health of nurses at work merely by virtue of their skill set, knowledge, and expertise. Chapter 5 highlighted how a nurse leader can set the tone and lay the foundation for nurses' workplace environments that can promote respect, collegiality, and safety. This chapter will build on that foundation for how nurse leaders can be instrumental and active in addressing workplace mental health issues and concerns for nurses.

PSYCHOLOGICAL JOB FIT

An appropriate level of challenge will engage and sustain one's interest and motivate one to do more as challenges increase in intensity over a period of time. Hence, nurses will feel good about themselves, valued, and driven to do more to achieve success. Asking them what further challenges they envision for themselves shows you care about their professional and personal development and growth.

PSYCHOLOGICAL SUPPORT AND PROTECTION

Nursing leaders pay a critical role in the provision of psychological support and protection for their nurses. The leader should have a regular and consistent presence in the nurses' workplace setting. This presence allows the nurse leader to become attuned to the atmosphere in the unit/setting, detect dynamics among nurses, and monitor for any injustices and conflict among them.

Through the use of respect, courtesy, consideration, and civility, leaders have to be psychologically supportive of their nurses. The value of psychological support and the ability of nurse leaders to recognize and use it are immeasurable because they result in greater job attachment, performance, commitment, satisfaction, and involvement (Guarding Minds @ Work [GM@W], 2012). Knowing that leadership support is present also reinforces nurses' positive mood, uplifts their spirits and attitudes, and increases their desire to stay with an organization. Finally, knowing that support is present and available often entices nurses to go that extra mile above and beyond their position description or role to complete something of great benefit to their organization and of much interest to the nurses involved (Sherman & Pross, 2010). "Psychological support occurs in a work environment where coworkers and supervisors are supportive of employees' psychological and mental health concerns and respond appropriately as needed" (Great-West Life Centre for Mental Health at Work, 2012).

The lack of leader psychological support permeates all corners of nursing. The organization is strained by increased costs, decreased productivity, and increased liability through more accidents, incidents, and injuries. Nursing staff members who are pressured, stressed, and absent from work leave colleagues short-staffed and contending with higher workloads. This situation can culminate in higher stress levels for the remaining nurses, who may provide inconsistent care and be divided and without the required knowledge, expertise, competency, and skill that seasoned staff took with them. Further, the risk for conflict increases, and physiologically nurses begin to feel the strain of stressors, which causes them to experience headaches, fatigue, burnout, and mental illnesses such as anxiety disorders and depression.

BOOSTING MORALE

In Chapter 2, we discussed how valuable morale is to a nurse's workplace and how in its absence a workplace of discontent, disrespect, and threat can grow. Given that leaders are often blamed for the low morale on the units they oversee

(Schuler, 2004), the leader's position is perhaps by default the most important place to begin. There are, however, many strategies that nurse leaders can practice to help build and boost the morale of nurses' workplaces.

Often, the very root of poor morale is what nurse leaders can focus on to overcome its effects. For example, many leadership competencies that contribute to issues of low nursing morale relate to inspiring trust, communicating vision, energizing staff, developing teams, and creating loyalty. Leaders need first to establish a culture of trust in the organization (Fink, 2007). A climate of trust exists when leaders do what they say they are going to do and are consistent in their actions (Goodman, 2013). "Leaders can earn trust and improve employee morale by being accessible, authentic, fostering openness, and by role modeling" (Dye & Garman, 2006). Further, leaders have the ability to shape and influence the organizational culture through role modeling, the way in which they allocate resources and reward employees, and the criteria they use for recruitment, promotions, and terminations (Shein, 1992). Communication that is clear and focused, delivers important information, and is frequent and meaningful but allows nurses to respond and discuss their concerns can contribute to increased morale, as everyone needs to be on the same page (Dye & Garman, 2006).

Energizing staff, or the activities leaders pursue to heighten levels of motivation in the people with whom they work, is another important leadership competency that can help boost nurse morale. Dye and Garman (2006) refer to energizing staff as the activities leaders pursue to heighten levels of motivation in the people with whom they work. The leader should energize staff by setting a personal example of a good work ethic and motivation, and by speaking and acting enthusiastically and optimistically about the future. This helps nurses recognize the importance of their work, makes work enjoyable, and is goal-oriented and ambitious. Leaders also need to be aware of what motivates individual employees, understand individual goals and priorities of employees, and recognize and celebrate nurses' successes. Simply writing thank-you notes, thanking nurses in person, or offering to cover an employee's workload to allow the employee to leave work early can go a long way when it comes to improving morale and preventing morale issues (Fink, 2007).

Building and maintaining an effective team is another important leadership-related competency linked to nurses' morale. To improve morale, leaders need to be proficient in developing the cohesiveness of the team by increasing the frequency of interaction, by providing opportunities to discuss group goals and how they can be best achieved, and by developing a healthy sense of competition against other teams. Further, the leader refers to him- or herself as a member of the team and builds a sense of "we" by including nurses in individual and team goal setting and by developing team-based incentive programs (Dye & Garman, 2006).

DUTY TO ACCOMMODATE

We discussed the duty to accommodate generically under the auspices of the organization, but a little closer to home, the leader also an important role to play. The "duty to accommodate" refers to the obligation of the employer to take steps to eliminate disadvantages to employees and prospective employees resulting from a policy, rule, practice, or physical barrier that has or may have an adverse impact on individuals or groups protected under the Canadian Human Rights Act or on designated groups under the Employment Equity Act (Government of Canada, 2012).

Just as individuals with physical disabilities may require physical aids in the workplace, individuals living with a mental illness often require organizational accommodations to be made. All efforts must be made to explore accommodation options without undue hardship and with operational requirements taken into consideration. A nurse who is experiencing stress beyond reconcilable limits may have to be accommodated at work. Similarly, for a nurse who is returning to work after being absent because of a mental illness, a workplace accommodation will in all likelihood be required. As a nurse leader, you have a role to play in making sure that the employee has genuine support and everything required to carry out assigned work.

There are many suggested ways that a workplace accommodation can be made. These may include flexible scheduling, flexibility at the beginning or end of working hours to accommodate the effects of medication or to allow time for medical appointments, part-time work (which may be used to return, or "ease back," as some organizations call it, to full-time employment a worker who has been away for a lengthy period of time), and more frequent breaks.

Nurse leaders can also employ some logistical measures to help. For example, they can modify the way instructions and feedback are given. Written instructions may help an employee focus on tasks, and weekly meetings between the supervisor and employee may help to deal with problems before they become serious. In addition, leaders can allow the employee extra time to learn tasks; set and monitor reasonable, objective standards of performance; provide clear instructions and expectations and realistic deadlines; exercise discretion over the day-to-day means and methods of work; ensure that the employee is treated as a member of the team and is not excluded from social events, business meetings, or other activities relevant to the job; encourage and praise of job performance if warranted; and recognize contributions. Finally, work space can be modified or location changed; an employee might be allowed to relocate to a quieter area where it is easier to concentrate or be allowed to work at home.

WORKLOAD MANAGEMENT

As follow-up to our previous discussion in Chapter 4 about the impact of workload management, this is an issue that can creep up on nurses, so that the nurse leader is required to step in. An organization's executives need to work closely with its frontline managers to monitor the acuity levels on the nursing units/pods. As was discussed previously, nurses often take on increasing workloads and responsibilities without "feeling" the associated increased levels of stress. Nurses, however, are not as immune to the effects of stress as they often think (Virginia, 2008), and therefore increased workloads can eventually jeopardize their mental health.

Workload management needs to include the monitoring and trending of workloads and acuity levels so that the health and well-being of both the patients and nurses are not jeopardized in any way, shape, or form. As such, a nurse leader needs to have some pot of resources upon which to call to ameliorate high workload levels and lift nurses' stress. A shift of patients can also occur in an effort to better balance the workload between two or more neighboring units/pods.

STRESS INTERVENTIONS LEADERS SHOULD USE

Nurse leaders can be very proactive and reactive when it comes to buffering the effects of stress on their nurses. To help nurses respond to the stress they face, leaders should invest in supportive, communicative, empathic, anticipatory leadership and should provide time-out facilities, cognitive behavioral interventions, and psychological counseling for nurses, especially those working in the emergency department (Adriaenssens, de Gucht, & Maes, 2012). A positive working environment is needed to maintain positive health outcomes of nurses, prevent job-related diseases, and better protect nurses who are already ill (Milutinovic, Golubovic, Brkic, & Prokes, 2012). In terms of stress and the impact that it can exert on nurses, it is important to recognize that many nurses are perhaps already ill as a result of stress, and they need support and protection to address it and to prevent its exacerbation (Milutinovic et al., 2012). For example, standard operating procedures and policies are needed for the nursing settings to bring consistency and cooperation. Security of the setting and adequate safety protection equipment are needed. Stress relief courses and even self-esteem training and coping skills programs that are supported by the nurse leader can potentially benefit nurses (Chen, Lin, Wang, & Hou, 2009).

OVERCOMING WORKPLACE NEGATIVITY

The nurse leader can also be an instrumental support person and advocate when workplace negativity begins to threaten nurses' workplace mental health. Nothing affects employee morale more insidiously than persistent workplace negativity. It saps the energy of an organization and diverts critical attention from work and performance. Negativity occurs in all realms of the workplace, such as in one's attitude and outlook, the talk of one department member, or a crescendo of voices responding to a workplace decision or event (Heathfield, 2013). Negativity often results from a loss of confidence, control, or community (Topchik, 2000).

Negativity and bad attitudes at work can spread to the point where they eventually affect performance and decision making. In the position of nurse leader, you are able to keep your fingers on the pulse of the organization to sense workplace negativity. It enables you to establish and identify early warning signals that all is not well (Heathfield, 2013). "Perhaps the organization made a decision that adversely affected staff. Perhaps the executive manager held a staff meeting and was perceived to threaten or ignore people asking legitimate questions. Maybe staff members feel insecure because concern exists over losing a product line. Perhaps underground rumors are circulating about an impending layoff. People may feel that they give the organization more than they receive in return. They may feel that a coworker was mistreated or denied a deserved promotion. Whatever the cause of the workplace negativity, you must address the issues. Or, like a seemingly dormant volcano, they will boil beneath the surface, and periodically bubble up and overflow to cause fresh damage" (Heathfield, 2013).

The actions a nurse leader can take to address workplace negativity are many. The best way to combat workplace negativity is to keep it from occurring in the first place; however, this is not always possible. Nurse leaders need to assess their own attitudes in relation to the workplace around them, identify sources of negativity, use principles to gain cooperation from negative people, use a process to disagree agreeably, and identify solutions for specific workplace negativity problems. Talking with employees is a must because it will help them understand the exact problems and the degree to which the problems are impacting their workplace.

Enthusiasm is one such action (Dale Carnegie, 2014). Enthusiasm and positive attitudes spread just as quickly as do negative ones and affect performance just as much, only this time in the right direction. Second, nurse leaders not only receive employee complaints but also do exit interviews with employees who leave, and so learn about the reputation of their organization in the community (Heathfield, 2013). Third, they watch the discussions on employee Intranets, manage the appraisal and 360-degree feedback process, and coach managers in appropriate staff treatment. This information helps them learn to identify the symptoms of negativity before its morale-busting consequences damage the workplace. It will also assists them in preventing and curing workplace negativity. Further, nurse leaders can provide opportunities for nurses to make decisions about and control/influence their own jobs, and to give input into policy and procedure development; nurse leaders provide timely responses to nurses' concerns, treat nurses fairly and consistently, do not stereotype and minimize the number of rules directing the behavior of working adults, provide the context for decisions, and communicate clearly, effectively, in a timely manner, and sincerely. The nurse leader can help nurses grow and develop, use rewards and recognition to make people feel valued, clarify work priorities, eliminate activities that are not essential, avoid perfectionism, promote nurse development, and encourage good relationships among team members (Morin & Forest, 2007; Shain, 2000).

Trust is the most important ingredient in gaining commitment from employees. Employees must feel that top management has the ability to continually balance the best interests of all of the stakeholders of the organization inclusive of patients, customers, employees, vendors, and shareholders. Truly good leaders understand that trust is a two-way street—it must be earned and it must be shared.

Conversely, distrust of leadership causes distrust among coworkers. Instead of cooperation and teamwork, there is competition. In this environment, employees become compliant. They do what they are told in the manner in which they were told to do it.

CONFLICT MANAGEMENT

Conflict is a natural phenomenon in all places of work. While it can be a catalyst for needed change and positive outcomes, it can also be detrimental to a workplace, work morale, personal and professional relationships, and work productivity. Conflict is defined as "disagreement in values or beliefs within oneself or between people that causes harm or has the potential to cause harm" (Yoder-Wise, 2011, p. 465). When nursing professionals come together for the greater good of clients, not always will you find 100% agreement among them. Conflict among individuals is a normal expectation and is inevitable, and it can actually increase productivity of a team (Daft, 2011).

All nurse leaders have the potential to demonstrate leadership in their professional roles. However, nurses in formal leadership positions who make decisions in the workplace have particularly important roles to play in the resolution of conflict. Nurses in formal leadership positions are responsible for supporting nurses in effective conflict management. For example, nurse administrators should establish systems that facilitate the development of conflict resolution skills for all members of the health care team.

Conflict has many advantages, but it also has many disadvantages. Although conflict can positively provide a catalyst for change, growth, and creativity, create a positive work environment, develop and deepen personal and professional relationships, contribute to creative problem solving, foster cohesiveness, and strengthen team spirit and motivation, it can also jeopardize productivity, cohesiveness, morale, quality patient care, communication, and satisfaction and increase absenteeism, liability, organizational costs, tension, and group division (Pangman & Pangman, 2010, p. 280; Yoder-Wise, 2011, p. 465).

Conflict that goes unresolved can weaken and destroy an organization and its people. When one colleague or peer believes that another's action, or intended action, threatens to harm his or her interests, it can be very stress-provoking, disrupt the flow of work, and infringe on personal and professional relationships to the point of creating a dysfunctional workplace environment.

Sources of conflict are many and varied. Sources of conflict in nursing include personality clashes and overactive egos, poor leadership (Lux, Hutcheson, & Peden, 2014), lack of honesty and openness (decreased transparency), ongoing personal and professional stress and stressors, and differences of values and opinions. Sources can also include a shortage of resources, unclear directives, and differences in goals to be achieved (Daft, 2011, p. 316). However, a nurse leader needs to be aware of the ways in which conflict can escalate and be prepared to prevent or manage it in the workplace. Nurses who effectively deal with conflict demonstrate respect for their clients, their colleagues, and the profession. It is the responsibility of any nursing college or association to help protect the rights to quality nursing services and patient care delivery (College of Nurses of Ontario [CNO], 2009).

Regardless of the source of conflict, be it patients, visitors, colleagues, or others, several strategies can be employed by a nurse leader to address workplace conflict. Chapter 5 was about preventing conflict; now let's investigate what a nurse leader can do to manage it. Using professional judgment, the nurse leader should remain calm and encourage the patient to express his or her concerns; implement a critical incident management plan; avoid arguing, criticizing, defending, or judging; focus on the client's or nurse's behavior rather than the client or nurse personally; involve the client and family in assisting with the behavior and developing solutions to prevent or manage it; state that abusive language and behaviors are unacceptable, if the nurse believes this will not escalate the client's behavior; step away from the client; and if necessary leave the situation to develop a plan of care with the assistance of a colleague. If a client intends to harm a nurse, staff members must protect themselves and other clients in abusive situations by withdrawing services, if necessary (CNO, 2009).

A strategy to address conflict resolution is a must for all health care organizations. Nurses work very closely with other health care disciplines toward the same goal of optimal patient care and recovery, so there is bound to be some difference of opinions and practices. Further, nurses work closely with one another for lengthy periods of time, typically 12-hour shifts, and therefore the opportunity for conflict to occur among them is increased. Intervention is indicated in situations such as the following: the people involved have tried unsuccessfully to come to an agreement, not resolving the conflict will have serious implications for the work unit, there is a pattern of conflict, and someone asks for your involvement (Warren Sheppell, 2002).

There are many strategies that the nurse leader can use to help address and deal with ongoing conflict in the workplace. These include creating and maintaining a positive work environment, being open to constructive suggestions and modeling the same, showing your interest, resolving conflicts with the least amount of escalation, and monitoring and constructively dealing with unacceptable interpersonal behavior (Warren Sheppell, 2002). Further, the nurse leader needs to recognize that all strategies are equally good and bad; there is no one right strategy. The leader should be responsive to the needs of the situation, tailor the response to the individual(s) involved, and be adaptable and flexible. Finally, nurse leaders can offer a confidential environment to encourage reporting without fear of retribution, deal with reports promptly and fairly, and ensure that follow-up procedures are in place, particularly for those who have been abused (CNO, 2009). Conflict that remains unacknowledged will not disappear. By actively resolving conflict among staff, nurses in leadership positions will help to establish equitable work environments for all members of the health care team. Finally, nursing leaders can promote conflict management among staff by establishing and using reporting processes that are fair and confidential.

Typically, there is a five-step negotiation model that can be used to help individuals navigate their way through a conflict resolution process (Warren Sheppell, 2002). These include an opening of the issue and intent; identification of facts and feelings by both parties; a "so what?" approach to identify interests and what is needed, wanted, and hoped; a "now what?" that comprises options and possible actions and next steps; and a closing to end the dialogue on a positive note and identify lessons learned in preparation for future dialogue.

There are also many different styles for handling conflict in the nurse's workplace. However, the manner in which one attempts to handle conflict depends on two unique aspects—one's level of assertiveness and one's level of cooperation. Some styles that nurse leaders can use to handle conflict include the following:

- Competing—uses assertiveness but not cooperation to get one's own way. This style is very important in emergencies or urgent cost cutback decisions.
- Avoiding—uses neither assertiveness nor cooperation when an issue is unimportant, there is no chance of winning, a delay is needed, or a disruption could be costly.
- Compromising—a moderate amount of cooperation and assertiveness is needed. Such a style may be best used when there is equal power on both sides and both

sets of goals are equally important, or when you can split the difference or need to agree on a temporary or expedient solution quickly.

- Accommodating—where there is increased cooperation and less assertiveness. It can occur if people realize they are wrong, the issues are important to others but not to you, cohesiveness is important to maintain, or you just wish to gather information and power for later discussions.
- Collaborating—increased cooperation and assertiveness increases the amount of discussion and negotiation, so both parties benefit (Daft, 2011, p. 317; Yoder-Wise, 2011, p. 469).

Remaining poised when tension is high is a difficult thing to do; however, nurse leaders need to diagnose conflict within their organization, find the hidden agenda that's really fueling the battle, analyze their own conflict response style, identify anger triggers and remain poised in conflict situations, encourage collaborative problem solving and gain consensus, and learn a variety of strategies for managing conflict (Dale Carnegie, 1984).

A PLETHORA OF PERSONALITIES

Nursing, like any other profession, attracts many different personalities. Being a nurse leader has many trials and tribulations, as we have seen thus far. When a group of individuals are brought together for a common purpose, such as a group of nurses in a specific nursing setting, it can be a very enriching experience for all involved, as they come from very different walks of life, backgrounds, histories, beliefs, values, and attitudes. The weaknesses and uncertainties of one nurse can often be offset by the strengths and confident competencies of another nurse, and vice versa. However, differing views, opinions, values, and attitudes can also create tumult. The diversity of a group of people with varying backgrounds and histories and with their own likes and dislikes can often be very counterproductive to achieving goals and tasks (Thorman, 2012) and can create much dissension and conflict among the ranks. Working with different personalities is not an easy task for many, and "one size does not fit all"; however, it is a reality in the world of nursing. Thorman (2012), a human resource specialist, has identified various approaches for how a leader can best work to build collegiality and respect in the workplace.

The trick to dealing with multiple personalities in the workplace is viewing each individual objectively, focusing on each person's strengths, promoting positive communication, and helping others do the same (Richards-Gustafson, 2013). The inclusion of the following steps is one referenced approach. First, give the nurse a feedback sandwich and start on a positive note ("I really like the work you've been completing"), continue with the potentially abrasive feedback ("but would love to see you meet deadlines"), and end on another positive note ("so we can continue the momentum on this project"). Second, figure out how your colleagues and managers enjoy working and try your best not to interrupt their work flow. Third, pick your battles, decide what your priorities are, and let everything else go—even if you know you're right. Do the costs outweigh the overall benefits? Fourth, realize you are on the same team; although the workplace has many personalities and opinions, everyone is working toward the same goal, and strong opinions may signify signs of a passionate team. Finally, you need to respect other people's expertise, as many would just like to be heard and validated. You don't know it all and you can't do it all. Do not undermine people's authority; instead, ask for their input, feedback, and advice when something comes up in their realm of expertise. They'll appreciate being consulted, and you'll learn something new.

People who become nurses are of all ages and come from all walks of life, backgrounds, and histories. However, when many different personalities are brought together in one workplace setting, it can make for a tumultuous work environment. There are many different strategies that can be undertaken by nurse leaders to help curb some of the potentially negative outcomes that can result when differing personalities meet. First, because younger employees tend to be a little more abrupt and less considerate of others, more time for guiding and training is needed (Teal, 2011). Showing them the ladder to success is often a way to increase their commitment and interest.

As a nurse leader, you need to know how best to deal with the different personalities in your workplace setting (Master Class Management, 2013). As suggested by Richards-Gustafson (2013), blending multiple personalities in a workplace can enhance creativity and lead to new ideas; however, it can also lead to communication barriers, conflicts, and lower productivity levels. The great work in this area by Masters Class Management (2013) suggests many interventions depending on personality type. First, the *considerates* are nice and calm, and they like to think things through. For them, the glass is optimistically half full. They are agreeable and cooperative, even though it may take them longer to get things done and they may need your input along the way, so be direct. However, their work is very thorough and will serve you well in a long-term, detailed project, so be sure to give them lots of praise and encouragement and spend time talking about other, lighter topics also. Second, the *aggressives* are controllers and doers, but don't let them control you. They are good at what they do, can produce great work, and can put out fires when needed; they know this, so they make decisions readily. They just sometimes need to be reminded of who is in charge. Be direct and straightforward, use a no-nonsense approach, and give them lots of praise when it is due. Third, the *analysts* play devil's advocate, criticize excessively and search for flaws, and procrastinate. If you say "yes, it's okay," they will say "maybe this way will work better." Listen to them, but if it isn't going anywhere, acknowledge their input and move on. These people are left-brain-dominant, concrete individuals who stick to the facts, avoid wasting time with small chitchat, and are good at troubleshooting and analysis. Fourth, the *sensitives* are nice, courteous, sincere, touchy-feely, and pleasant, but they can take comments and remarks personally, even if they aren't meant to be. They are very cooperative and compliant, so give encouragement, not direct orders, because they can't make decisions well. Fifth, the *talkatives* are feeling-oriented and emotional. They like people, can be social butterflies, and like making decisions with the group majority, so take a light-hearted approach and humor to get your point across. Sixth, the *brainiacs* use knowledge and sarcasm to get what they want and avoid decision making by avoiding the topic. They are easily distracted and derailed, so make them repeat themselves and let them collect the data. Seventh, the *quiets* are the ones who very rarely talk at meetings, seem to have low self-esteem, and are continually subconscious of their actions, yet they may have some great ideas and so need to be pulled out of their shell; seek them out. Eighth, the *results-drivens* focus solely on the data results but sometimes can't see the big picture. They can excel in one area of the job and be lacking in another, so be direct and emphasize the importance of common sense. They have a very narrow focus and so are more suited for simple, straightforward tasks that do not require thinking outside the box. Ninth, the *loners* just want to do the job and not get involved with company picnics, break room conversations, or any nonwork-related subjects. You need to emphasize the value of teams and relationships in the workplace because they need to be supportive and reliable. They may have to be moved to another task if they can't do teamwork, but still work to bring them out of their shell. Tenth, the *overly confidents* know everything and can do no wrong, even if the reverse is true. Be very direct, but compliment them periodically. They should repeat back instructions and be monitored closely for progress. Eleventh, the *curmudgeons* believe they are more competent than others, don't take supervision well, and are often grumpy and sarcastic. Their glass is half-empty, so be firm and direct, stick to the facts, and give clear directions with a matter-of-fact approach. Twelfth, the *mean-spiriteds* are not often happy with work or the people at work because of other, nonwork-related issues. They compromise morale, so the value of teamwork needs to be emphasized. Finally, those with a *bad attitude* are a major problem because they lower morale, which is unacceptable, so let them know this.

Dealing with conflicts between employee personalities is challenging for the nurse leader. One of your jobs is perhaps to become the arbitrator of the department. This means that you have to have the ability to hear both sides and choose the option that is best for the customer and the company. Your choice can sometimes fall between the two sides, but often it becomes a matter of choosing one over the other. You have been made a manager because you have the ability to be decisive. Use this skill heavily in this area. Employee conflicts usually arise because each person wants his or her way to prevail. You risk becoming an enemy to one or both, but that goes along with your title. Letting the employees settle it themselves rarely ever works. Be a manager, make the call, and deal with the consequences of the choice. Most of the time, bad attitudes cannot prevail unless they are allowed to continue unchecked. Being a decisive manager will help keep bad attitudes away from the workplace (Teal, 2011). Richards-Gustafson (2013) adds that asking clarifying questions instead of making assumptions about the reasons and motives behind employees' actions and words allows for some autonomy. As long as employees meet deadlines and consistently perform well, it may be beneficial to allow some autonomy in how they approach projects. As a nurse leader, you should also promote open, constructive communication and be nonjudgmental to allow the flow of ideas and the expression of suggestions, constructive criticism, and concerns. Finally, embrace your employees' personality differences and strengths, and encourage other staff members to do the same. When employees recognize and understand one another's differences, they can act more respectfully toward one another and play to one another's strengths when completing projects.

CHANGE MANAGEMENT

Change is a natural occurrence, not only in an organization but also in the nursing profession. Many often resist and shudder at the thought of possible change, but it can be implemented in such a way as to help alleviate some of the anxiety, tension, and conflict that it tends to create. While there are numerous change management frameworks in existence, they all tend to highlight a similar series of steps that can help implement change successfully and smoothly. All serve a similar purpose to introduce, implement, and encourage the acceptance of change. We briefly touched upon change management in Chapter 5, but I provide here now some more detail and structure related to how best to deal with change. As an example, I highlight here John Kotter's Model of Change Management for the purposes of illustration. Directly from John Kotter (2012) himself, his model of change is as follows:

Step 1: Establishing a sense of urgency. Help others see and understand the need for change, and they will be convinced of the importance of acting immediately.

Step 2: Creating the guiding coalition. Assemble a group with enough power to lead the change effort, and encourage the group to work as a team.

Step 3: Developing a change vision. Create a vision to help direct the change effort, and develop strategies for achieving that vision.

Step 4: Communicating the vision for buy-in. Make sure as many as possible understand and accept the vision and the strategy.

Step 5: Empowering broad-based action. Remove obstacles to change, change systems or structures that seriously undermine the vision, and encourage risk taking and nontraditional ideas, activities, and actions. Some people will have doubts.

Step 6: Generating short-term wins. Plan for achievements that can easily be made visible, follow through with those achievements, and recognize and reward employees who were involved.

Step 7: Never letting up. Use increased credibility to change systems, structures, and policies that don't fit the vision; also hire, promote, and develop employees who can implement the vision; and finally reinvigorate the process with new projects, themes, and change agents.

Step 8: Incorporating changes into the culture. Articulate the connections between the new behaviors and organizational success, and develop the means to ensure leadership development and succession.

CRITICAL INCIDENT STRESS DEBRIEFING

As not all conflict can be identified, prevented, or curtailed, there will be times when conflict can escalate into a critical incident or crisis situation. After a critical incident has taken place, it is important for the nurse leader involved to collaborate with the health care team to debrief about the situation. Debriefing allows nurses to reflect on and learn from what has occurred. This can provide insight into the conflict's contributing factors, as well as contribute to its future prevention and management. *Critical incident stress debriefing* (CISD) is defined as "any situation faced by emergency personnel that causes them to experience unusually strong emotional reactions having the potential to interfere with their ability to function at the scene or later" (Rubin, 1990). Further, it is often a short-term, adaptive, psychological helping and healing process that focuses on the immediate or acute series of traumatic events and aims to return individuals to their previous normal level of functioning. While *normal* is different for everyone, critical incidents raise stress levels dramatically in a short period of time and establish a new *normal*. The purpose of the intervention process is to establish or set the new *normal* stress levels as low as possible.

The goal of CISD is to reduce psychological "casualties" among emergency personnel (Iacono, 2002). Iacono adds that "CISD consists of semi-structured interventions designed to decrease initial distress and prevent ongoing problems, concerns, and negative or destructive behaviors. The emphasis is always on keeping people safe and returning them quickly to more *normal* levels of functioning. Staff may experience emotional numbing, hostility, anger, withdrawal, or sleep problems. CISD promotes emotional processing through ventilation (verbal acknowledgement) and normalization of reactions to trauma, stress, disasters, and critical incidents. It also prepares the staff for possible future experiences." Nurse leaders can engage in many different interventions to help their nurses through the process of CISD. Some of these interventions include the following: consulting with those involved about the meaning of their experiences during the incident with the intent to heal themselves and the client and family; reviewing and reflecting on the responses, and recommending future strategies based on team members' actions and reflections on their own behavior, which may have unintentionally affected the nurse–client relationship; helping the client understand how his or her behavior negatively affected the therapeutic nurse–client relationship; developing communication strategies with the client so the client can express his or her feelings appropriately; using best-practice strategies to develop a care plan for dealing with the client's behavior; using anticipatory planning to develop a consistent approach to addressing the client's behavior in the future (CNO, 2009); and defusing, debriefing, and follow up. Defusing (done the day of the incident) is designed to reassure the person(s) involved that their feelings are normal, tell them what symptoms to watch for over the short term, and offer them a lifeline in the form of a telephone number where they can reach someone whom they can talk to. Debriefing (done within 72 hours of the incident) gives the individual or group members the opportunity to talk about their experience and how it has affected them, brainstorm coping mechanisms, and identify individuals at risk, and it informs the individual or group members about services available to them in their community. The final step is to follow up with them the day after the debriefing to ensure that they are safe and coping well, or to refer the individual(s) for professional counseling. All these are critical interventions the nursing leader can implement.

ENHANCING STAFF ENGAGEMENT

In Chapter 5, we learned how important staff engagement really is. According to Culture Consultancy (2013), fixing low employee engagement does not happen overnight. It will take some time and much effort to succeed because there is a change in attitude that has to occur. First, as a nursing leader you have to make sure everyone is still on the same page with the same goals; this collective identity makes staff feel included and valued and not forgotten about. To achieve this takes active "listening and responding effectively to staff issues or complaints, setting up systems to improve communication, and creating rewards initiatives for staff that perform well." Most importantly, you need to keep up the engagement of the nurse and not lose sight of its importance. Over time and even after an event has unfolded on your unit, pod, or facility, you need to continue to let your nurses know how valuable they are by involving them in making decisions for the unit and patient population and listening attentively to their concerns expressed. As a leader, you are the most valuable resource person for them to look up to and obtain support from, so keeping them engaged in your corner should help you continue to achieve a mentally healthy workplace for all.

DEALING WITH PROBLEM EMPLOYEES

Problem employees not only can jeopardize and sabotage the mental health of others and create a poisonous atmosphere but can also literally destroy a workplace. They can destroy the morale of the workplace and the integrity one's existence and become an organizational liability. According to Fischer (2013), there are several actions the nurse leader can take, which include not ignoring the problem employee; this is not someone having an off day. While some people "need a little push, others need a swift kick in the hindquarters." Nip this in the bud as soon as you see it; the majority of your nurses will thank you for it. Second, decide whether the problem is training or attitude. "Retraining is easy if the person wants to do [his or her] job properly, but when you have a behavior issue, it could mean termination may be around the corner." Third, take the employee aside and point out exactly what he or she has been doing wrong and why work performance is not up to acceptable standards. Tell him or her what was done wrong and how to correct it. You really need to be frank and open. Fourth, document, document, document, and have them sign the documented notes taken during your interaction. You will need these to resort to later during possible disciplinary measures. Fifth, follow up and revisit the behavior at a later date. Follow-up emphasizes the importance of this action or event, so you need to follow through on this. Finally, as a leader you may have to terminate the nurse, but make sure you have all the facts first, as you want to do this without any negative ramifications to yourself, the nurses, the patients, or the organization.

DEALING WITH BACKSTABBING COLLEAGUES

"Back-stabbers, also known as back biters or back attackers, might seem easygoing, even complacent, with a 'don't worry' attitude, but don't let them deceive you. Their strategy is to be nice to your face and act like your best friend, lulling you into a false sense of security that tricks you into revealing information you really don't want them to have. They fish for some morsels of ammunition to fire back when you're unsuspecting; then they attack you behind your back, bad mouthing or implicating you. They may lie and deny their involvement, even by pointing fingers at others as the source of their malicious mischief. By calling them on their game, you take away their satisfaction with their own cleverness and prevent them from exulting in their sense of power (false though it may be). When dealing with them, be vigilant and watch your back!" (Sanow, 2011). Although we briefly chatted about this in Chapter 12 for how you as a nurse can deal with such people, there is also a role for the nursing leader to play. Sanow (2011) suggests that as a leader you need to gather your evidence with concrete examples and intimate detail to give you a stronger stance against an individual instead of relying on gossip and hearsay. Next, you need to discuss the remarks openly with the person while using a calm, gentle tone and ask the person to specify whatever accusations have been made. Third, you can give the person a graceful exit, as he or she probably will deny it; you can identify it as perhaps an exaggeration or a subtle warning that you are aware of his or her behaviors and act, and don't argue if he or she denies intent to harm. Next, identify the professional level of behavior that you expect of your nurses in this facility, unit, or pod. Finally, you can also make mistakes, so if this is the case, apologize as it shows a sign of strength, not weakness.

As highlighted by writer Karen Salmansohn (2013), "People don't hate you for your weaknesses, they hate you for your strengths." When you think about it, this makes much sense. How true it is that when you attempt to set the record or practice straight, you are met with opposition by a select few. This opposition is reflected by peers who are often jealous or scared and perhaps see you as a threat to an environment where they have already established much control with followers. Whether you like it or not, some people just cannot be trusted, and the nursing leader is often one of the individuals who gets a true sense of this when it happens, or should I say "after" it happens.

There are other important points to remember, as outlined by Salmansohn (2013). She points to the realities of saying less to protect you more, so don't say anything in private that you would not want to be repeated in public. Also, in times of change, always keep eyes in the back of your head, as layoffs and cuts may make people desperate to look out for themselves at the expense of others. Next, leaders can backstab as well, so be on the alert and keep yourself in the grapevine traffic. Keep on doing good deeds to create a more positive workplace and "love thy neighbor," so try and surround yourself with the people you trust the most, as you need friends at all levels. "Don't just work to create good relationships with your boss and colleagues, but also become friends with secretaries and assistants." As a leader, you also need to better read someone like a book, as actions speak louder than words, so pay attention to someone's body language. People who cannot look you in the eye are sending a message.

POWER AND POLITICS

Nurse leaders are becoming aware of the need to become more politically active and that power is a central concept of politics. From a political standpoint, nurse leaders can be effective at promoting political support for nurses, but they can also exert a positive influence on the dysfunctional politics that can occur at work.

A leader's ability to gain and wisely use power is critical to his or her success. Leaders must be able to identify the resources needed and legitimately manipulate them to best meet organization change, the demands of a nurse's work environment, and patients' care needs. Nurse leaders who are able to bridge or minimize power gaps, build their own personal base, and address the dysfunctional politics of the organization are the most successful leaders.

The use of legitimate (position power), reward (promotions and praise), expert (skill, ability, knowledge, expertise), and referent (charisma and connected relationships) power helps nurses to become effective leaders and handle the politics at work. However, they have to tread carefully because they can lose power just as quickly as they gained it, such as occurs when workplace politics becomes divisive and corrupt, associated with gossip, rumors, and other unethical innuendos (e.g., workplace harassment, bullying, and violence). It is this political climate at work that can impact success and failure. In order to deal with the most influential and powerful group in the health care system, nurses must take advantage of the knowledge they have and the attributes they possess, and part of that means being an effective leader.

In the workplace, nurse leaders are often confronted with the negativities that politics can bestow upon them, threatening nurses' moral fiber. The politics of work is often unavoidable, so you need to be aware of and understand it to cope with it. Politics of this nature represents the behaviors of individuals as they attempt to acquire, develop, and use power and other resources to obtain their preferred outcomes in a situation in which there is uncertainty about choices. It is frequently characterized by relationships within an organization that determine how a person will act in a given situation. While closely associated with power, this type of politics can be to the detriment of the individual nurse, the leader, and the workplace respect and morale in general. Rosenberg McKay (2013) suggests that in order to succeed at any game, you must know the rules and office politics, as this can be the most competitive game you will ever play.

Leaders spend a great deal of time addressing the politics of the workplace (Rosenberg McKay, 2013). The dynamics, the culture, and the workplace atmosphere and environment all impact the output and productivity of an organization, especially in the area of health care delivery for patients. Leaders spend approximately 18% of their time or the equivalent of 9 weeks per year addressing workplace politics and the employee conflict that comes with it, leaving less time for other tasks.

Across disciplines, Kreindler (2013) provided a divisive foundation upon which the completion of patient-centered goals was argued. What is typically seen as a "seemingly benign concept of patient-centered care" became a "weapon on an intergroup battlefield" as each discipline argued over who did what and to what degree over the other. Kreindler adds that understanding this dimension may actually help leaders address the intergroup tensions that precipitate conflict and prevent patient-centered care.

The concepts of power and politics are closely related, and both are integral components of how nurses can become effective leaders. While power is defined as the ability to influence another to conform in accordance with one's wishes, politics is the art of using power wisely. A leader's ability to gain and wisely use power is critical to his or her success. Leaders must be able to identify the resources needed and recognize the need to legitimately manipulate resources to best meet organization change and the demands of nurses' work environment and patients' care needs. Nurse leaders who are able to bridge or minimize power gaps, build their own personal base, and address the dysfunctional politics of the organization are the most successful leaders.

In many ways, a paradigm shift has occurred in nursing with respect to power. Power in nursing has come a long way from historical times. Power was once perceived as a threat and alien to the caring and compassionate profession of nursing. What was characteristically found was that there was power "sharing," not one person seeking power "over" another. Today, power takes many forms, some bad and some good. If power is used in a beneficial, positive manner, nurses can help transform organizations and the delivery of patient care. They can achieve this by bringing a vision of their own, where power is used and fostered to embrace the caring and quality that organizations aim to achieve. An effective nurse leader has the capacity and know-how to mobilize and focus energy or resources in a productive manner to achieve what needs to be achieved for the organization and the patients/clients.

Without the strength to move others, one cannot compete with the managerial elite for scarce funds, scarce personnel, scarce space, and expensive materials. In order to deal with the most influential and powerful group in the health care system, we must take advantage of the knowledge we have and the attributes that we possess, and part of that means being an effective leader.

DEALING WITH COMPLACENCY

Just as there are difficult personalities, bullies, and others making the workplace difficult, there are also a cohort of workers who are really not interested in working and hence become complacent. In essence, they are not performing and completing their duties as needed or in as timely a manner as is needed. According to HCPro (2008), to deal with complacency, a leader can hold people accountable for their actions, work assignments, and tasks. An accountability framework would help in such matters to support and enforce the leader's efforts. Reorganizing nurses from shift rotations and units is another way to be creative, lessen the risk for nurses' work becoming monotonous and nurses becoming disinterested, increase the flexibility of all nurses as they learn new and different aspects of nursing, invest in your nurses for new or different training and education, and comply with performance reviews to identify gaps in skills and knowledge (HCPro, 2008). Further, complacent nurses often know their jobs very well, so bring them on board in more responsible roles, such as training other nurses.

ENCOURAGING A JUST AND BLAMELESS CULTURE

It is very tempting and so easy to blame others for what has unfortunately occurred. The focus needs to be not on pointing a finger at the person who is suspected or known to have been the cause, but instead on how the situation can be rectified and prevented from happening again. This creates an atmosphere of trust and encouragement, and it rewards people for providing essential safety-related information. The American Nurses Association (ANA) would refer to this "just culture" as an alternative to a debunked punitive system. The model "seeks to create an environment that encourages individuals to report mistakes so that the precursors to errors can be better understood in order to fix the system issues" (ANA, 2010).

LAWSUITS, LITIGATION, AND ALTERNATE DISPUTE RESOLUTION

The nurse leader will play a significant role in any lawsuits and litigations that may arise when the mental health of a nurse is sabotaged or jeopardized because of a work-related incident that the leader and/or organization knew about and took no action to address. Allegations of nursing malpractice are adjudicated under the civil law system known as tort law. Tort law requires that an injured party prove four elements: duty, breach, causation, and injury (Miller, 2011). However, as found by Miller (2011), "tort law continues to promote an adversarial relationship between clinicians and patients without providing compensation in a fair and just manner. It results in undue stress for clinicians and does nothing to promote improved relationships with patients" and colleagues; "rather, it fosters distrust and thwarts attempts at transparency."

However, alternate (or external, as referred to in Australia) dispute resolution (ADR) is an option that can similarly help to address such matters. In this process, several techniques are used as a medium through which an agreement can be reached or a conflict can be settled by parties in disagreement; a third party or ombudsman may be involved. ADR can occur through five different tribunals: negotiation, mediation, collaborative law, arbitration, and conciliation, but the primary goal is conflict resolution. Although ADR is often used in labor dispute issues and cases of professional incompetence in which patient safety was jeopardized, I assert here that it can also provide a means for resolving conflict between colleagues, which can equally jeopardize nurse, colleague, and patient safety. The many benefits of ADR include the following: suitability for multiple-party disputes, flexibility of the procedure/process, lower costs for all parties, simplicity, parties' ability to choose a neutral third party (and therefore expertise in the area of dispute) to direct negotiations and adjudicate, more timely and efficient settlements, tailored and individualized solutions, maintenance of confidentiality, and preservation of long-standing relationships.

DUE DILIGENCE

Nurse leaders are also responsible for completing due diligence when they know that a potential or volatile situation between staff nurses or colleagues is escalating to dangerously high and threatening levels. Due diligence is "the level of judgment, care, prudence, determination, and activity that a person would reasonably be expected to do under particular circumstances" (Canadian Centre for Occupational Health and Safety [CCOHS], 2013). From an occupational health and safely perspective, it means that employers shall take all reasonable precautions, under the particular circumstances, to prevent injuries or accidents in the workplace.

To establish due diligence, there are many conditions that apply. From the CCOHS (2013), these include the following: The employer must have in place written occupational health and safety policies, practices, and procedures that demonstrate and document that workplace safety audits to identify hazardous practices and hazardous conditions were conducted and necessary changes were made to correct these conditions, and that employees were provided with information to enable them to work safely. Second, the employer must provide the appropriate training and education to the employees so that they understand and can carry out their work according to the established polices, practices, and procedures. Third, the employer must train the supervisors to ensure they are competent persons, as defined in legislation. Fourth, the employer must monitor the workplace and ensure that employees are following the policies, practices, and procedures. Written documentation of progressive disciplining for breaches of safety rules is considered due diligence. Fifth, workers also have a responsibility to take reasonable care to ensure the safety of themselves and their coworkers; this includes following safe work practices and complying with regulations. Sixth, an accident investigation and reporting system should be in place. Even "near misses" should be reported and investigated in which any findings are incorporated into these policies and practices. Next, the employer should document, in writing, all of the above steps so that a history is kept to reflect progress over time and to provide up-to-date documentation in the defense of any charges.

It is important also to remember that the process of due diligence should be in place before any accident or harm occurs, as it reflects proactive measures and the continued monitoring of what should be kept in place so as to promote a mentally healthy work environment for nurses.

TERMINATION OF A NURSE

It is no easy task to terminate one of your nurses. However, as a nurse leader you know it may have to be done at some point in time. If, in spite of one-on-one discussions, performance appraisals and evaluations, support, and education, the nurse is still breaching standards of nursing practice, is involved in professional misconduct, or continues to place patient safety and care in jeopardy, then it is perhaps time to let the nurse go.

As suggested by Balovich (2006), "the manager should have a very blunt talk with this individual about [his or her] ability to perform and fit into the company's culture." If specific training is needed, the nurse's behavior should be monitored to ensure it has changed. "If the employee cannot adapt, [he or she] must be released from employment so [as not to] continue to disrupt the rest of the workplace. Terminating a disruptive employee shows respect not only for the people who are meeting the company standards but also the person who does not fit in. The terminated employee is not wrong for being who [he or she is]; [he or she] simply must be shown that [his or her] attitude and work style is not appropriate in the organization." Further, the termination of a nurse who has been very disruptive and unsafe in nursing practice shows an incredible amount of respect for the nurses who remain working there.

An exit interview with the outgoing nurse is another option for the leader. An exit interview will better inform the nurse leader about many of the events that have occurred, provide feedback on his or her own leadership skills, and finally provide the outgoing nurse a last opportunity to voice concerns, perceived unfairness, and any unjust processes and experiences he or she feels have been experienced.

SUMMARY

A leader is in a pivotal position to bolster all efforts to help address a toxic workplace environment for nurses. The mere description of the position's roles and responsibilities speaks loudly as to how a leader can employ various strategies and make some very key decisions so that good mental health is promoted in the workplace.

Although nurse leaders may experience challenges of their own with how they engage and direct nurses, their astute knowledge, skills, and expertise as leaders can help them deal with some of the most challenging elements of a negative workplace.

DISCUSSION QUESTIONS

1. What are some of the various strategies a nurse leader can use to create a mentally healthy workplace?
2. What roles do duty to accommodate, workload management, conflict management, and change management have in helping a leader to respond to nurses' stressors and foster a mentally healthy workplace?
3. Why is it important for nursing leaders to deal with problem and backstabbing employees?
4. How can complacency, politics, and different personalities jeopardize the mental health of nurses at work?
5. Why are due diligence, stress debriefing, and sometimes the termination of a nurse needed to maintain a mentally healthy workplace for nurses?

REFERENCES

Adriaenssens, J., de Gucht, V., & Maes, S. (2012). The impact of traumatic events on emergency room nurses: Findings from a questionnaire survey. *International Journal of Nursing Studies, 49*(11), 1411–1422. doi:10.1016/j.ijnurstu.2012.07.003

American Nurses Association. (2010). *Position statement: Just culture.* Retrieved from http://nursingworld.org/psjustculture

Balovich, D. (2006). *Respect in the workplace.* Retrieved from http://www.creditworthy.com/3jm/articles/cw81706.html.

Canadian Centre for Occupational Health and Safety. (2013). *Due diligence.* Retrieved from http://www.ccohs.ca/oshanswers/legisl/diligence.html

Chen, C. K., Lin, C., Wang, S. H., & Hou, T. H. (2009). A study of job stress, stress coping strategies, and job satisfaction for nurses working in middle-level hospital operating rooms. *Journal of Nursing Research, 17*(3), 199–211.

College of Nurses of Ontario. (2009). *Conflict prevention and management.* Retrieved from http://www.cno.org/Global/docs/prac/47004_conflict_prev.pdf

Culture Consultancy. (2013). *What is employee engagement?* Retrieved from http://www.cultureconsultancy.com/links/should-i-worry-about-employee-engagement/#sthash.YfLKHkRb.dpuf

Daft, R. L. (2011). *The leadership experience* (5th ed.). Mason, OH: Cengage Learning (South-Western Publishing Co.).

Dale Carnegie. (1984). *How to win friends and influence people.* Hauppauge, NY: Dale Carnegie and Associates.

Dale Carnegie. (2014). *5 tips for overcoming workplace negativity with enthusiasm.* Retrieved from http://www.dalecarnegie.com/5_tips_for_overcoming_workplace_negativity_with_enthusiasm

Dye, C., & Garman, A. (2006). *Exceptional leadership.* Chicago, IL: Health Administration Press.

Fink, N. (2007). *The high cost of low morale: How to address low morale in the workplace through servant leadership.* Retrieved from http://www.roberts.edu/Academics/AcademicDivisions/BusinessManagement/msl/Community/Journal/TheHighCostofLowMorale.htm

Fischer, K. (2013). *How to deal with a problem employee.* Retrieved from http://www.ehow.com/how_4838320_deal-problem-employee.html#ixzz27UFObMCE

Goodman, B. (2013). *Leadership and management in nursing: A critical approach.* Retrieved from http://www.academia.edu/4710241/Leadership_and_Management_in_Nursing_-a_critical_approach

Great-West Life Centre for Mental Health at Work. (2012). *Psychological support.* http://www.gwlcentreformentalhealth.com/images/agenda/pdf/1_Psychological_Support_EN.pdf

Guarding Minds @ Work (2012). *A workplace guide to psychological health and safety.* Retrieved from http://www.guardingmindsatwork.ca/info/index

HCPro. (2008). *Distracting environments: Mitigating complacency.* Retrieved from http://www.reliability.com/healthcare/articleshcp/aug_08_diestractive%20environments%20Mitigating%20complacency.pdf

Heathfield, S. M. (2013). *Tips for minimizing workplace negativity.* Retrieved from http://humanresources.about.com/od/workrelationships/a/negativity.htm

Iacono, M. (2002). Critical incident stress debriefing: Application for perianesthesia nurses. *Journal of PeriAnesthesia Nursing, 17*(6), 423–426.

Kotter, J. (2012). *The 8-step process for leading change.* Retrieved from http://www.kotterinternational.com/our-principles/changesteps/changesteps

Kreindler, S. A. (2013). The politics of patient-centred care. *Health Expectations: An International Journal of Public Participation in Health Care and Health Policy.* doi:10.1111/hex.12087

Lux, K. M., Hutcheson, J. B., & Peden, A. R. (2014). Ending disruptive behavior: Staff nurse recommendations to nurse educators. *Nursing Education in Practice, 14*(1), 37–42.

Master Class Management. (2013). *Managing different personalities.* Retrieved from http://www.masterclassmanagement.com/ManagementCourse-ManagingPersonalities.html

Mental Health Commission of Canada. (2012). *Mental health first aid.* Retrieved from http://www.mentalhealthcommission.ca/English/system/files/private/document/MHCC_MHFA_Improve_Mental_Health_Workplace_ENG.pdf

Miller, L. A. (2011). Health courts: An alternative to traditional tort law. *Journal of Perinatal and Neonatal Nursing, 25*(2), 99–102. doi:10.1097/JPN.0b013e318215926e

Milutinovic, D., Golubovic, B., Brkic, N., & Prokes, B. (2012). Professional stress and health among critical care nurses in Serbia. *Arhiv za Higijenu Rada i Toksikologiju, 63*(2), 171–180.

Morin, E. M., & Forest, J. (2007). Promouvoir la santé mentale au travail: Donner un sens au travail. Retrieved from *Promouvoir la santé mentale au travail* [in French only].

Pangman, V. C., & Pangman, C. (2010). *Nursing leadership from a Canadian perspective.* Philadelphia, PA: Lippincott Williams & Wilkins.

Richards-Gustafson, F. (2013). *How to deal with multiple personalities in the workplace.* Retrieved from http://smallbusiness.chron.com/deal-multiple-personalities-workplace-19294.html

Rosenberg McKay, D. (2013). *Office politics: A rude intruder.* Retrieved from http://careerplanning.about.com/od/workplacesurvival/a/politics.htm

Rubin, J. (1990). Critical incident stress debriefing: Helping the helpers. *Journal of Emergency Nursing, 16*, 255–258.

Salmansohn, K. (2013). *Ten tips for dealing with backstabbing coworkers.* Retrieved from http://www.divinecaroline.com/life-etc/career-money/ten-tips-dealing-backstabbing-coworkers

Sanow, A. (2011). *5 ways to deal with backstabbers.* Retrieved from http://www.leadersbeacon.com/5-ways-to-deal-with-back-stabbers/#sthash.8cgxg3nI.dpuf

Schuler, A. J. (2004). *Turning around low morale.* Retrieved from http://www.schulersolutions.com

Shain, M. (2000). *Best advice on stress risk management in the workplace.* Retrieved from http://www.mentalhealthworks.ca/sites/default/files/stress-part-1_e.pdf

Shein, E. H. (1992). *Organizational culture and leadership* (2nd ed.). San Francisco, CA: Jossey-Bass.

Sherman, R., & Pross, E. (2010). Growing future nurse leaders to build and sustain healthy work environments at the unit level. *The Online Journal of Issues in Nursing, 15*(1). Retrieved from http://nursingworld.org/MainMenuCategories/ANAMarketplace/ANAPeriodicals/OJIN/TableofContents/Vol152010/No1Jan2010/Growing-Nurse-Leaders.html

Teal, A. (2011). *How to manage different personality types in the workplace.* Retrieved from http://voices.yahoo.com/how-manage-different-personality-types-workplace-8798833.html?cat=31

Thorman, R. (2012). *How to successfully work with different personalities.* Retrieved from http://money.usnews.com/money/blogs/outside-voices-careers/2012/11/08/how-to-successfully-work-with-different-personalities

Topchik, G. S. (2000). *Managing workplace negativity.* Los Angeles, CA: AMACOM Books.

Virginia, J. (2008). *Nurses must learn to take care of themselves.* Retrieved from http://allnurses/com/general-articles-about/nurses-must-learn-300832.html

Yoder-Wise, P. S. (2011). *Leading and managing nursing* (5th ed.). St. Louis, MO: Elsevier-Mosby.

Warren Shepell. (2002). *Workplace trends linked to mental health crisis in Canada.* Retrieved from http://www.warrenshepell.com/newsroom/pr-nov152002.asp

14

Meeting the Mental Health Needs of Employees: An Organizational Approach

The achievements of an organization are the results of the
combined effort of each individual.
—Vince Lombardi

LEARNING OBJECTIVES

By the end of this chapter, the learner will be able to:

1. Identify the importance that a mental health champion can have in building positive mental health in an organization.
2. Discuss how conflict management, change management, and disability management can help an organization promote and foster good mental health.
3. Identify the role that professional associations/colleges and unions can have in an organization to help deal with workplace mental health issues.
4. Understand and discuss why it is important for organizations to uphold the duty to accommodate.
5. Discuss the purpose of employee assistance programs in organizations for how they help address workplace mental health issues.
6. Identify pertinent legislation for how it can help organizations structure a workplace with good mental health.
7. Discuss some generic organizational responses that can help show employees that the organization really does care about their mental health.

In Chapter 4, we discussed in depth the role of an organization/employer in creating a work environment that is supportive of good mental health for its nurses. The chapter focused on much of what can be done to foster a workplace environment that promotes mental health well-being for all. Chapter 4 was based on the belief that a proactive, not a reactive, approach should be taken to prevent any challenges to nurses' mental health from occurring in the workplace. However, nurse mental health challenges cannot always be prevented, nor can precipitating factors always be identified. As was highlighted earlier, an organization is only as good as the people who work there, so if nurses' mental health becomes compromised or

353

jeopardized, the source needs to be addressed. This chapter therefore will address how an organization can best respond when employees' mental health becomes compromised in the workplace as a result of the workplace environment and the people working there.

INVOLVEMENT AND INFLUENCE

Involvement and influence are important in fostering a mentally healthy workplace for all nurses, and they carry the same importance in addressing these concerns. Only this time, the involvement and influence need to come from the top or executive personnel.

Top executives, inclusive of chief executive officers, vice presidents, and others, are truly the figureheads of an organization. Their stance, opinions, input, and status are taken seriously by everyone and are often well-known to everyone, particularly the media, as the voices of the health care organization. However, the same stance, position of authority, and figurehead status will also carry weight to confront the evils lurking in the organization. These are the evils we refer to when we are talking about events, people, and an environment that jeopardize nurses' mental health in the workplace; however, it is how these evils are addressed by executives that makes people stand up and take notice. Executives are representatives of the philosophy of any health care organization. To be effective in taking action against unacceptable people and unfavorable events, executives and leaders at all levels need to demonstrate a "Broken Windows" Theory approach. This is a sociological theory that often applies to the occurrence of violence. However, it can also apply to other wrongdoing and unacceptable behaviors and events.

The basic premise of the Broken Windows Theory is one example of how time and visibility are important in achieving goals. When organizations respond to wrongdoing and people who challenge nurses' mental health, they must respond in a manner that is immediate and visible. If negative behaviors, events, and people's actions are tolerated without being addressed, this begins to foster an environment that encourages increasingly negative actions, behaviors, and events. For example, tolerating workplace bullying without the person responsible being reprimanded or penalized allows such behaviors to grow in intensity and the level of threat to increase because a message is clearly being sent that such behavior is tolerated and therefore is accepted and can continue. In the Broken Windows approach, such bullying is identified and caught quickly, and it is confronted and addressed in a manner that is visible so that all can witness. This then sends a message that such behavior is not going to be tolerated and there is something being done actively to address this unacceptable behavior (Hasketh et al., 2003). The clear message that should be sent is that all actions, behaviors, people, and events that do or can potentially jeopardize others' mental health or cause an increasingly stressful workplace environment are taken very seriously by the organization and executives and hence are actively and immediately addressed.

MOBILIZING MENTAL HEALTH CHAMPIONS

In Chapter 4, we talked in detail about the value of having a mental health champion. Here, I would just like to reiterate the value of mobilizing these champions to the benefit of the organization and workplace. As these persons would typically be altruistic, sincere, and kind, they should be instrumental in addressing any conflict or adverse situation afterward. Using their characteristic capacities of credibility, respect, fairness, pride, and camaraderie, they can translate their knowledge and know-how into influence, passion, and collegiality to build a workplace that prides itself on good mental health (Great-West Life Centre for Workplace Mental Health, 2013).

PSYCHOLOGICAL JOB FIT

As we identified in Chapter 4, poor psychological job fit basically means a disconnect between a nurse's skill mix, knowledge, competencies, and experience and the job the nurse is expected to fulfill. Although an organization may promote the necessity of ensuring psychological job fit for its nurses, this may not always occur. At times, a nurse's job fit is not attended to until it is too late. When attention is not paid to a nurse's psychological job fit, the nurse's mental health can become challenged. This disconnect results in increased stress levels, emotional exhaustion, frustrations, and decreased motivation and energy, which can jeopardize the nurse's mental health to the extent that intervention or modifications are needed. The organization must take responsibility and respond to best meet the needs of the involved nurse. The organization should involve all required personnel immediately and become instrumental in completing a psychological job fit for the nurse. For the individual nurse, work has to meet a particular level of comfort and competence. For the organization, time is money, and a nurse who is frustrated, discontented, and exhausted because of a job misfit is a possible cost liability that needs to be rectified.

THE DUTY TO ACCOMMODATE

The duty to accommodate is significantly related to psychological job fit. The duty to accommodate is a well-recognized term and strategy employed by most large health care organizations. It reflects an effort and obligation of the organization to do its best to accommodate employees and provide them with work settings and conditions that are compatible with their limitations, be they physical or mental. For example, a nurse who is experiencing a severe anxiety disorder and is easing back into work would most likely be placed in a work setting that is perhaps not as stressful or acute as the one where the nurse worked when he or she first became ill. Placing the nurse in a somewhat slower and less acute workplace setting, such as a long-term care unit as opposed to an acute and very busy emergency department, would be one way in which an accommodation could be achieved. The Americans With Disabilities Act requires organizations to make "reasonable accommodation" for employees with disabilities (Williams, 2012).

It is important for managers to be aware of what may be necessary or prudent when providing workplace accommodations. There is a legal duty to offer reasonable accommodation when an employee has a disability. Even when the law is not engaged, reasonably accommodating staff can provide opportunities for maximizing productivity. Knowing their strengths and limitations will allow managers to be as effective as possible with all employees. In a nutshell, these include assessing the situation, planning for success, implementing the plan, and evaluating the outcomes. Supervisors may not fully understand how to carry out their duty to accommodate, and this lack of understanding can lead to stress for all concerned.

Most people with mental health issues will find their own path to recovery. If you feel that the employee is not progressing well toward recovery, you may want to advocate for enhanced treatment approaches. The employee may rely on your expertise and connections to be pointed in the right direction. Most organizations have specific processes and documentation that are required as part of the return to work and accommodation related to a disability.

The accommodation of an individual can occur through many different interventions. For example, flexible scheduling can be implemented with flexible work hours, part-time or split shifts, more frequent breaks, or a return-to-work program.

A change in a leadership style may also occur. For example, maybe instructions and feedback need to be written down as opposed to being given verbally. Further, brief weekly meetings may help everyone keep on track and give them an opportunity to discuss any issues.

Changes in training modalities may need to occur, such as allowing the nurse extra time to complete tasks and providing one-on-one training if needed. Similarly, modifying job duties can help accommodate a nurse. This can take the form of reassignment of tasks. For example, if maintaining stamina is a challenge, vary the tasks, consider job sharing, allow a self-paced workload, and provide for regular breaks. To build concentration, focus on the essential aspects of the job, increase natural lighting, and break down large tasks into small ones. When dealing with deadlines that are challenging, ask for reminders from your manager/leader, arrange regular meetings for follow-up, and use electronic reminders. If memory is an issue, ask for things in writing and write down what is important. If working relationships are a challenge, outline clear expectations and what defines collegiality, and ask for honest feedback. Handle stress and emotions as they occur, deal with change when needed, and let your leader know if you feel anxious; ask the leader to keep communication open.

As a leader, you need to find out what it is that you do that is considered supportive to the employee and what it is that you do that may inadvertently make the employee's symptoms worse. As a leader, you do need to recognize that from a legal perspective, the duty to accommodate does not mean that a disabled employee is guaranteed a job. If a person cannot perform the essential requirements and duties of a job after being accommodated, there will be no finding of discrimination. Whether employees must be able to perform all the essential duties or just some duties of the position, there is a clear expectation that they must perform useful and productive work. When the employer can show that accommodation will enable the employee to perform only substandard work, or work of no real value to the employer, a refusal to accommodate will not be discriminatory.

POLICY ENFORCEMENT

In Chapter 4, we talked about the importance of having in place policies and programs that can help foster the development of a respectful workplace. In response to issues that infringe on nurses' mental health at work, we now focus in on enforcing such policies and doing whatever it takes for an organization to ensure that policies are followed, respect is maintained, and a mentally healthy workplace is sustained.

The consistent application and enforcement of workplace policies are typically the responsibility of the supervisor/manager and the human resources department. In order for organizations to succeed in making their policies effective, the policies have to be enforced consistently and in a timely manner. "Companies that pick and choose which policies to enforce when are setting themselves up for failure, not to mention exposing themselves to potential liability for employee complaints about unfair treatment" (Mayhew, 2013). To promote the use of policies to ensure their utmost effectiveness, organizations need to do the following: publish and distribute employee policy handbooks or post them on their website for all to see; provide training to supervisors and managers on workplace policies, and designate mandatory training in policies regarding equal employment opportunity to avoid potential supervisor liability for allegations of unfair employment practices; construct disciplinary review and corrective action forms that contain a comprehensive list of policies and consequences for violations; train supervisors and managers in how to apply workplace policies in a fair and consistent manner; and explain workplace policies to every group of new hires during orientation (Mayhew, 2013). Further, organizations need to develop and maintain programs to implement their policies and to provide information and instruction to workers on the contents of these policies and programs.

THE ROLE OF UNIONS

Unions are the bodies that advocate for and represent employees when it comes to labor issues, contract development, and negotiation. They also help to ensure fair and equitable treatment of all in the workplace. Nurses' unions are no different. Several shop stewards are strategically placed throughout hospitals and health care organizations to monitor nursing activities and practice. The primary role of these shop stewards is to be someone who is on the ground with the nurses that can help advocate, support, and counsel nurses so that their labor rights in the workplace are respected. Workload is one example of how nurses' unions become involved. If union shop stewards are hearing many concerns expressed that the nurses of any particular area are being subjected to increased workloads and unwarranted stressful situations or criticism, then the union will play an active role to advocate for better working conditions for the nurses. The main part of their active role is to ensure that their membership is being respected and supported in the workplace, and that conditions that could possibly impact their work negatively, such as the environment, are addressed and confronted. In the case of a nurse's mental health becoming jeopardized as a result of workplace conditions, it would be smart and prudent for the health care organization to work with the nurses' union collaboratively to develop solutions to help resolve such stress-provoking situations.

THE ROLE OF PROFESSIONAL ASSOCIATIONS

Nurses' professional associations serve to monitor the practices of nurses and are responsible for overseeing and governing nurses' practice. They have a key role to play for nurses who may be experiencing mental health issues as a result of work or who are being subjected to or are targets of standards violations by other nurses. As part of that mandate, they also help to monitor and ensure that nurses meet their professional standards of practice. However, nurses are not able to maintain those standards of practice if their mental health is potentially being jeopardized because of workplace factors. A workplace environment that is filled with hostility, professional misconduct, and unsafe practices obviously challenges the fulfillment of nurses' standards of practice. Therefore, it now becomes a workplace safely issue as well. An association will help to address negative issues involving specific nurses who are the perpetrators of hostility, violence, and labile work conditions that hinder other nurses from achieving nursing standards of practice. An association will also address the behavior and unacceptable practices of nurses who are breaching standards of practice. Again, just as it would be prudent for organizations to collaborate with unions, it would also be prudent for them to collaborate with nurses' professional associations. Health care organizations need to share with association leaders any pertinent documentation or video footage needed to best address any issues that jeopardize the safety of nurses' workplace environments.

Most nursing associations are affiliated with legal nursing protective societies and also maintain their own internal alternate dispute resolution programs to deal with nurses who breach nursing standards of practice. The alternate dispute resolution programs are a significant part of any nurses' professional association. They exist to ensure that the right course of action is taken for a nurse who has breached standards of nursing practice.

DISABILITY MANAGEMENT

A well-designed, progressive disability management program can shorten or even prevent employee absences, reduce costs, and maintain productivity. The most effective approach combines integrated disability management with prevention and health promotion. Disability management is a proactive, employer-centered, systematic, and goal-oriented process that coordinates the activities of management, unions, insurance carriers, health care providers, and vocational rehabilitation professionals for the purpose of actively minimizing the impact of impairment or disability on an employee's capacity to participate actively in the work environment and successfully perform his or her job. Mental health is the fastest-growing segment of disability claims—accounting for 30% to 40% of claim volume. Mental health claims cost twice as much as physical health claims, with the average mental health claim costing $18,000 Cdn. (Ontario Hospital Association, 2013). In the United States alone, national health expenditures for mental health services were estimated to be over $100 million (Centers for Disease Control and Prevention, 2014). For example, "depression is estimated to cause 200 million lost workdays each year at a cost to employers of $17 to $44 billion" (Stewart, Ricci, Chee, Hahn, & Morganstein, 2003).

Organizations can help assist in disability management in several ways, such as the following: mental health education and awareness sessions with a focus on depression and anxiety, access to resources for staying well and accommodating disabilities, manager training in the identification of indicators of mental illness, effective interventions for accommodations and plans for remaining at work/returning to work, manager consultation and coaching in workplace mental health issues, and facilitation with managers and employees to develop plans for remaining at work/returning to work (Health Canada, 2011).

Certain criteria can be used to optimize a disabled nurse's return to work. These include the work itself, the nurse's presence in the workplace, the nurse's meaningful performance of tasks, and a workplace that is welcoming and free of harassment and other pressures that might delay recovery. Involving the nurse and asking what is needed, setting benchmarks in the form of realistic goals, and leading by example are all valuable components of making a return to work and disability management successful.

Evaluating a nurse's performance relative to these criteria is also important and includes monitoring of the nurse's symptoms and their severity, the effectiveness of treatment, the employee's resilience, the employee's ability to prevent a relapse (by identifying and avoiding issues that lead to relapses), and the level of mental acuity and stamina the job requires. Typically, some segment of the organization's human resources department concerned with employee wellness would oversee the implementation of a disability management program.

CONFLICT MANAGEMENT

Conflict is the last thing you want when you are trying to return to work a nurse who has been absent with a disability, particularly a mental disability. Employers can promote quality practice settings in which nurses are encouraged to understand conflict and employ strategies to mitigate it. Employers can institute reporting systems to help nurses acknowledge when conflict has occurred. A fair and efficient reporting system encourages communication among staff members by helping nurses identify underlying causes of conflict. Open communication and understanding will promote an atmosphere of trust and respect within the health care team. Employers can (a) provide a system that promotes the reporting of incidences of workplace conflict, protects nurses from reprisal, and deals with reports fairly and efficiently; (b) routinely assess the incidence of workplace conflict and implement strategies for corrective action; and (c) institute clear policies and consequences for those who breach policies aimed at preventing conflict and abuse (College of Nurses of Ontario [CNO], 2009). Further, "Corporations that have developed collaborative conflict management systems report significant litigation cost savings: Brown and Root reported an 80% reduction in outside litigation costs, Motorola reported a 75% reduction over a period of six years, and NCR reported a 50% reduction and a drop of pending lawsuits from 263 in 1984 to 28 in 1993" (Ford, 2000).

CHANGE MANAGEMENT

During times of change, there is much an organization can do to limit the negativity or perceived negativity that threatening change can sometimes bring. The following, proposed by the National Institute for Occupational Safety and Health (NIOSH; 2008), is one organizational change intervention model that can be used. It advocates that the most effective way of reducing occupational stress is to eliminate the stressors by redesigning jobs or make organizational changes. Organizations should take the following measures (NIOSH, 2008):

1. Ensure that the workload is in line with workers' capabilities and resources
2. Clearly define workers' roles and responsibilities
3. Give workers opportunities to participate in decisions and actions affecting their jobs
4. Improve communication
5. Reduce uncertainty about career development and future employment prospects
6. Provide opportunities for social interaction among workers

The most commonly implemented organizational interventions in health care settings include team processes, multidisciplinary health care teams, and multiple-component interventions.

Team process or worker participatory methods give workers opportunities to participate in decisions and actions affecting their jobs. Workers receive clear information about their tasks and roles in the department. Team-based approaches to redesign patient care delivery systems or to provide care (e.g., team nursing) have been successful in improving job satisfaction and reducing turnover, absenteeism, and job stress. Multidisciplinary health care teams (e.g., composed of doctors, nurses, managers, pharmacists, psychologists, and others) have become increasingly common in acute, long-term, and primary care settings. Teams can accomplish the following:

1. Allow services to be delivered efficiently, without sacrificing quality
2. Save time and promote efficiency (a team can perform activities concurrently that one worker would need to provide sequentially)
3. Promote innovation by exchanging ideas
4. Integrate and link information in ways that individuals cannot

Multiple-component interventions are broad-based and may include the following (NIOSH, 2008):

1. Risk assessment
2. Intervention techniques
3. Education

Successful organizational stress interventions have several things in common when it comes to implementing change without much disagreement and resistance. These include the following (NIOSH, 2008):

1. Involving workers at all stages of the intervention
2. Providing workers with the authority to develop, implement, and evaluate the intervention

3. Significant commitment from top management and buy-in from middle management
4. An organizational culture that supports stress interventions
5. Periodic evaluations of the stress intervention

The NIOSH (2008) suggests that without these components (in particular, management support), it is not likely that the intervention will succeed. Further, you need to address the "human side" systematically and start at the top because the leaders themselves must embrace the new approaches first, both to challenge and to motivate the rest of the institution; however, be sure to involve every layer of the organization and its accompanying staff. Next, a formal case needs to be presented as to why this change is needed, along with a road map of how you expect to get there. Finally, the organization needs to create ownership of the change by engaging nurses, communicating the message and keeping communication clear and regular, assessing the cultural landscape, and addressing the existing culture for any barriers that may exist. It also has to prepare for the unexpected, as no project moves forward seamlessly when a large number of people are involved.

As identified earlier for leaders, organizations should follow the same change management framework set forth by Kotter (2013). Basically, if organizations increase urgency and inspire people to move, make objectives real and relevant, build the guiding team, get the vision right, communicate for buy-in, empower action, create short-term wins, don't let up, and make change stick, they will be able to implement change successfully without jeopardizing the mental health integrity of the involved nurses and nurse leaders.

EMPLOYEE AND FAMILY ASSISTANCE PROGRAMS

An employee (and family) assistance program (EAP) is a confidential, short-term counseling service for employees with personal problems that affect their work performance. EAPs grew out of the industrial alcoholism programs of the 1940s. They should be part of a larger company plan to promote wellness that involves written policies, supervisor and employee training, and, where appropriate, an approved drug-testing program (CCOHS, 2013). EAPs are a valuable resource that can help employees cope with critical issues in an increasingly complex and challenging world. There is a relationship between an organization's own interests and the ability of employees to work to their full potential. Marital and family problems, conflicts among coworkers and managers, depression and other psychological conditions, substance abuse, legal and financial issues, and child and elder care needs—these are just some of the personal issues and problems that have a direct impact on employee well-being and, as a result, an organization's bottom line. While most EAPs offer a wide range of services, they often refer employees to other professionals or agencies that can offer more or extended care in particular areas. The range of services that can be provided by an EAP relate to personal issues: job stress, relationship issues, elder care, child care and parenting, harassment, substance abuse, separation/loss, work–life balance, financial troubles, and family violence. A referral to an EAP can typically be a self-referral; an informal referral made by a supervisor/leader, friend, or colleague; or a formal referral based on a job performance issue. The success of most EAPs is based on their concepts of confidentiality; involvement of families as well as employees; supported policies; recognition and commitment by managers, unions, and associations; and the use of both formal and informal referrals.

STAFF DEBRIEFING

In the aftermath of a large-scale disaster, organizations need to address the issues that can follow such traumatic events. When 9/11 occurred in New York City, what was targeted was the workplace of thousands of Americans. The noises of crashing and people screaming and the horrific feelings of impending doom posed tremendous challenges to both employees and employers that will never be forgotten. How employers respond to such events and prepare for future ones will have critical consequences for the health and well-being of both their employees and their organizations. At this critical juncture, there are actions employers can undertake to help minimize and mitigate the psychological impact of terrorist violence.

In such troubling and critical times, there is ample opportunity for organizations to intervene to help their employees deal with such horrifying events and the surrounding feelings of fear and anxiety. Good leadership is one necessity. Organizations need to stay strong and monitor employee well-being. The most effective leaders are visible, convey a sense of hope and optimism while being realistic, and are calm and calming, all the time communicating both what is known and what is not known. Further, they will often involve their employees in developing disaster and recovery plans and profoundly affect outcomes when they ensure that organizational supports are in place and that they themselves are accessible, supportive, and empathic. Further, they need to reduce any uncertainty, if at all possible. With the uncertainty of "how did this happen to us?" comes the belief that personal safety and security, which were formerly taken for granted, have been eroded. This is of real concern for both the individual employee and the organization, as uncertainty has been linked to employees' physical and psychological problems, and to poorer organizational performance. Leaders must therefore do all within their power to convey useful and timely information, including what is not known, and must do so in a manner that is specific and avoids ambiguous messages. The development of a response plan is a good starting point to get people involved. It is important for leaders and organizations to remember that although bridging the perceived gaps after a traumatic event is difficult, it can be done.

EMERGENCY RESPONSE

All organizations should have in place an emergency response plan or crisis management plan, either of which is frequently used. This plan is a guide to providing a response to a major crisis or emergency that occurs in the workplace. It also includes all personnel designated to carry out specific responsibilities, and as such they are all expected to know and understand the policies and procedures outlined in this plan (Lewis & Clark College, 2003). The purpose of a crisis management plan is to coordinate resources and personnel to address the situation and help workers to recover from the crisis that is occurring or has just occurred. The event triggering a response should be of a magnitude beyond what can be controlled through routine institutional measures. Many templates exist to help develop a crisis management plan. However, some critical elements include sitting down with your staff to discuss possible scenarios and what would need to be done in each case; identifying any limitations; preparing statements that would have to be sent to all employees, families, and the media; creating an emergency contacts call list; getting to know the first responders; and once the crisis is over, reaching out to and supporting those employees who need your help (Bhattarai, 2013). Some items on your emergency response checklist should include staying calm by taking deep, slow breaths; listening attentively; maintaining eye contact; being courteous and patient; keeping the situation in your control if you can; maintaining a calm, quiet tone of voice; signaling for help; and calling security.

DUE DILIGENCE

The term *due diligence* first came into common use as a result of the U.S. Securities Act of 1933, which included a defense in Section 11, referred to as the due diligence defense, to address perceived inadequate disclosure and avoid liability. Due diligence takes different forms depending on its purpose, and in nursing and health care it can be an investigation of current practices of process and policies. For example, in a court of law, a hospital may have to prove that it did everything possible to prevent something from happening. It is not enough that it exercised the normal standard of care in its industry—it must show that it took every reasonable precaution, such as is the case where there is a suspected violation of human rights. Within an organization dealing with the lives of vulnerable populations, even stress personnel and nurses need to ensure prudent, responsible practice.

WHISTLE-BLOWER LEGISLATION AND POLICY

The development of whistle-blower legislation is making great progress in the area of health care delivery, but the legislation remains today not quite as completely integrated as it should be. Simply defined, whistle-blowing is the disclosure of information about perceived wrongdoing in an organization, or the risk thereof, to individuals or entities believed to be able to effect action (Transparency International, 2009). The legislation for whistle-blowing is enacted by governments and other authority bodies to enforce the tenets of whistle-blowing. For psychiatric nurses, such legislation provides something of a safety net to support them in those often intimidating cases in which they have seen or witnessed wrongdoing or are aware of wrongdoing and feel apprehensive about coming forward to identify what they know for fear of negative ramifications. However, whistle-blowers can play an essential role in detecting fraud, mismanagement, and corruption. Their actions help to save lives, protect human rights, and safeguard the rule of law. To protect the public good, whistle-blowers frequently assume a high level of personal risk, and psychiatric/mental health nurses are no different.

Most countries develop and implement some form of legislation requiring that workplaces be safe and healthy. This legislation is not "nice to know," it is "need to know." Acts or statutes are imposed and enforced by governments, and it is mandatory for the states, counties, provinces, and other geographical jurisdictions of a country to obey them. Although such legislation and organizational policy are a welcome development, the debate still continues about when the whistle should be blown (Huston & Brox, 2004).

OTHER ORGANIZATIONAL RESPONSES AND STRATEGIES

In addition to the development of policies and enactment of legislation, there is much more an organization can do to help maintain a workplace that creates positive mental health for its nurses. For example, it can engage in information and awareness campaigns about workplace mental health, and even about bullying, violence, and respect. Further, it can promote and ensure employee and manager training, take action against bullying and discrimination, tackle identified sources of workplace stress, implement policies to support people if they develop mental health problems, and use recruitment practices that do not discriminate against people with mental health problems (Knifton et al., 2011).

Organizations need to ensure that they follow up and follow through on all concerning issues. In most circumstances, things can slip again, problems can resurface, or new problems can arise, so planning for the healthiest approach to relapse is important. Similarly, you should consider that the stressors of the workplace may still have an impact on employees; all is not necessarily resolved once the stressor is identified and removed. The communication problems that might have contributed to the problems may occur again, coping strategies may not be well developed, or skills may have gotten rusty. If you simply turn a blind eye until the situation once again reaches the crisis point, you risk making the original issue worse and reducing trust in the process.

SUMMARY

An organization has a very important role to play in the delivery of safe and competent patient care services, and it also has the responsibility and liability to promote workplace safety for its nurses. There is much that an organization can do to help support and foster strength for its nurses in its endeavors to build a respectful and positive mental health environment. Given that nurses are often the backbone of many health care organizations, the maintenance of their mental health is critical. As long as organizations are aware of required legislation; address conflict, change, and disability in a timely and efficient manner; and work with professional associations and unions to achieve this goal, then a collegial and respectful workplace for nurses can be maintained.

DISCUSSION QUESTIONS

1. What is the importance of a mental health champion in building positive mental health in an organization?

2. How do conflict management, change management, and disability management help to promote and foster good mental health?
3. What role do professional associations/colleges and unions have in an organization to help deal with workplace mental health issues?
4. Why is it important for organizations to uphold the duty to accommodate?
5. What purpose do employee assistance programs have in organizations for how they help address workplace mental health issues?
6. What legislation exists to help organizations structure a workplace with good mental health?
7. What are some generic organizational responses that can help show employees that the organization really does care about their mental health?

REFERENCES

Bhattarai, A. (2013). *How to create a crisis management plan.* Retrieved from http://articles.washingtonpost.com/2013-07-21/business/40713622_1_crisis-management-plan-social-media-business-owners

Canadian Centre for Occupational Health and Safety. (2013). *Employee assistance programs.* Retrieved from http://www.ccohs.ca/oshanswers/hsprograms/eap.html

College of Nurses of Ontario. (2009). *Conflict prevention and management.* Retrieved from http://www.cno.org/Global/docs/prac/47004_conflict_prev.pdf

Ford, J. (2000). *Workplace conflict: Facts and figures.* Retrieved from http://www.mediate.com/mobile/article.cfm?id=95

Great-West Life Centre for Workplace Mental Health. (2013). *Championing a healthy workplace.* Retrieved from http://www.gwlcentreformentalhealth.com/display.asp?l1=4&l2=55&l3=58&d=58

Hasketh, K. L., Duncan, S. M., Estrabrooks, C. A., Reimer, M. A., Giovannetti, P., Hyndman, K., et al. (2003). Workplace violence in Alberta and British Columbia hospitals. *Health Policy, 63,* 311–321.

Health Canada. (2011). *Environmental and workplace health.* Retrieved from http://www.hc-sc.gc.ca/ewh-semt/occup-travail/empl/support-eng.php

Huston, J. L., & Brox, G. A. (2004). Professional ethics at the bottom line. *Health Care Management (Frederick), 23*(3), 267–272.

Knifton, L., Watson, V., Gründemann, R., Dijkman, A., den Besten, H., & Have, K. T. (2011). *A guide for employers to promote mental health in the workplace.* Retrieved from https://webgate.ec.europa.eu/sanco_mental_health/public/openAttachment.html?id=1341&fileName=Mental%20health%20Employers_TNO.pdf

Kotter, J. (2013). *The 8-step process for leading change.* Retrieved from http://www.kotterinternational.com/our-principles/changesteps/changesteps

Lewis & Clark College. (2003). *Crisis management plan.* Retrieved from http://www.lclark.edu/offices/human_resources/employee_resources/policies/institutional/general/crisis_management_plan

Mayhew, R. (2013). *How to enforce policies consistently at work.* Retrieved from http://smallbusiness.chron.com/enforce-policies-consistently-work-10970.html

National Institute for Occupational Safety and Health. (2008). *Exposure to stress: Occupational hazards in hospitals.* Retrieved from http://www.cdc.gov/niosh/docs/2008-136/pdfs/2008-136.pdf

Ontario Hospital Association. (2013). *Disability management.* Retrieved from http://www.oha.com/SERVICES/HEALTHSAFETY/DISABILITYMANAGEMENT/Pages/DisabilityManagement.aspx

Stewart, W. F., Ricci, J. A., Chee, E., Hahn, S. R., & Morganstein, D. (2003). Cost of lost productive work time among US workers with depression. *Journal of the American Medical Association, 289*(23), 3135–3144.

Transparency International. (2009). *Resolution on the protection of whistleblowers.* Retrieved from http://www.transparency.org/files/content/activity/2009_ResolutionProtection Whistleblowers_EN.pdf

Williams, R. B. (2012). *The silent tsunami: Mental health in the workplace.* Retrieved from http://www.psychologytoday.com/blog/wired-success/201209/the-silent-tsunami-mental-health-in-the-workplace

Index

absenteeism, 87–88
abuse and neglect as form of workplace
    violence, 245
accountability. *See* transparency and
    accountability
active listening, 147
addiction, 263–284
    adverse outcomes, 280
    background, 263–264
    code of silence, 281–282
    disciplinary recommendations, 275–276
    history, 265
    legal/ethical responsibility of nurses, 274
    physiology, 268
    predisposition for nurses, 272–274
      accessibility, 273
      knowledge, 273–274
      self-medication, 273
      stressful work, 272
    prevalence rates, 264–265
      background, 264
      subspecialty impact, 265
    professional associations, role of, 277
    responses to, leaders and organizations,
      277–279
      alternatives to discipline, 277–278
      random drug screening, 279
      recognition of, 277
      ten-step strategy, 278–279
    risk factors, 265–267
      biological, 265–266
      environmental, 267
      physical, 266
      psychosocial, 266–267
    signs and symptoms, 268–270
      behavioral, 268–269
      financial consequences, 269–270
      physiological, 269
      social ramifications, 269
      specific to nursing, 270–272

attendance, 271
    diversion of medication, 271–272
    work performance, 271
    treatment, 280–281
addressing conflict, 322
adrenocorticotropic hormone (ACTH), 8–9
adverse outcomes, addiction, 280
aging workforce, workplace, as source of
    stress, 42
Alzheimer's disease, 12
anxiety, 17
    chronic disorder, 18
    disorders, 301–302
    severe, 17–18
assertiveness, 324
atmosphere, workplace, as source of
    stress, 51
attitude, workplace, as source of stress,
    52–53
attributes, effective leader
    active listening, 147
    clarity, 147
    communication, 146–147
    concern and respect for others, 144–145
    eager, positive, uplifting, 147
    energy and enthusiasm, 145
    engaging, 147–148
    influential, 146
    innovative and creative, 146
    insightful, flexible, adaptable, 145–146
    intelligent, 148
    role models, 148
    synergy, 148
    vision, 145
autonomy and control enhancement, role of
    leaders in developing, 169

backstabbing colleagues
    personal approach, 322–323
    professional approach, 344–345

367